MOBILIZING MERCY

McGill-Queen's/Associated Medical Services Studies in the History of Medicine, Health, and Society

SERIES EDITORS: J.T.H. Connor and Erika Dyck

Volumes in this series have financial support from Associated Medical Services, Inc. (AMS). Associated Medical Services Inc. was established in 1936 by Dr Jason Hannah as a pioneer prepaid not-for-profit health care organization in Ontario. With the advent of medicare, AMS became a charitable organization supporting innovations in academic medicine and health services, specifically the history of medicine and health care, as well as innovations in health professional education and bioethics.

MOBILIZING
MERCY

A History of the Canadian Red Cross

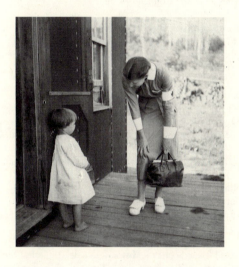

Sarah Glassford

McGill-Queen's University Press
Montreal & Kingston • London • Chicago

© McGill-Queen's University Press 2017

ISBN 978-0-7735-4775-9 (cloth)
ISBN 978-0-7735-4831-2 (ePDF)
ISBN 978-0-7735-4832-9 (ePUB)

Legal deposit first quarter 2017
Bibliothèque nationale du Québec

Printed in Canada on acid-free paper that is 100% ancient forest free
(100% post-consumer recycled), processed chlorine free

This book has been published with the help of a grant from the Canadian
Federation for the Humanities and Social Sciences, through the Awards to
Scholarly Publications Program, using funds provided by the Social Sciences
and Humanities Research Council of Canada.

McGill-Queen's University Press acknowledges the support of the Canada
Council for the Arts for our publishing program. We also acknowledge the
financial support of the Government of Canada through the Canada Book
Fund for our publishing activities.

Library and Archives Canada Cataloguing in Publication

Glassford, Sarah Carlene, 1978–, author
Mobilizing mercy : a history of the Canadian Red Cross / Sarah Glassford.

(McGill-Queen's/Associated Medical Services studies in the history of
medicine, health, and society ; 45)
Includes bibliographical references and index.
Issued in print and electronic formats.
ISBN 978-0-7735-4775-9 (cloth).– ISBN 978-0-7735-4831-2 (ePDF).
– ISBN 978-0-7735-4832-9 (ePUB)

1. Canadian Red Cross Society – History. I. Title. II. Series: McGill-
Queen's /Associated Medical Services studies in the history of medicine,
health, and society ; 45

HV580.C33G53 2017   361.7'6340971   C2016-907480-3
                                                  C2016-907481-1

CONTENTS

ILLUSTRATIONS

ACKNOWLEDGMENTS

There is a general consensus among historians of humanitarian organizations that one of the biggest obstacles to preserving and sharing humanitarian history is the organizations' intense focus on meeting the present emergency: too often the past simply falls off their radar. I would therefore like to start by thanking Robert Gourgon, Ann Butryn, and their predecessors for being the guardians and preservers of the Canadian Red Cross National Archive through its many moves and incarnations over the past century. I especially thank Robert for his support, cooperation, and trust in me. It began with archival access and photocopying privileges in 2004, evolved into friendship, and enabled me to contribute historical content to two important projects: the revamped Canadian Red Cross website in 2012, and the 120th anniversary Canadian Red Cross digital history exhibit in 2016. It has been a real pleasure to know him over the years. I am also grateful to the Canadian Red Cross as an organization for allowing me and other scholars to access their private archive. Our ability to tell the story of Canada's humanitarian history is infinitely richer and better balanced as a result. However, the interpretations and arguments in this book are solely my own, and I assume full responsibility for their accuracy.

My thanks also go to all the public and university archivists and staff who helped make my archival experiences in Calgary, Toronto, Ottawa, Halifax, and Charlottetown both pleasant and productive. At the other end of the process, I am more grateful than I can adequately express to editor Kyla Madden of McGill-Queen's University Press for her many years of encouragement and good advice. This is the book I wanted to write when I first began my doctoral studies, but it took everything I learned between then and now to become the historian and writer capable of producing it. I hope the result repays Kyla's patience and Robert's trust. Many thanks also to copyeditor Kate Merriman for applying the final polish to the manuscript.

My personal experience of how voluntary organizations work and my interest in Red Cross history largely grew out of four stints as a summer student with the Windsor-Essex County branch of the Canadian Red Cross. I am grateful to my Grandma Lucienna Jones Pattison (a volunteer at the branch) for encouraging me to apply, to the branch for taking a chance on me (since I had zero relevant job experience), and to the oft-maligned Human Resources Development Canada for funding the job. Together, they set my feet on a path of historical inquiry I have yet to leave.

I was extremely fortunate to receive research and travel funding from the Ontario Graduate Scholarship program, the Social Sciences and Humanities Research Council of Canada, the University of Western Ontario, York University and its Ramsay Cook Research Fellowship fund, the Toronto Loyalist League, the University of Ottawa, and the University of Prince Edward Island. The University of New Brunswick Department of History generously paid for indexing. I am financially solvent today largely because of these institutions; I trust they will consider this book a good return on their investment.

York University's graduate program in history was a vibrant and dynamic place at which to study Canadian history during the first decade of the twenty-first century, and I am proud to be a product of its heady mix of scholarship and sociability. Although we no longer meet at Historian's Craft or appear in the pages of *Document*, I deeply appreciate the past and present support of the friends and colleagues I met there. Special thanks go to Kristine Alexander, Tarah Brookfield, Kristin Burnett, Tom Crawshaw, Chris Dooley, Jenny Ellison, Christine Grandy, Natalie Gravelle, Jarett Henderson, Greg Kennedy, Sean Kheraj, and Ian Mosby. I also want to once again express my gratitude to the members of my dissertation committee for their help in getting me from proposal to defence: H.V. Nelles and Kathryn McPherson (both of whom I also thank for their unfailing post-PhD support), the late Georgina Feldberg, and the late Myra Rutherdale. Cynthia Toman, my postdoctoral supervisor and mentor at the University of Ottawa, helped make the transition from graduate student to junior scholar a smooth one, for which I sincerely thank her.

It took many more years than I like to admit to research and write this book, but along the way I met (in addition to those I have already mentioned) many amazing teachers, colleagues, and friends at six universities, who offered help, encouragement, and support. A huge "thank-you" to: Erin Black, Claire Campbell, Caron Daley, Mike Dunn, Catherine Kilbride, Shannon LaBelle, Matt McKean, Amy Shaw, Craig Simpson, Tim Syer, and Jonathan Vance, from the University of Western Ontario; Laura DeCamillis, Christine DeLuca, Alison Norman, Jennifer Polk, Jill Rutherford, and the whole Toronto Area Women's Canadian History Group, in Toronto; everyone at the Associated Medical Services Nursing History Research Unit at the University of Ottawa but especially Jayne Elliott, and the academic and public historians of the National Capital Women's History Reading Group; Dominique Marshall and Will Tait at Carleton University; from the University of Prince Edward Island the entire Department of History but especially Susan Brown, Lisa Chilton, Ed Mac-Donald, and James Moran, plus Nia Phillips, the Faculty of Arts Writing Group, and the talented creative writers in ENG 382 and ENG 486; and finally, at the University of New Brunswick, the Department of History and the Gregg Centre for the Study of War and Society, particularly Cindy Brown, Jeff Brown, Erin Morton, and Lisa Todd.

While writing this book my non-academic life would have been emotionally poorer and a lot less fun without these special people: Jason and Moura Avey, the Bateman/Atkinson family, the Bolt/Brace family, Cvita Delac and Terry Warne, Lindsay DenBoer, Linh and Randy Drexler, Kerry Fegyverneki, the Friesen family, the MacIntyre/Jones family, Glenn and Pam Mooney, Jennifer Palmer, Mario Spagnuolo, Jenn Sullivan, Shannon Wilmot, the Wiseman/Eberhardt family, all of my church friends, my Glassford and Jones relatives, and my brother-in-law Ryan Kirkby.

This extra-special last paragraph is reserved for the family into which I was born. Their long-distance love and support keep me going in hard times and make the good times sweeter. I could fill a book with all the reasons I love them, but I hope a few words each will help them understand the things I'm not saying: Ian, thank-you for putting up with me every time I accidentally broke your Lego creations; Rachel, thank-you for wanting to play Barbies and for listening to my stories in our room-sharing years; Dad, thank-you for dragging us to countless historic sites and museums on every family vacation; Mom, thank-you for still crying every time I leave home. It took me many long, self-doubt-filled years to finish this book, while the rest of my life unfolded around it. The four of you always believed I could do this, and now here it is in your hands. This one's for you.

ABBREVIATIONS

Organizations

AMOMC	Association of Medical Officers of the Militia of Canada
ANRC	American National Red Cross
ARC	American Red Cross
BDS	Blood Donor Service
BNAS	British National Society for Aid to the Sick and Wounded in War
BRCS	British Red Cross Society
BTS	Blood Transfusion Service
CAMC	Canadian Army Medical Corps
CEF	Canadian Expeditionary Force
CH&RA	College Heights and Rosedale Association
CIDA	Canadian International Development Agency
CPF	Canadian Patriotic Fund
CPFA	Canadian Patriotic Fund Association
CRC	Canadian Red Cross
CRCS	Canadian Red Cross Society
CUARF	Canadian United Allied Relief Fund
CUSO	Canadian University Service Overseas
CWC	Canadian Welfare Council
DSCR	Department of Soldiers' Civil Re-establishment
FEWT	Far East Welfare Team
ICRC	International Committee of the Red Cross
IODE	Imperial Order Daughters of the Empire

IRC   International Red Cross
LRCS   League of Red Cross Societies
NATO   North Atlantic Treaty Organization
NCWC   National Council of Women of Canada
NSS   National Selective Service
NWPS   National Women's Patriotic Society
NWS   National War Services
OHSC   Ontario Hospital Services Commission
OSJJ   Order of St John of Jerusalem
RCAMC   Royal Canadian Army Medical Corps
RCMP   Royal Canadian Mounted Police
RLSS   Royal Life Saving Society
SJAA   St John Ambulance Association
SJAB   St John Ambulance Brigade
TGH   Toronto General Hospital
UN   United Nations
UNRRA   United Nations Relief and Rehabilitation Administration
VON   Victorian Order of Nurses
WCF   War Charities Funds
WHO   World Health Organization
YMCA   Young Men's Christian Association
YWCA   Young Women's Christian Association

Archives and Citations

AMCM   Archived Minutes of Commissioners' Meetings
AMNOM   Archived Minutes of National Officers' Meetings
AO   Archives of Ontario
BRCMA   British Red Cross Museum and Archive
CC   Central Council
CRCNA   Canadian Red Cross National Archive
CTA   City of Toronto Archives
DCB   Dictionary of Canadian Biography
EC   Executive Committee
ECAMB   Executive Committee and Central Council Archived
Minute Book

GMA   Glenbow Museum and Archives
LAC   Library and Archives Canada
ns   new series
NSARM   Nova Scotia Archives and Records Management
PPC   Postwar Planning Committee
UPEI   University of Prince Edward Island

Terms

HIV/AIDS   human immunodeficiency virus/
acquired immunodeficiency syndrome
POW   Prisoner of War
VAD   Voluntary Aid Detachment

MOBILIZING MERCY

INTRODUCTION

On an oppressively humid southwestern Ontario afternoon in July 1995, a quiet, bookish sixteen-year-old in a Red Cross smock refills several plates of cookies and makes another pot of coffee in the small refreshment area of the open-concept donation room in her local, permanent blood donor clinic. The space is bright, modern, and scrupulously clean, kitted out with comfortable reclining seats and all the technological apparatus of late-1990s blood collection. She shyly chats with donors as they pause for post-donation refreshments and thanks them as they leave. Despite having attended the mandatory orientation session for all volunteers, she has not thought deeply about the Red Cross and its history. She feels vaguely positive about its ideals of humanitarian service, but above all she is happy to be getting some volunteer work experience in a pleasant environment.

Fast-forward to another humid southwestern Ontario summer afternoon, this time in July 2000. The same young woman, soon to begin her fourth year of an undergraduate arts degree, is back at her hometown Red Cross, now as an employee in the Field Operations office. She makes photocopies, stuffs envelopes, helps with fundraising efforts, and occasionally fills in for the coordinators of local programs like the Home Health Equipment Service. Talking with her fellow staff and volunteers has expanded her knowledge of the Red Cross movement a little, but she is still grossly uninformed. More than anything else she is happy to be able to cover half her university tuition costs by helping an organization whose work seems to do a bit of good for others.

On this particular afternoon, a retired teacher and long-time volunteer named Doreen O'Brien walks into the open-concept office and stands

beside the young woman's desk. "I've been sitting in that storeroom crying over a bunch of old letters," she announces, thrusting a handful of
yellowed pages at the summer student, whom she knows is a history
major. "They're from women who went overseas in the Second World
War." The student sets down her work and reads the letters eagerly,
quickly drawn into their wartime narrative. She is officially hooked on
Red Cross history.

I was this young woman. My association with the Red Cross began
with the casual thoughtlessness of youth, but the letters Doreen un-
earthed that afternoon inspired me to start asking questions which, over
the following decade, inspired both my doctoral dissertation and this
book, which grew out of it. How did ordinary volunteers and staff members like me fit into the institutional story of the Red Cross? What motivated Canadians to be part of this organization and its work, and did
those motivations change over time? And most befuddling of all, how
did an organization founded in mid-nineteenth-century Europe to provide battlefield aid in wartime, then established in 1896 Canada for similar purposes, end up supplying raised toilet seats, teaching swimming
lessons, and (until the late-1990s) collecting blood for civilian use in
Windsor, Ontario? This book tries to answer those questions.

✚

During the highly politicized Tainted Blood Scandal of the 1990s, some
observers predicted the end of the Canadian Red Cross. The findings of
the Royal Commission of Inquiry into Canada's Blood System (also
known as the Krever Inquiry) led to a complete overhaul of the Canadian blood system, and in the process the Canadian Red Cross relinquished its longstanding, high profile role as the public face of that
system. How, observers wondered, could the Red Cross survive such a
blow? What they failed to recognize was that the organization already
had a long history of innovation and transformation: from its inception,
the Canadian Red Cross Society fought an ongoing battle against ir-
relevance. Between 1896 and 1914 it struggled to establish itself as a
wartime agency in a country most often at peace. During two world
wars it battled long distance, government regulation, criticism, and rumours of mismanagement to create and maintain a role for voluntary aid

in the context of increasingly state-organized total war. In 1918–19 it overturned its own wartime mandate to ward off obsolescence, and subsequently forged its way into new peacetime public health territory in the face of open hostility and resentment from other organizations. It struggled against severely reduced financial means and overwhelming need in order to maintain a skeleton structure and provide what programs it could during the Great Depression. During the Second World War the society rose phoenix-like from its own ashes to reach the pinnacle of its achievement, then continued its struggle to remain relevant in the challenging postwar context, a process in which the nationwide Blood Transfusion Service played an integral part. By the time the blood service was fully established in the 1960s, the Canadian Red Cross had demonstrated its resilience through numerous permutations. A blood-less Canadian Red Cross after 28 September 1998 was merely the latest incarnation of an ever-evolving organization.

How and why did the Canadian Red Cross travel the distance from its late-nineteenth-century roots in military medicine to its role as the public face of Canada's domestic blood system a century later? Understanding how the Red Cross rose from obscurity to become Canada's leading humanitarian organization is essential for making sense of the directions it has subsequently travelled. The society's survival and successful adaptation prior to 1970 rested upon four pillars, the first of which was its ability to tap into contemporary currents of militarism, patriotism, and maternalism in order to mobilize first military and medical men, then middle- and upper-class white women, and eventually as wide a swath of the Canadian population as possible. The second pillar was the vision of Red Cross leaders who constructed and exploited openings for the society in military medicine, women's wartime service, Canadian health and welfare provision, and global disaster relief. Pillar three was the society's decision to regionalize, nationalize, and internationalize, creating a nation-building mission for itself in the broadly defined health realm, entrusting the future of the national organization to the initiative and activity of local and provincial branches, and increasing the society's role in international relief efforts. The flat-out refusal of a long line of volunteers and staff to let the society slip into oblivion constituted the final pillar. The organization George Sterling Ryerson founded with his friends at a meeting held in his home in 1896[1] was not necessarily destined to become the country's leading humanitarian organization. Nor did it become one of Canada's most enduring charities by chance.

A tension between renewal and obsolescence therefore characterizes the entire history of the Canadian Red Cross. Since its inception, the organization's ability to adapt to a society that keeps changing around it, while maintaining a core identity (helping the vulnerable) as it drifts ever further from its original mission, has been the key to the Canadian Red Cross's survival and longevity. After an initial period in which a failure to adapt nearly led to the demise of the organization, adaptability became the defining element of the first century of Red Cross work in Canada. Many factors contributed to this adaptability – for instance, the importance of voluntarism is a given, throughout – but militarism, patriotism, and gender were equally important forces contributing to the creation and endurance of the Red Cross in Canada.

Maple Leaf Mercy: Why Voluntary Organizations Matter in Canadian History

Canadians have a long history of voluntary action and charitable giving, through religious tithing, community barn raisings and work bees, fraternal and mutual aid societies, social welfare organizations, recreational and youth groups, international humanitarian aid, disaster relief efforts, and political activism, to name but a few.[2] Like people around the globe, Canadians have banded together and offered their resources in support of a wide variety of causes and mutual goals. Some of these organizations and causes arise under particular circumstances, flourish for a time (or do not), and subside, giving way to other efforts more relevant to the changing times. Others put down deep roots, taking hold in society and outlasting the circumstances of their birth. Some organizations toil quietly and on a small scale. Others rise to local, national, or even international prominence. Some focus on a single need or issue; others cast their nets more widely. At their best, they can contribute positively to the functioning of a democratic society by offering citizens the opportunity to support causes dear to their hearts and fight injustices that move them.[3] Voluntary and charitable organizations – and people's propensity to create and support them – have contributed significantly to the development of Canadian society, and have often pioneered endeavours, filled gaps, and otherwise responded to changes in the local, national, and global community. While governments and other official bodies are usually slow and ponderous, and often reluctant to take on new (and perhaps politically charged) responsibilities, voluntary organizations – while often flawed in their own ways – can be swift and decisive.[4] Armed with the power of a noble cause, a visionary and impassioned leadership, a body of like-minded volunteers and donors, and public support, voluntary organizations can accomplish enormous feats.

But it does not always work out that way. Noble causes fail to capture public interest, leaders lose their vision – or their followers – and other issues and events compete for limited money, media attention, and volunteers. Needs cease to be needs, organizations drift from their original missions, governments intervene, and high ideals are shaken or co-opted for different purposes. What is manageable when small can cease to be manageable when swelled by an outpouring of public support. Not all volunteers prove reliable or trustworthy; not all recipients of aid prove worthy of help. Donors fail to donate; volunteers fail to volunteer; scandals and rumours spring up; leaders fail to lead. When people join together of their own accord to achieve a goal without state coercion or monetary reward, the results can be inspiring – or heartbreaking.[5]

Voluntary organizations are important. They were crucial to the functioning of Canadian society in the past, and they remain a key, if sometimes overlooked, element of Canadian society at the beginning of the twenty-first century. If we would understand where we are today as a society and how we got here, it is vital that we pay attention to the story of these organizations. They offer a window into the dreams, ambitions, fears, and concerns of Canadians past and present; they highlight the ways in which our attitudes toward individual and government responsibilities have changed over time, as well as when, why, and how. They can also illuminate a society's conceptions of its duty to help and its role in the wider world: at a given time, who is worth helping – where, why, and how?

In her influential 1995 article "The Mixed Social Economy as a Canadian Tradition," Mariana Valverde asserts that, in Canada, the traditional distinction between public and private, state and civil society, has never existed – at least not in a clear-cut fashion. Instead, using Ontario as a case study, she argues that the "modern" inclination toward mixed public-private forms of service provision is in fact a longstanding feature of Canadian life.[6] On one level, *Mobilizing Mercy* serves as a further, extended case study, examining this proposition. State intervention in Canadian society grew dramatically between 1885, when the first hints of Red Cross activity appeared in Canada, and 1970, when this book's substantial narrative concludes; during the same period, the activities of the Canadian Red Cross were repeatedly transformed in their own ways. Mapping the subtle shifts in the relationship between these two evolving bodies – government and voluntary/charitable organization – therefore offers valuable insights into the applicability of Valverde's argument. Seen over the long term, the history of the Canadian Red Cross Society paints a complex portrait of a mutually dependent relationship between the state and the voluntary sector. Each has leaned on the other to supplement its own deficiencies in different times and contexts, thereby creating and participating in the "mixed social economy" put forward by Valverde.

The Canadian Red Cross Society, on the grounds of its longevity and national scale alone, is an object worthy of study. But added to those aspects are its international roots and connections, its complicated and ever-changing relationships with different levels of government, its roles in both wartime and peacetime, its symbolic power, its multi-levelled governance that long mirrored Canada's federal system, its shifting relationships with the British and American Red Cross organizations, its integral role in Canada's postwar blood donation system, and the sheer scope of its activities between the late-nineteenth century and the present. The result is a case study in the evolution of a single voluntary organization that offers a window into major events and developments in twentieth-century Canadian history ranging from Canadian military engagements to the development of the modern health care system; from youth citizenship education to the changing roles of women. To trace the history of the Canadian Red Cross is, in many ways, to trace the history of twentieth-century Canada.

Idea, Movement, Organization: The International Red Cross

The Red Cross idea originated in a very specific set of circumstances, but grew into a transnational movement and a powerful, multi-faceted organization active around the world. Over the course of the nineteenth century, European wars became increasingly destructive, and observers noted that many deaths came not from the actual battles but from sickness and wounds. Moved by the carnage and grossly inadequate medical care he witnessed during the Battle of Solferino in 1859, Swiss citizen Henry Dunant wrote a small volume entitled *A Memory of Solferino* and sent copies to royalty and politicians throughout Europe. His memorable descriptions included "bleeding, muddy, vermin-covered bodies" suffering in a "scorching, filthy atmosphere in the midst of vile, nauseating odours, with lamentations and cries of anguish all around." Dunant proposed that voluntary aid societies be set up and allowed to assist the sick and wounded during war,[7] an idea that gained him the active and able support of fellow Swiss citizen Gustave Moynier. In 1863 they assembled a group of Swiss men to advance Dunant's ideas.

Calling themselves the International Committee, Dunant and Moynier's group organized an international conference in Geneva that same year, which aimed to "civilize" war by setting rules of conduct and treatment for the sick and wounded. A second conference in 1864 formally codified the first Geneva Convention to ameliorate the condition of wounded armies in the field. These first two conferences in Geneva provided for each signatory state to have a committee ready to aid (but not displace) army medical services in caring for the sick and wounded, and established a symbol to indicate the neutral status of volunteers on the battlefield: the now-iconic white armband bearing a red cross. The International Committee renamed itself the International Committee of the Red Cross (ICRC), and most of the principal European nations of the 1860s and 1870s subsequently set up national aid societies that they enthusiastically put to work. The idea of providing special aid to the sick and wounded in war was not new, but it gained fresh currency among European nations in the late nineteenth century. European states came to realize that if they wished to maintain popular support for their territorial wars they must appear to care about the fates of their citizen-soldiers. Official indifference was no longer an option in the new world of conscripted citizen armies, sanitary reform movements, and developments in communication that allowed war news to be widely and rapidly dispersed. The resulting movement to regulate war – of which the Geneva Conventions were an integral part – reached its highest peak between 1870 and 1914.[8]

The ICRC continued to play a key role in facilitating the development of international humanitarian law even after the creation of the 1864 Geneva Convention. Chief among the ICRC's efforts over the course of the twentieth century were the conferences it initiated and hosted in order to revise the Geneva Conventions in response to new developments in warfare and conflict. As a result, the international community revised or added to the Geneva Conventions in 1906, 1929, 1949, and 1977.[9] As Geoffrey Best notes, the idea of regulating and restraining warfare "bristles with paradox," but the international community repeatedly attempted to do just that, beginning in the late nineteenth century. The paradoxical spirit which characterized the nineteenth century is evident in its simultaneous peace and war movements: the strident militarism that marked the century was matched by a longing for international harmony and cooperation that manifested itself in (among others) a series of major international expositions, the creation of the Nobel Prize, the Olympic revival, and the creation of a Permanent Court of International Justice.[10] Caroline Moorehead points out that, within this context, European leaders of the 1860s "wanted 'civilized' and 'humane' war, which could be invoked or set aside as a political instrument." The Red Cross idea sprang directly from this period of paradox, and the great irony of the Red Cross as a movement is that by mobilizing civilian populations through its work to alleviate the physical suffering caused by war (thereby returning soldiers to battle, and/or boosting civilian morale) it inadvertently made it easier for countries to wage war.[11] The Red Cross movement's acceptance of the existence of war and determination to alleviate suffering in that context make it the classic example of what Michael Barnett calls "emergency humanitarianism" – providing relief in the immediate crisis within a framework of neutral, impartial independence – as opposed to "alchemical humanitarianism" which tries to alter the underlying conditions which produce humanitarian crises, and is more likely to become political in the process.[12]

By the 1870s national Red Cross societies had become a means by which civilians unable to fight could "serve almost as directly by caring for their fighters," thus inherently undermining the purported neutrality of national Red Cross societies. The 1906 Geneva Conventions acknowledged this fact by making the Red Cross societies of belligerent nations subject to military laws and regulations for the duration of the particular conflict in which they were engaged. This move effectively brought national Red Cross societies under the authority of their respective national military organizations during times of war, allying them with one side of the conflict in spite of their putative neutrality.[13] However, the ICRC and Red Cross societies not belonging to a belligerent nation in a given conflict retained their independence of action and could exercise something akin to true neutrality.

Dunant's original idea for voluntary humanitarian aid in wartime eventually produced three distinct branches of Red Cross activity. Today they are known collectively as the International Red Cross (IRC), an umbrella term encompassing the International Committee of the Red Cross, the International Federation of Red Cross and Red Crescent Societies, and the many national Red Cross, Red Crescent, and Red Crystal organizations.[14] None of these three distinct components has control over any of the others. The founding organization of the Red Cross movement, the ICRC, remains an elite committee of Swiss citizens who serve as the guardians of the Geneva Conventions. Red Cross activity that requires strict neutrality, such as inspecting prisoner-of-war (POW) camps or tracing persons missing because of war or disaster, takes place under the banner of the ICRC. The tasks themselves are undertaken by individuals from around the world but because the ICRC's claim to neutrality is predicated on Switzerland's traditional neutrality, the committee itself maintains a Swiss-only membership. This neutrality has often allowed the ICRC to gain access to soldiers and civilians which is denied to explicitly partisan groups, and the ICRC's self-proclaimed non-political approach is a model that hundreds of subsequent non-governmental organizations have followed.[15]

Today's International Federation of Red Cross and Red Crescent Societies was created in 1919 as the League of Red Cross Societies, in an attempt to turn the combined power of national Red Cross societies (flush with money, volunteers, and influence) to the task of European relief and worldwide public health promotion following the First World War. Today the federation continues to act as a coordinating body that encourages international Red Cross/Crescent/Crystal cooperation, co-ordinates international disaster relief efforts, and assists in the exchange of information and expertise among the national organizations.

National Red Cross/Crescent/Crystal organizations exist as auto-nomous, officially recognized wartime voluntary aid agencies in their re-spective countries, and undertake whatever range of peacetime activities they wish, usually in the fields of public health and disaster relief. By the time of the First World War, national Red Cross societies had largely lost their original role of providing volunteer battlefield assistance to the sick and wounded. Reforms carried out within most belligerent nations' mil-itary medical services had rendered such a role unnecessary, and instead national Red Cross societies largely became channels through which civil-ians could provide gifts of medical supplies and comforts to sick and wounded combatants.[16] No country or empire may have more than one officially recognized national Red Cross/Crescent/Crystal, but most of the national organizations are internally subdivided by region, province, state, and/or locality, with all sub-branches ultimately responsible to the national organization. Canadians were relative latecomers to the Red Cross movement but they created the first colonial branch of the British Red Cross Society within the British Empire. The Canadian Red Cross Society in turn divided itself into provincial divisions and local branches (now replaced by a system of zones, regions, and local branches). Na-tional Red Cross/Crescent/Crystal organizations require the official recognition of the International Committee of the Red Cross in order to qualify for protection under the Geneva Conventions and representation at International Red Cross conferences. However, beyond this initial re-quirement the ICRC has no control over national Red Cross/Crescent/Crystal societies, which have historically been influenced primarily by their respective national contexts. The 1975 Tansley Report commis-sioned by the IRC identified this autonomy and general lack of cohesion among national Red Cross societies as being among the greatest weak-nesses of the IRC, but the national organizations themselves have tradi-tionally cherished their freedom.[17]

Selling Humanitarianism: The Red Cross as a
Not-for-Profit Brand

While the IRC developed over the course of a century and a half into the form it takes today, a less concrete but nonetheless powerful parallel development was underway: the "branding" of the Red Cross. In her bestselling book *No Logo*, Naomi Klein describes how the brand mania of the 1990s produced companies whose businesses came to rely not on physical products, but on names and logos, so that "Brand X is not a product but a way of life, an attitude, a set of values, a look, an idea."[18] The red cross emblem is perhaps one of the earliest and most successful non-corporate examples of branding in modern history: although designed specifically to represent two particular groups during wartime – members of army medical corps on the field of battle and members of voluntary aid societies helping the sick and wounded – it quickly became widely recognized and associated with a vast range of activities. Beginning with the creation of the ICRC and the first Geneva Convention, the red cross emblem was associated with a powerful idea: neutral, humanitarian aid to the sick and wounded. The precise form that such assistance took was always less important than the larger idea it represented. Ambulances, bandages, POW parcels, health pamphlets, district nurses, disaster relief workers, and international family messages could all display the red cross emblem and thereby be marked as belonging to an organization that stood for certain principles and values.

Red Cross organizations have always promoted themselves as something more than simply charities: since its earliest days the Red Cross has been a "Movement," an "Idea," and the product of a revered founder's vision ("Dunant's Dream," as Caroline Moorehead titled her history of the International Red Cross). For this reason, a cartoon history of the origins of the International Red Cross used by the Canadian Red Cross at the end of the twentieth century was called simply "The Story of an Idea."[19] The Seven Fundamental Principles of the IRC adopted in 1965 – humanity, impartiality, neutrality, independence, voluntary service, unity, and universality – further emphasize the idea that the Red Cross is more than a mere charity.[20] One can also speak of "Red Cross" in a general sense without specifying the International Red Cross, the International Committee of the Red Cross, the League of Red Cross Societies/

International Federation of Red Cross and Red Crescent Societies, or a national, provincial, or local Red Cross organization. Like Disney or the United Nations, "Red Cross" has become an overarching entity encompassing many component parts, which collectively stand for certain values and possess a distinct and recognized identity.

"Red Cross" initially evolved as a brand on a global scale because of four overlapping developments: first, the range of activities undertaken in its name during wartime; second, the international movement's large-scale expansion into peacetime work after the First World War; third, the public's frequent failure to distinguish between the activities of various national Red Cross societies; and fourth, the public's corresponding failure to distinguish between medical personnel wearing the emblem for protection under the Geneva Conventions and those wearing the emblem as members of a national Red Cross society. "Helping" is a common theme throughout Red Cross history, and Red Cross work quickly came to be associated with attributes such as caring, generosity, self-sacrifice, kindness, humanity, love, and service. A diverse range of products and services took on the Red Cross name after the first Geneva Convention (prior to legislation designed to reserve the name and emblem exclusively for the two purposes for which it was intended), as companies attempted to capitalize on the early establishment of "Red Cross" as a name – and the Geneva-style red cross as an emblem – linked to helping and health. Nor did the appeal of the Red Cross stop there. From the beginning, citizens of many countries used the Red Cross and its work in order to express their patriotism, serve state purposes, socialize, or find adventure. Canada was no exception.

Beyond the Brand: History, Historiography, and the Red Cross

The global branding of the Red Cross and its association with ideas, fundamental principles, and generic "helping" have often overshadowed the movement's historical development, making it seem as if it has been unaffected by the currents of contemporary thought and circumstance. This serves the international organization well, since it relies on its emblem to grant protection to medical personnel and aid workers under the Geneva Conventions, but it obscures the unique histories of the various

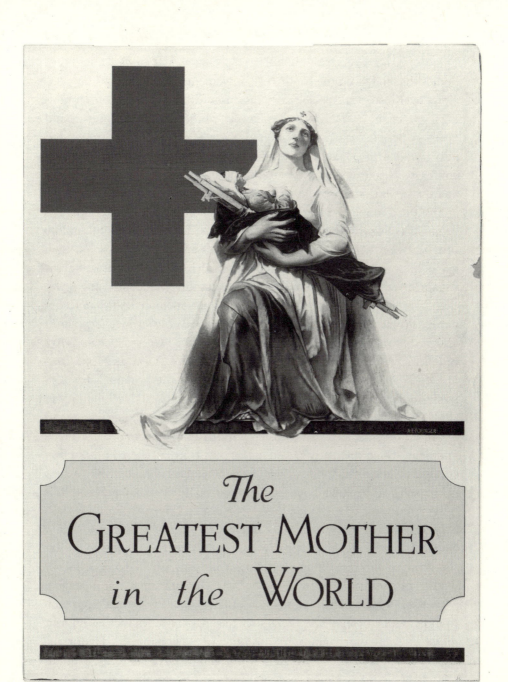

The
GREATEST MOTHER
in the WORLD

Figure 0.1
As this iconic American Red Cross poster illustrates, during the First
World War the Red Cross "brand" became associated throughout the
English-speaking world with maternal attributes like love and care.

bodies that make up the Red Cross movement. This emphasis on principles over historical specifics also disguises the fact that the lofty founding ideals of the Red Cross movement (and others that governments and ordinary people foisted on the organization at various points) translated into a wide array of activities and attitudes, and played out in national contexts of fundraising competition, inter-agency squabbling, government intervention, wartime hysteria, and peacetime apathy.

Sustained scholarly interest in the history of the Red Cross movement began in 1989 with the publication of the late John Hutchinson's mildly provocative article "Rethinking the Origins of the Red Cross." It then gained momentum during the 1990s, likely because newer humanitarian organizations with different mandates (notably Médecins Sans Frontières) and tainted blood scandals in a number of countries began to undermine the Red Cross's reputation as a "sacred cow" above criticism.[21] Older accounts produced by those within the Red Cross, such as Pierre Boissier's *From Solferino to Tsushima* and André Durand's *From Sarajevo to Hiroshima*, had already capably traced the principal developments in the history of the Red Cross at an international level, but newer studies by Nicholas Berry, Caroline Moorehead, Jean-Claude Favez, and David P. Forsythe, as well as further work by Hutchinson, deconstructed and demystified the often secretive IRC and ICRC.[22] These authors persuasively argued that, lofty principles notwithstanding, the Red Cross movement was deeply influenced by the social, intellectual, political, and military currents that shaped the nineteenth and twentieth centuries. In his 2011 volume *Empire of Humanity: A History of Humanitarianism*, Michael Barnett demonstrates that such influences have moulded the entire modern Western humanitarian aid movement.[23] Excellent recent studies of the American Red Cross (ARC) by Julia Irwin and Marian Moser Jones have pioneered the work of applying this critical approach to individual national Red Cross societies: Moser Jones focuses on ARC disaster relief, and Irwin on early ARC international aid.[24] Historians Melanie Oppenheimer and Margaret Tennant have similarly brought analytical rigour to new centennial histories of, respectively, the Australian and New Zealand Red Cross societies, while Ian Willis dissects the intersections of class and gender in a local study of Australia's Camden District Red Cross during both world wars.[25]

John Hutchinson's 1996 monograph *Champions of Charity: War and the Rise of the Red Cross* is unquestionably the most influential of the newer, more critical works. Hutchinson argues that internationalism and humanitarianism alone did not produce the rise and survival of the Red Cross movement, and he demonstrates how the spread of the Red Cross and its internationalist agenda in the latter part of the nineteenth century was inextricably entwined with the fierce nationalism of the day. National governments frequently supported the development of their respective Red Cross societies because they saw them as a means of mobilizing populations, imposing voluntary taxation, and financing operations (care of the sick and wounded, for example) that the state itself ought to be financing. The Red Cross seed successfully sprouted in so many countries, Hutchinson argues, because each autonomous national Red Cross society retained the freedom to determine its own methods of applying Red Cross principles. In essence, internationalism could be adapted to individual national agendas. Hutchinson also elaborates on Geoffrey Best's earlier concept of "the militarization of humanitarianism"[26] in nineteenth-century Europe – it becomes "the militarization of charity" in Hutchinson's work. Hutchinson follows this idea beyond Best's observation that Red Cross societies took on the tone of the war movement, to uncover what he calls "Red Cross patriotism." The militarization of charity led to a situation in which "working for the national Red Cross society became both an outlet for, and a measure of, a citizen's patriotic enthusiasm."[27]

Hutchinson's arguments regarding the Red Cross at an international level offer an important framework for understanding the Red Cross in Canada. The Canadian Red Cross Society (CRCS – often referred to as simply "the Society" until the later twentieth century, when the "Society" part of its full name was gradually dropped), its history, and its work, are very much the products of their historical contexts. As is the case with many voluntary and community organizations, individuals associated with the society and proud of its humanitarian accomplishments have produced the majority of existing accounts of Canadian Red Cross history. They generally revolve around the society's work in times of war or disaster.[28] In the absence of more comprehensive and critical works, McKenzie Porter's 1960 CRCS-approved and largely anecdotal

To All Men: The Story of the Canadian Red Cross has now served as the
standard work on the history of the CRCS for over half a century.[29] Most
of these surveys of CRCS history (including Porter's) were written within
a few decades after the end of the Second World War (1939–45). Tinged
with the triumphant glow of the war years, they tend to see all CRCS activity before 1939 as a mere prelude to the society's massive Second
World War effort, and/or to the subsequent expansion of its peacetime
program and creation of the national Blood Transfusion Service. One
aim of this book is to reduce the society's Second World War work to a
more appropriate proportion of the society's history and place it within
a much broader canvas of Red Cross activity in Canada. A related aim
is to explain how the CRCS became responsible for Canada's blood collection system, and how that program fit into the overall scope of the society's work in Canada during and after the Second World War.

Despite the absence of a comprehensive scholarly study of Canadian
Red Cross history, Canadian scholars have produced insightful micro-
histories of select portions of the CRCS's work – research that has facilitated *Mobilizing Mercy*'s attempt at a broad overview and synthesis. In
the mid-1980s the first of these scholars, Nancy M. Sheehan, began considering the CRCS's role in interwar Alberta drought relief, and examined
the role of the Junior Red Cross in prairie school curricula.[30] In the mid-
1990s Richard H. Kapp outlined the origins of the Second World War
blood program, and in her MA thesis Deanna Toxopeus investigated a
1951 agreement between the CRCS and the St John Ambulance Association as a case study in Canadian Cold War civil defence efforts.[31] The
first decade of the twenty-first century has produced further research:
Jayne Elliott's and Linda Kealey's work on outpost nurses,[32] Linda J.
Quiney's research into women's voluntary and paid work for the Red
Cross during the First World War and interwar years, Jennifer Ann
Polk's MA thesis on the CRCS mission to Siberia (1918–21), Douglas
Baldwin and Gillian Poulter's work on Mona Wilson and the CRCS in
Newfoundland during the Second World War, and studies of the society's
POW work during the Second World War by both Jonathan Vance and
Daniel Pomerleau.[33] Ian Mosby's analysis of Red Cross food work in
the Second World War and my own studies of women's Red Cross work
in war and peace and the First and Second World War Red Cross work

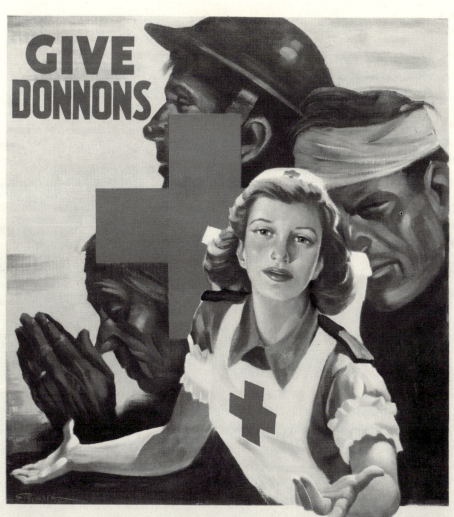

GIVE
DONNONS

THE CANADIAN RED CROSS
LA CROIX ROUGE CANADIENNE

Figure 0.2
Visually memorable wartime artifacts like this fundraising poster,
reproduced in CRCS publications and on the internet, reinforce the dominance of the
Second World War in both institutional and popular memory.

of Canadian children have added to this patchwork body of knowledge.[34] Each micro-history offers crucial insights into the complexity of the Red Cross's relationships with its volunteers, donors, and staff; the Canadian military; various levels of government; and the Canadian public it served. Since these micro-histories have focused on CRCS work during and after the First World War, another aim of this book is to highlight the importance of many distinct experiences and formative developments during the often-overlooked preceding twenty-nine years (from 1885 to 1914). This earlier period saw the society take shape and establish certain patterns and assumptions which would fundamentally influence its work throughout the twentieth century.

To this point, critical studies of the international Red Cross movement have primarily considered the development of leading countries' Red Cross societies, such as those in Germany, France, Britain, Russia, Japan, and the United States. Recognizing the ways by which the history of the Red Cross in smaller countries either mirrors or diverges from the history of the Red Cross in these great powers contributes to a fuller understanding of the Red Cross's development around the world. Oppenheimer, Willis, and Tennant have begun this work with regard to Australia and New Zealand; in turn, *Mobilizing Mercy* offers a more nuanced sense of what is "Canadian" about the Canadian Red Cross, and broadens our ability to compare the development of Red Cross societies in countries sharing a heritage as white settler colonies of the British Empire. These international comparisons can be fruitful: for instance, not every founder of a Red Cross Society had battlefield experience, but many did. Henry Dunant was inspired to found the entire Red Cross movement after seeing the sick and wounded suffering on the battlefields of Solferino. John Furley saw firsthand the plight of the wounded in the Prusso-Danish war in 1864 and went on to spearhead the effort to form an active British Red Cross Society. Clara Barton's experiences working with the sick and wounded during the American Civil War eventually led her to create the American Red Cross.[35] Many core members of the original Canadian Red Cross (including founder G.S. Ryerson) served as either combatants or medics in the 1885 Northwest campaign. The mounting evidence therefore suggests that direct experience of battlefield casualties and illness was a major contributor to many individual founders' enthusiastic embrace of the Red Cross idea, regardless of their national contexts. Beyond the Red Cross movement, adding the history of the CRCS to the histories of other international humanitarian and human rights organizations, such as Oxfam, Save the Children Fund, Amnesty International, or Médecins Sans Frontières, similarly offers an opportunity to more fully understand Canadians' roles in twentieth-century humanitarian aid efforts and an evolving sense of global community and responsibility.[36]

International comparisons aside, this study contributes first and foremost to our knowledge of one of Canada's oldest and most prestigious voluntary humanitarian organizations, and its role in Canadian society during the late-nineteenth and twentieth centuries. It also widens our understanding of the history of voluntary labour in Canada, particularly during wartime, and of volunteers (largely women) themselves. From 1899 onward, women were the heart and soul of Red Cross voluntary work, and over the course of the twentieth century they held many leadership roles within the society. Yet the fact that the society drew on the efforts of men as well as women, and children as well as adults, meant that gendered understandings of both labour and childhood shaped the organization and its work. This study therefore makes a significant contribution to the somewhat sparse literature on Canadian women's and children's important voluntary action during the South African War, First and Second World Wars, and Korean War, and contributes to the already rich literature surrounding women, children, and work.[37] Shirley Tillotson's 2008 book *Contributing Citizens* illuminates the crucial role of twentieth-century charitable organizations in pioneering efficient, rationalized fundraising methods, thereby contributing to the rise of the Canadian welfare state. Many of the fundraising practices she discusses were also used by the CRCS in both war and peace. Considering the CRCS's domestic efforts, therefore, adds to our emerging understanding of the role of voluntary organizations in Canada both before and after the advent of the welfare state. Exploring the society's peacetime public health efforts in particular enriches our knowledge of how voluntary organizations pioneered health services later taken up by governments.[38]

This study blends institutional history with social history in order to portray not only the evolution of the Canadian Red Cross Society as an organization but also its place in Canadian society more broadly. Sources detailing the history of the CRCS and its work between 1885 and 1970 vary widely depending on the years under examination. *Mobilizing Mercy* therefore draws on a combination of primary sources including memoirs, journals, personal papers, contemporary newspapers and magazines, photographs, House of Commons Debates and Sessional Papers, the Statutes of Canada, and federal government records, but it relies most heavily on institutional records: CRCS Executive Committee minute books, limited surviving correspondence between the British and Canadian Red Cross organizations, CRCS annual reports, and CRCS publications such as newsletters, advertising material, and health propaganda. Materials produced by the CRCS must be read particularly critically since they often paint the brightest possible picture in order to court or maintain public donations, volunteer enthusiasm, and government support. Yet these materials also contain useful statistics, financial records, and reports on national, provincial, and overseas activity, while other aspects of the CRCS, such as its attitudes toward Britain and the British Red Cross Society, can be gleaned from the language and illustrations used. They therefore lend themselves well to an investigation of the society's voluntary and fundraising efforts and how the CRCS imagined and portrayed itself and its work.

What these institutional sources do not reveal very clearly is the broader context in which the CRCS operated – for example, the precise division of responsibilities for medical provisioning between government and voluntary organizations in wartime, and how well these arrangements did or did not work. CRCS sources also offer an incomplete picture when it comes to criticism of the society's work. The society's wartime *Bulletin* and *Despatch* publications mention efforts to combat rumours, for instance, but the rumours themselves have left no documentary record as to where and when they originated, who spread them, who believed them, and of what exactly they consisted. This points to a broader challenge of this study: the frequent difficulty of finding non-CRCS sources with which to corroborate the claims made by the society. Haphazard record-keeping practices by both governments and voluntary organizations have limited what sources survive, as have accidental losses and policies of deliberately destroying records (such as those that affected the archival holdings of the British Red Cross Society).[39] During the Second World War the federal government established a Department of National War Services specifically to regulate and supervise war charities, but during the period 1885 to 1939 the CRCS, like other voluntary organizations, undertook its activities largely without regulation or government supervision. As a result there are far fewer government records relating to the CRCS prior to 1939 than there are for later periods.

Accessing the ways ordinary Canadians – especially women – experienced and felt about Red Cross work poses particular difficulties, but the First World War writings of prominent middle-class women like Nellie McClung, L.M. Montgomery, and Adelaide Plumptre, bolstered by information from the women's pages of contemporary newspapers and the letters and memoirs of Second World War Canadian Red Cross Corps members, provide a basis for informed speculation about how some women understood their wartime work for the Red Cross. (The fact that famous women like McClung and Montgomery were deeply involved with the CRCS when they had many other demands on their time highlights its omnipresence in wartime.) *Mobilizing Mercy* focuses on the national level of an organization headquartered in Toronto, and acknowledging the many regional and local varieties of Red Cross work that existed in Canada involves further challenges. Local and provincial Red Cross histories help address this issue, while for the years after the First World War a relative wealth of archival materials from the Nova Scotia and Alberta provincial divisions allows some comparison between the society's work in the eastern and western regions of the country.

It proved difficult to access francophone voices, and their silence in the early chapters reflects their conspicuous absence from most CRCS activity before the Second World War rather than a decision to exclude or ignore them in the course of my research. Not until the Second World War did the CRCS make any concerted effort – either nationally or within the Quebec Division specifically – to work in the French language or to attract francophone leaders and ordinary volunteers. French Canadians' money was always welcome, but the explicitly imperial slant of early CRCS propaganda and the society's unofficial policy of publishing its materials only in English until halfway through the twentieth century seem to have counteracted much of the humanitarian appeal which might otherwise have drawn French-Canadian volunteers on a scale comparable to that of their English-Canadian compatriots. The dearth of sources relating to francophones' experiences within the CRCS before the Second World War is lamentable, and is directly responsible for the absence of francophone voices from most of this study.

Collectively, these sources paint a picture of CRCS history that is as monumental and colourful as Canada itself, the canvas dominated by figures engaged in meaningful and sometimes dramatic acts of humanitarian mercy. Filling the background, however, is a compelling and inescapable clash between the forces of renewal and obsolescence. *Mobilizing Mercy* tells the story of the Canadian Red Cross Society's ongoing battles against obsolescence by tracing its development through the uncertain early decades (chapters 1 and 2), the heady years of the First World War (chapter 3), two turbulent decades of interwar peacetime work (chapter 4), a return to power and prominence during the Second World War (chapter 5), and the tensions of a rapidly changing Cold War-era Canada (chapter 6).

Beginning with a consideration of the context in which the Red Cross idea took root in Canadian soil, chapter 1 explores its beginnings during the Northwest Uprising of 1885 and in the late-nineteenth-century quest to improve Canada's military medical service. Chapter 2 examines the society's first successful wartime effort during the South African War and considers the implications of that conflict for subsequent Red Cross wartime responses. Together these two chapters reveal how the society's British-inspired wartime mandate both fostered the organization's creation and hindered its early development. Chapter 3 examines the society's transformation from a small and unimportant Toronto-based organization to a nationwide, leading Canadian humanitarian agency during the First World War, as it tapped into powerful currents of patriotism and maternalism, Christian impulses, and social expectations. By bridging the gap between Canadians at home and Canadian citizen-soldiers abroad, the CRCS made a lasting positive impression on both groups. The society's pragmatic 1918 decision to take on peacetime public health work, the First World War's influence on that work, and the role of that work as part of a vast nation-building project, are the subjects of chapter 4. Chapter 5 traces both the triumphs and challenges that marked the society's massive Second World War effort, arguing that the conflicts and difficulties that appeared during those six years were forerunners of the challenges which would face the society in an altered postwar world. The years between 1946 and 1970 are the focus of chapter 6, which traces the society's growing international involvement, its movement into water safety and blood collection, and the challenges it faced in a rapidly changing postwar society. The conclusion considers the society's position at the opening of the 1970s, peers ahead briefly into the blood scandal of the 1980s and 1990s and its aftermath, and draws broad conclusions about the CRCS and its place in Canadian society since 1885.

From Myth to History: Seeing beyond Dunant

Surveys of the history of the Canadian Red Cross Society typically gloss over the early years of the society in Canada and instead emphasize the European story of Henry Dunant. The mythology surrounding Dunant, the ICRC, and the Geneva Conventions is central to the way the Red Cross movement as a whole understands itself and its role in the world, and the Canadian Red Cross has historically looked to Dunant for its identity as well. Certainly without Dunant and the ICRC there would be no Canadian Red Cross. But as Hutchinson and Moorehead demonstrate, the establishment and subsequent development of the ICRC – and in turn, each of the national Red Cross/Crescent/Crystal societies – was by no means inevitable. Each organization took root and flourished (or did not) within a particular set of historical circumstances.[40] As Roger Cooter rightly insists, one cannot "separate the theatres of war and medicine from the social and economic contexts of which they are a part."[41] In the Canadian case, CRCS wartime work and public health activities were influenced by the aims and goals of the international Red Cross movement, as well as by the British and American Red Cross societies to which it sometimes looked for models. Yet the history of the Red Cross in Canada is also unique: it has been profoundly shaped by the people, places, and preoccupations of this country.

The Canadian Red Cross has its own founding mythology separate from the story of Henry Dunant. This "flag on a wagon" story begins with Dr George Sterling Ryerson hoisting a red cross flag on a wagon during the Northwest Uprising (1885), as though Dunant's dream of neutral Red Cross organizations magically crossed the Atlantic Ocean and patiently waited to be applied in Canada. Eleven years later, in 1896,

Ryerson (for little apparent reason) then forms a Canadian branch of the British Red Cross Society, and sometime later there is (conveniently) a war, which allows the Canadian Red Cross to flourish ever after.

Although there is a measure of truth to this tale, it oversimplifies and omits a great deal. That is what myths are supposed to do, as they attempt to crystallize the muddiness of history into a more useable past. But there is another story to be told. As it has unfolded over the course of more than one hundred years, the history of the Canadian Red Cross Society is a long and complicated one, full of intriguing characters and unexpected twists and turns. It is a story that begins in the late nineteenth century, in a large, sparsely populated country still in its infancy, where the military medical system is a shambles and a handful of elite men want to fix it. This, then, is where we shall begin.

I

MEN, MEDICINE, AND MILITIA, 1885–1896

The Métis settlement of Batoche was usually a peaceful place of enormous blue sky, prairie fields interspersed with bush, and humble wooden frame homes, along the tranquil broad expanse of the South Saskatchewan River. But on 12 May 1885 it was instead the site of a pitched battle between the Canadian militia and skilfully constructed Métis defences. This fourth day of battle at Batoche would finally see the government's 800-strong Northwest Field Force achieve a clear-cut victory over the weakened Métis defenders, but neither side knew this as the crack of rifle fire, the cries of men and horses, and the smoke of battle filled the air. Amid the noise and confusion, Dr George Sterling Ryerson, an assistant surgeon with the ambulance corps of the Tenth Royal Grenadiers, sought to distinguish himself and his stretcher-bearers from combatants of both sides as they collected and attended to wounded militiamen. What he needed was a symbol – a visible one. Ryerson hastily sewed two strips of red cloth onto a large white piece of cotton, producing a rough approximation of a Geneva red cross, and hoisted his flag above the ambulance wagon that he and his men used to carry stretchers and other medical equipment.[1] One problem solved; one Canadian Red Cross Society (CRCS) born on the field of battle.

Or so the story goes. The founding myth of the CRCS is not, strictly speaking, untrue. But it does not tell us anything about how Ryerson knew of the Red Cross, or whether anyone else on the battlefield understood what his flag meant. It gives the impression that Ryerson acted alone and it fails to explain why it took another eleven years for Ryerson to get around to actually founding (as he did) an official Canadian Red Cross Society. Similarly, this story omits any explanation of why such a society seemed useful or necessary in late-nineteenth-century Canada. It has in common with the founding myth of Amnesty International (studied by Tom Buchanan) a focus on one man's flash of inspiration, and a large measure of good timing.[2] But as with the Amnesty myth, the Canadian Red Cross Society's "flag on a wagon" story is not particularly helpful in understanding where the organization came from, or how it grew and developed from these origins. On a symbolic level, however, it remains a powerful narrative. The story of Ryerson's "flag on a wagon" includes the three elements that worked together to inspire the creation, and foster the earliest development, of the Red Cross in Canada: namely, men, medicine, and the militia.

After the establishment of the International Committee of the Red Cross in 1863, the Red Cross idea slowly spread to Canada and took tenuous root. Unofficial Red Cross activity during the 1885 Northwest Uprising was followed in 1896 by the creation of an officially recognized Red Cross branch in Canada, when it appeared that the organization might offer a solution to the rather dismal state of the country's military medical service. The Canadian Red Cross Society which would, in time, come to be best known for women's caring labour in wartime and peacetime public health work for the civilian population, owed its origins to an elite circle of British-Canadian men concerned about the state of medical provision in the Canadian militia. At this early point in the organization's life, the ideals of humanitarianism and neutrality that distinguished the international Red Cross movement were barely on the radar.

Early Glimpses of the Red Cross in Canada

The existence of an International Committee of the Red Cross and the ratification of the original Geneva Conventions in 1864 and 1868 initially had a limited impact on Britain's North American colonies. British military officers who came to British North America in the mid-1860s likely brought with them some knowledge of the Geneva Conventions' provisions relating to the treatment of the sick and wounded on the field of battle. It therefore seems reasonable to imagine that the idea of national aid societies was casually discussed over mess hall tables and across club smoking rooms by those in military and medical circles. In the broader public sphere, Toronto's major daily newspaper the *Globe* drew its readers' attention in a perfunctory way to the 1864 and 1868 international congresses that produced the Geneva Conventions. However, no evidence has survived to *prove* that military men discussed the idea, and the *Globe* appears to have been the only major British North American newspaper to take note of the events in Switzerland. These early developments, therefore, made little impression on civilian British North Americans at the time.[3]

While the Swiss founders of the Red Cross rallied support for their idea in European capitals and gathered delegates for the 1864 convention, politicians in the British North American colonies were occupied in Charlottetown and Quebec City, hammering out the confederation agreement that would create the Dominion of Canada. The British signature on the first two Geneva Conventions automatically bound all British colonies to observe their provisions, but Canada itself had no role in the creation or acceptance of the early Geneva Conventions. The American Civil War (1861–65) brought large-scale modern warfare to North America and created particular difficulties for British maritime colonies with long-standing economic, social, and kinship ties to the United States,[4] but the absence of any equivalent major military engagements for the Canadian militia between 1864 and 1885 considerably lessened the Geneva Conventions' relevance for Canada. The same pattern can be seen in Australia and New Zealand: although the emblem became well known, young British dominions did not need Red Cross societies when war was something that generally happened elsewhere.[5]

Neither of Canada's two chief influences, Great Britain and the United States, was at the leading edge when it came to the creation of officially recognized national aid ("Red Cross") societies, but by the 1870s both had begun to make efforts in this direction. Some Canadians may have noted the organization of the British National Society for Aid to the Sick and Wounded in War (BNAS) in 1870, and word of BNAS activities during the Franco-Prussian War may have filtered back to Canada. Meanwhile, the expansion of the American National Red Cross founded by Civil War heroine Clara Barton was considered newsworthy by the *Globe* in 1882, seven years after the organization's 1875 creation. These examples aside, proof of the Red Cross idea's migration to Canada and its gradual integration into contemporary culture is most clearly demonstrated by the fact that, from the 1880s onward, "Red Cross nurse" was a frequent costume choice for Canadian young ladies at fancy dress balls and skating parties – an association of the Red Cross with nursing that reflects the contemporary public prominence of nursing pioneer Florence Nightingale. Nightingale strongly opposed the idea of Red Cross societies, believing that governments should take responsibility for the health of their sick and wounded soldiers. Nevertheless, in many people's minds Nightingale's work during the Crimean War linked her – and nurses more generally – with the emerging Red Cross movement, an erroneous association that continues today.[6]

In subtle ways such as these (difficult, in the absence of sources, to reconstruct a century and a half later), the Red Cross idea took root in Canadian soil. Several notable Red Cross moments during the 1885 Northwest Uprising offer the first clear evidence that the Red Cross idea had gained some recognition within Canadian military medical circles. Independent of one another, Torontonians raised a Red Cross corps, and no less than three homemade red cross flags were hoisted on the field of battle. These undertakings were unofficial, in the sense that they were not sponsored by or affiliated with any national Red Cross society. But in each instance the symbol of the Geneva red cross was deliberately claimed as an identifying mark and emblem, presumably under the assumption it would be recognized and understood. A *Globe* editorial about the formation of the Red Cross corps stated that explaining the aims and virtues of the Red Cross Society would be "superfluous" – implying that at least a rudimentary knowledge of the international organization was already in circulation among the Canadian reading public by 1885. "Suffice it to say that the work is one of the noblest and most self-sacrificing in which a man can engage," the editor concluded.[7]

Red Cross Moments in the 1885 Northwest Uprising

The event that led to this sudden, homegrown interest in the Red Cross was a second uprising in Canada's western territories, as the Métis rallied once again under the leadership of Louis Riel (as they had done previously in 1869–70), this time in conjunction with Aboriginal allies. The federal government swiftly dispatched the Canadian militia west along the new Canadian Pacific Railway, determined to crush the resistance and permanently secure the prairie West for continued white settlement and economic expansion. By early April news reached Canadians of the sufferings of the militia volunteers as they marched through snowstorms in sub-zero temperatures between sections of the incomplete railway. Casualties were expected from the battles to come. In Montreal one concerned citizen wrote anonymously to the *Gazette* to ask what preparations were being made for aiding the sick and wounded of the militia.[8] As this anonymous letter suggests, suddenly the Red Cross idea had practical applications for Canada. Little surprise, then, that a number of men apparently familiar with its outlines put it to use.

The first recorded use of a red cross flag in Canada is attributed to Lieutenant-Colonel Alfred Codd, a McGill University graduate in medicine who ran a surgical practice in Ottawa before being appointed as a surgeon to the First Ontario Rifles of the Wolseley Expedition (which responded to the first Métis uprising at Red River) in 1870. Codd and his wife subsequently settled in Winnipeg and raised a family. He worked as a recruiting medical officer for the North West Mounted Police until 1885, when he was once again called into action. The forty-two-year-old Codd was serving as a surgeon for the Winnipeg Field Battalion under General Middleton when he sewed together his own improvised red cross flag (the cross decidedly Christian in proportion, rather than the shorter-limbed Geneva version) to use during the battle of Fish Creek on 24 April 1885.[9]

Unofficial Red Cross activity in the Northwest went beyond flags to include personnel. Some of the regiments called up for service in 1885 provided their own ambulance corps, and Darby Bergin, the newly appointed surgeon-general of the Canadian militia,[10] arranged for two fully staffed field hospital units, a group of female nurses, and requisite medical supplies to be sent to the front. In addition to these arrangements, Bergin also accepted the offer of a privately raised "Red Cross corps" from Edwin Wragge, local Toronto manager of the Grand Trunk Railway. Wragge secured government support for the venture in the form of official permission, transportation, and rations, then solicited public subscriptions and recruited an independent unit of medical volunteers to

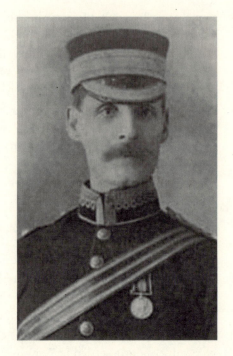

Figure 1.1
Dr William Nattress, Toronto surgeon
and member of the Queen's Own Rifles,
led the (unofficial) red cross ambulance
corps to the Northwest in 1885.

provide first aid and stretcher-bearing services on the battlefields and in
the rear hospitals. Wragge's Red Cross corps consisted of twelve young
men, nearly all of them newly minted physicians and surgeons, under the
direction of thirty-three-year-old Dr William Nattress, a lifelong temperance advocate and son-in-law of Toronto chief magistrate Colonel
George Taylor Denison. Like many (and perhaps all[11]) of the volunteers
in the corps, Nattress also belonged to the Queen's Own Rifles, a fashionable Toronto regiment called up for service in 1885.

After an enthusiastic and well-attended public send-off at Toronto's
Union Station on 16 April, the gray-uniformed Red Cross corps volunteers and their stores of medical supplies and provisions (each crate or
valise stamped with a large red cross) travelled to the Northwest territory.[12] The corps joined Colonel Otter's force on its way to Battleford,
and earned Otter's praise for its work under enemy fire at Cutknife Hill
on 2 May. While dealing with the casualties from that engagement, the
corps, which had been given the status of "dressers" in a temporary field
dressing station unit, is reported to have "hastily collected some cotton

sheets and red flannel and made up a Red Cross flag which was flown over their 'Station.'" Dr Nattress described the wounds treated by the corps, and the benefits he believed patients gained from the fresh air of the Northwest, in a paper for the Canadian Medical Association after his return to Toronto, but little other evidence survives of the corps' experience in the Northwest. Newspaper correspondents, men invalided back from the expedition, and Surgeon-General Bergin united in offering glowing praise for the assistance it rendered.[13]

Meanwhile, the highly effective Métis defences at Batoche (in present-day Saskatchewan) cost General Middleton and his militia five dead and twenty-five wounded in the course of the militia's first clear-cut victory of the campaign, on 12 May.[14] During the battle, Dr George Sterling Ryerson, assistant surgeon with the Tenth Royal Grenadiers, sought to distinguish his medical work in the chaos of battle. In a now well-established pattern, he created and hoisted a homemade red cross flag (the third red cross flag to be flown in the Northwest) as he and his stretcher-bearers undertook their dangerous work.[15]

Since the Métis warriors were not part of the Euro-Canadian military establishment, it is questionable whether they would have recognized or understood the neutrality and medical non-combatant status these red cross flags were meant to confer. But given that "Flags (red cross)" were among the items sent from Winnipeg to the militia's field hospitals, one would expect that at the very least Canadian militia members appreciated their meaning. Since all three reported cases of red cross flags used in 1885 indicate that the flags were improvised, hand-made versions, one can only surmise that either medical personnel were unaware of the red cross flags sent among the official supplies, or no one could find them when they were needed. In Ryerson's memoirs and in later Canadian Red Cross histories, Ryerson's flag took on mythic proportions, but at the time each of these flag-raisings – Ryerson's, Codd's, and the Red Cross corps' – was a minor incident in the confusion of battle. Both Codd and Ryerson preserved their flags, and they are now on display in Canadian Red Cross offices in Regina and Ottawa respectively.[16] Yet in 1885 it was the now-forgotten Red Cross corps which excited the most interest, and it was not until years later that either Codd's or Ryerson's flags attracted significant notice. In addition to this documented flag and corps activity, it is possible that a BNAS commissioner was sent to the Northwest – something tantalizingly referred to in a *Globe* article from 1896 – but nothing is known of this hypothetical person's activities or identity.[17]

When "Volunteer Surgeon" wrote to the Montreal *Gazette* regarding medical provisions for militia members in the Northwest, he or she called for some ladies' aid association to begin rolling bandages and furnishing comforts, urging "Above all, let the women be heard from on this sick-comforts question."[18] Perhaps aware of efforts undertaken under the Red Cross banner during European wars of the past few decades, Surgeon-General Bergin similarly recommended that women in urban areas "be invited to form Red Cross Societies for the purpose of supplying medical comforts."[19] Yet the first unofficial Red Cross activity in Canada is notable for women's absence, rather than their presence. The flags, corps, and mysterious BNAS commissioner all offered examples of men (primarily military men) helping tend other men, by collecting and treating the wounded and providing materials for their care. Observers called the work of the Red Cross corps noble and self-sacrificing, words later associated with women's Red Cross work, but when it came to describing the corps volunteers themselves, reporters highlighted what they perceived as the masculine nature of the work, emphasizing the volunteers' manliness and athleticism.[20]

Women contributed to the public charitable response to the Northwest Uprising, but their efforts largely took place outside any Red Cross affiliation. Among the ninety individual and corporate donors of money and supplies to the Red Cross corps, only two women are listed: a Mrs Worthington and a Mrs Ellis. A small number of women went west to nurse the sick and wounded, while many women at home rolled bandages and prepared parcels for the men of the militia, but they did not do so in conjunction with any official Red Cross organization, or understand it to be "Red Cross work," as would later generations of women caught up in war.[21] Even if women *had* formed Red Cross branches, Bergin's rudimentary medical and surgical department lacked any means of officially recognizing societies such as the St John Ambulance and Red Cross, as the surgeon-general noted in his 1886 report to Parliament.[22] Female involvement in these first Red Cross forays in Canada was therefore limited to a cheerleader role, such as the "large numbers of ladies [who] were on hand to show their deep sympathy" for the work of the Red Cross corps when it departed Toronto for the North-west on 15 April.[23]

While the letter from "Volunteer Surgeon" indicates that citizens of Montreal, then Canada's largest city, were concerned for the fate of the sick and wounded of the 1885 campaign, Toronto was clearly the centre of (unofficial) Red Cross activity at this time. The city and its surrounding area provided the bulk of support for the Red Cross corps in 1885 and would continue to be the beating heart of Red Cross interest and activity in Canada for many years to come.

George Sterling Ryerson and the Quest for Military Medical Reform

The Northwest Uprising signalled a need for reform in the Canadian militia broadly, including its military medical provisions. As Colour Sergeant C.F. Winter, a participant in the 1885 campaign, later recalled, before 1885 "the Defence Forces had never been treated seriously, nec-essary funds for their maintenance had been voted grudgingly, and the real up-keep of the units left to the enthusiasm and devotion of a few." Winter added that "No real reserve of arms, ammunition, or the most essential military supplies of clothing and equipment existed, and there was no practical organization of the Medical, Ordinance, and Supply Departments, absolutely necessary for a force to take the field."[24] The 1885 campaign was the first military campaign to be undertaken by Canadians on their own (with the exception of a few British officers at-tached to the militia), and many arrangements for transport, supply, and medical services had to be created from scratch.[25] The Red Cross corps and multiple homemade red cross flags were the kind of improvised so-lutions to unforeseen problems that characterized the entire campaign.

Highly efficient contemporary military organizations such as that in Prussia had by this time found it in their best interest to support and foster the development of a strong national Red Cross society as a corol-lary to their normal military operations.[26] In contrast, the Canadian mili-tia (which had not faced the kind of serious wars that were frequent in Europe) possessed insufficient infrastructure of many varieties, and mil-itary medical provisions were nowhere near the top of the priority list.

The 1885 campaign merely highlighted these deficiencies. In his 1924 memoir, George Sterling Ryerson wrote, "My experiences in the North-West Rebellion ... impressed upon my mind the necessity for reform in the Medical Service of the Militia," and although this statement may be coloured by Ryerson's subsequent role in founding the Canadian Red Cross Society, he was not the only participant in the 1885 campaign to recognize the need for change.[27] Most notably, in his official report on the medical aspects of the campaign, Surgeon-General Bergin made numerous recommendations for reform, including the replacement of regimental ambulance corps with a new (pan-)Army Medical Department to be established by the militia. As Bergin's report suggests, when military surgeons and politicians talked about reforming the military medical service in the late nineteenth century, they seem usually to have meant *creating* one: a brand-new, permanent, centralized, well-trained, staffed, and fully supplied medical branch of the Canadian militia. At the time, Canadian practice was to temporarily cobble together a medical service in times of war from the unevenly (perhaps indifferently?) trained medical personnel attached to individual militia regiments, and order supplies at the last minute. Despite the need for reform identified by Bergin in 1886, political inertia set in. The medical service so hastily organized for the Northwest campaign disappeared again shortly thereafter, and Bergin's recommendations went unheeded by the federal government until 1899.[28]

In the meantime, military medical men continued to think and talk about the reforms they wished to see. For Dr George Sterling Ryerson, reforming the military medical service, as he wrote in his memoir thirty-nine years later, became "the idea which almost obsessed me."[29] Others shared his concern, some of whom, like him, eventually envisioned at least a partial solution via the Red Cross. For instance, Dr Thomas Roddick of Montreal, a renowned surgeon and leading Canadian proponent of antisepsis whom one colleague described as "the leading figure in Canadian medicine of his generation," served in the Northwest as deputy surgeon general in 1885, and in this post he helped bring the Red Cross corps into being. Despite an increasingly busy and illustrious career in politics as well as the practice and scholarship of medicine and surgery, Roddick found time to take an active leadership role in the Quebec branch of the Red Cross after 1896.[30] Other founding Canadian Red

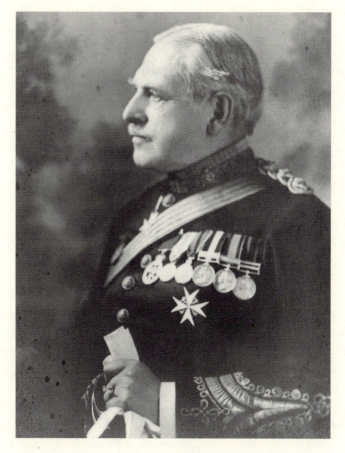

Figure 1.2
Dr George Sterling Ryerson, founder and champion of the CRCS,
looking every inch the elite Tory defender of the British Empire.
This is how he wished to be remembered.

Cross members with 1885 connections included Dr Nattress, who led the Red Cross corps to the Northwest and went on to write a popular and influential textbook on physiology for schoolchildren; and Captain James Mason, who reportedly led his company "with great dash" until he was seriously wounded at Batoche, but survived and went on to a long military career.[31] Men like Roddick, Nattress, and Mason would play important roles in the development of the Red Cross in Canada, but it was Ryerson whose obsession with reform and evident belief in the power of voluntary associations took him and his peers down the particular path that led to the creation of the Canadian Red Cross Society.

George Ansel Sterling Ryerson (who usually omitted his second name) was what one biographer has called "an archetypal Toronto Tory" – and thoroughly proud of it. The Methodist Ryersons of Upper Canada, whose name was attached to Ryerson Press and Ryerson University in Toronto, were George Sterling's Ryersons. His grandfather Joseph was a distinguished Loyalist, his father George was a noted clergyman, and his uncle Egerton famously shaped Ontario's system of public education. Having begun his education at a grammar school in Galt (now Cambridge), George Sterling Ryerson moved on to Toronto's Trinity Medical College. Ryerson's favoured position as the only son of an elite Upper Canadian family made itself apparent when, as a twenty-one-year-old recent graduate, he was able to leave Toronto in 1875 and sail for Europe to continue his medical studies. This was a relatively common practice for young physicians of his social class at the time, but nonetheless required, as he put it, "self-sacrifice" on the part of his parents.[32]

Between 1875 and 1879 the young Ryerson studied, worked, and travelled widely, including lengthy work/study stays in Edinburgh, Paris, London, Vienna, Munich, and Heidelberg, and tourist visits to Belgium and the Italian states. In doing so he participated in two trends of his time for North Americans of means: the European Grand Tour, and study in Europe, particularly in the German universities and, for medical students, Edinburgh. His time in Austria coincided with the Austrian Army's occupation of Bosnia and Herzegovina in 1878, and Ryerson, who had joined the Queen's Own Rifles at the age of fifteen "for a lark," temporarily attached himself as a military surgeon to the Austrian Army's military base hospital.[33] It seems likely that Ryerson first became familiar with the Red Cross movement during his time with the Austrian Army medical service in Bosnia, or perhaps during his stay in the German states of Baden and Bavaria. Austria had signed the Geneva Convention in 1866, while Prussia had been a key supporter and innovator of the Red Cross movement since its inception. By the time the Franco-Prussian War broke out in 1870, Berlin was directing the work of 2,000 Red Cross committees spread out across the various German states. Over the course of the 1870s and 1880s, the movement to codify and enforce laws of war gained further momentum. As both a doctor and a military man, Ryerson could hardly have failed to pick up on these currents swirling through Europe during his years on the Continent.[34]

George Sterling Ryerson was acutely aware of his status as a member of the old-Ontario elite: his penchant for name-dropping in his memoir makes it clear he was a well-connected individual from the day he was born. Upon his return to Canada in January of 1880, he began to put to work his connections and his genuine talents as a physician, in order to establish himself both in his profession and in Toronto society. In his professional life he set up a practice in the city, became a professor at Trinity Medical College, worked as a surgeon at Toronto General Hospital, and undertook innovative work in the field of colour blindness, so that by 1885, when his battalion was called up for the Northwest campaign, he was a well-respected specialist and instructor in eye, ear, and throat diseases. He was financially secure enough to wed Mary Amelia Crowther by 1882, and worked to cement and further extend the connections he had inherited as a Ryerson by remaining active in fashionable militia units and joining the Masonic Order, the Toronto Hunt Club, the Royal Canadian Yacht Club, and the Canadian Military Institute.[35]

Dr Ryerson's experience in the Northwest opened his eyes to the need for reform in Canadian military medicine, and although his professional and social involvements kept him otherwise occupied for some years, the issue stayed with him. The nineteenth century in Canada was an "Age of Organization" for both men and women, during which, as Darren Ferry writes, "an extremely vibrant movement of highly fractured and secluded class interests" created a plethora of voluntary associations running the gamut from agrarian organizations and mechanics' institutes to literary societies and temperance groups. Such organizations "bridged a significant gap between the limited social services offered by the developing colonial society of the early nineteenth century, and the origins of the Canadian welfare state nearly a hundred years later."[36] True to his age, Ryerson eventually found in voluntary associations an outlet for his concern over the state of the Canadian military medical service.

In the spring of 1892 Dr Ryerson took a leading role, along with fellow medical officers on the Militia List, in founding the Association of Medical Officers of the Militia of Canada (AMOMC). With the approval of the minister of militia and defence, and Surgeon-General Darby Bergin as honorary president, the AMOMC was created in order to foster discussion about improving the efficiency of the Canadian military medical service. The first annual meeting in June 1892 featured papers, ambulance drill demonstrations, and enthusiastic resolutions calling for change. The influence of the international Red Cross movement is evident in the fact that, despite its emphasis on government- and militia-led change, the constitution and by-laws of the AMOMC also envisioned a place for voluntary humanitarian aid in the broad scheme of military medical provision. Unfortunately for the reformers, after this first meeting the general officer commanding at Ottawa, Ivor Herbert, denounced the AMOMC's discussions as subversive to discipline – particularly its complaints about "antediluvian" equipment. Forbidden to meet, the AMOMC would not reconvene until 1906. The reformers' hopes for change from within had, for the time being, come to nought.[37]

Ryerson and his colleagues were not ready to give up. In 1892, the same year as the ill-fated AMOMC experiment, Ryerson was appointed an honorary associate of the Order of St John of Jerusalem (OSJJ) in England, a Christian order of chivalry that had roots in the humanitarian work of the Knights of St John during the Middle Ages. The OSJJ was officially revived in England in 1858, and boasted an exclusive male membership primarily composed of aristocrats and elite professionals (including but not limited to noted physicians like Ryerson). The 1885 Northwest campaign had highlighted the need for a reliable supply of trained men for Canada's military medical service, and in 1895 Ryerson began corresponding with a branch of the OSJJ in hopes of addressing that need. He (and perhaps others) believed the St John Ambulance Association (SJAA), headquartered at St John's Gate, London, might be used to create a reserve of trained stretcher bearers upon which the Canadian military medical service could call in times of emergency. In addition to the practical benefits of the SJAA as an organization dedicated to the teaching of first aid, it had the added prestige of being, along with the St John Ambulance Brigade, one of only two active bodies associated with the OSJJ. For an elitist like Ryerson, the St John Ambulance Association therefore held a double appeal, and in 1894 he requested permission to establish a branch of the SJAA in Canada. With the blessing of St John's Gate, in November 1895 an Ontario centre of the SJAA was launched and Ryerson was appointed to the positions of general secretary and medical director. Ryerson's personal social connections, as well as his 1895 appointment as deputy surgeon-general of the Canadian militia, no doubt helped secure him the active support of Ontario lieutenant governor Sir George Kirkpatrick and his wife Lady Kirkpatrick. Sir George was persuaded to serve as the first president of the new organization.[38]

The SJAA began spreading across eastern Canada in 1896, but although it taught useful first aid skills, it was not a real solution to the problem of military medical reform. Under the terms of the Geneva Convention, St John Ambulance could provide trained personnel but could not take part in active hostilities under its own auspices – a role at that time reserved exclusively for national Red Cross societies. As a civil organization, the SJAA also had to be subsidiary to the Red Cross in wartime. For this reason Ryerson and some of his peers became convinced that Canada needed a Red Cross Society. Since the Geneva Convention of 1864 stipulated that there could be only one officially recognized aid society per country or empire, and Canada was a self-governing colony of the British Empire, this meant once again appealing to Britain for help. In 1896, therefore, Dr Ryerson – perhaps on his own initiative, or perhaps deputized by his fellow reform-minded military medical colleagues – mixed business with pleasure on his return from a holiday in Spain. En route to Toronto he stopped in London, England to meet with Secretary James G. Vokes and President Lord Wantage of Britain's Red Cross organization, to discuss the possibility of establishing a Canadian branch.[39]

Unlike Prussia and Japan, Britain had not initially embraced the Red Cross idea or recognized its potential service to the state. In 1865 British representatives signed the first Geneva Convention, but a further four years elapsed before members of the OSJJ initiated the creation of a national aid society for Britain. After this slow start the British National Society for Aid to the Sick and Wounded in War (BNAS, also known colloquially as the British Red Cross Society) successfully took shape and enlisted prominent Britons to its cause. It then went on to provide assistance to the sick and wounded of the Franco-Prussian and Turco-Serbian wars, as well as those of various British military engagements in the last decades of the nineteenth century. After meeting with Ryerson in July, Vokes, Wantage, and their fellow BNAS Council members con-

sidered his proposal. In August of 1896 they granted Ryerson permission
to start a Canadian branch of the BNAS.[40] The year 1896 proved an
eventful one for Ryerson: in addition to his Red Cross and St John work,
he continued a controversial climb to the top of the Canadian military
medical establishment by being promoted to surgeon-major and sur-
geon-lieutenant-colonel – both on the same day.[41]

The Canadian Red Cross Society Is Born

On his return to Toronto, Dr Ryerson hosted an organizational meeting
for his new Red Cross branch, which set the tone for the agency's early
years. The twenty-three "gentlemen" elected to the presidency, vice-
presidency, and council of the new organization reflect the importance
of Ryerson's personal and professional connections to this first official
Red Cross incarnation in Canada. In addition to the family and professional ties already discussed, by this time Ryerson had political ties as
well: he won election to the Ontario legislature as a Conservative member of the legislative assembly (MLA) in 1892, and held the seat until
1898. The members of the new Canadian Red Cross were drawn from
the medical, legal, business, and political professions. In addition to
Ryerson (doctor, politician, and militia-member) they included at least
ten doctors, seven political figures (elected or appointed), one lawyer,
one bank manager, and one journalist/publisher. Dr John G. Hodgins
was a well-known supporter of Toronto charitable organizations who
had worked as deputy minister of education under G.S. Ryerson's uncle
Egerton Ryerson for thirty-three years. Major John Bayne MacLean, a
wealthy journalist and publisher (whose name lives on in *Maclean's* magazine) was at one point a member of Toronto's Tenth Royal Grenadiers
(Ryerson and Mason's regiment). Three of the group were surgeons-major,
and several were veterans of the 1885 Northwest campaign (including
Ryerson, Roddick, Nattress, and Mason). Surgeon-Major Frederick
Grasett's younger brother Henry had commanded the Tenth Royal Grenadiers in the 1885 campaign before going on to become chief constable of
the Toronto police force, while Frederick Grasett himself was a colleague
of Ryerson's at Trinity Medical College, as well as president of the

Ontario Medical Association. Lawyer Edward H. Smythe was Queen's Counsel, a militia veteran who had served in the 1866 and 1870 Fenian Raids, and a former mayor of Toronto. Dr Charles O'Reilly, active in the field of public health and superintendent of the Toronto General Hospital (TGH) from 1876 to 1905, likely encountered Ryerson through the latter's work as an examiner for Trinity Medical College and through Ryerson's work at TGH. Dr Frederick Montizambert (a physician and civil servant who spent his career bringing Grosse Île and other Canadian quarantine stations into the scientific age) and Dr Charles Hodgetts (a Toronto physician and medical inspector for the Ontario Board of Health) were, like Ryerson, Mason, MacLean, and O'Reilly, actively involved in the St John Ambulance Association.

Most of the men had a history of militia involvement. This is not surprising for a period when militia units were social institutions offering members a wide range of recreational and leisure facilities, a pleasant amount of pomp and circumstance, and the so-called "right" kind of company in an all-male environment.[42] Many of the members, including Ryerson (who had left Methodism to revert to his grandfather's Anglicanism), had served in the fashionable Queen's Own Rifles at some point, were members of the Church of England, and voted Conservative. Given the social and professional importance of the Masonic Order at the time, many were likely Masons. Most of the core members and officers of the fifteen-man council lived in southern Ontario (and Toronto in particular), although Ottawa, Quebec City, and Montreal were also represented.[43]

The elite status of early Red Cross supporters was not limited to the active membership of the council. Among the provincially representative individuals appointed as vice-presidents were senior statesman Sir Charles Hibbert Tupper for Nova Scotia and Conservative Member of Parliament (MP) and Cabinet minister the Hon. Hugh Macdonald (son of first Canadian prime minister Sir John A. Macdonald) for Manitoba. Dr Frederick Borden, the new reform-minded minister of militia, agreed to serve as honorary president. The newly elected president, Lieutenant Colonel J.M. Gibson, was a lawyer, businessman, member of numerous provincial Reform governments, lieutenant governor of Ontario, and veteran of the Fenian Raids, whose "philosophy of public service had always been voluntarism." Inaugurating a tradition of vice-regal support for the

Canadian Red Cross, the Earl of Aberdeen, then governor general of Canada, consented to serve as patron to the new society. The next governor general, the Earl of Minto, succeeded Aberdeen as patron.[44]

The gentlemen who joined Ryerson on the first council of the "Canadian Branch of the British National Society for Aid to the Sick and Wounded in War" (as it was officially named) therefore capably fulfilled BNAS Secretary Vokes's direction that Ryerson should assemble a council whose members (no gender specified) were "of sufficient influence to give public confidence."[45] The 1896 Canadian organization did not include women, which was a notable departure from the examples set by the French, Russian, and American Red Cross societies, where women played visible and significant roles in the initial creation and establishment of their respective organizations, but in keeping with German and British precedents.[46] The Canadian Red Cross Society originated from within military circles, in response to the deplorable state of the Canadian military medical service. Women were not part of that military world.

On behalf of the BNAS, J.G. Vokes wrote that the new Canadian branch should focus on aiding the sick and wounded in war and offer supplemental assistance to three groups: the Army Medical Department of Canada, the BNAS (if England should be engaged in war), and the belligerents of other countries at war who recognized Red Cross neutrality and expressed a willingness to accept assistance. The Canadian society was advised to keep its work "entirely distinct from any branch of the St John Ambulance Association in Canada," and to be mindful of the need to reserve the red cross emblem only for approved use under Article 7 of the 1864 Geneva Convention. Although the Canadian Red Cross Society was officially a branch of the BNAS, it would have complete autonomy in all domestic affairs, "such as enrolling members, collecting subscriptions, appointing officers, training nurses, etc."[47] At a council meeting held 1 December 1896, the BNAS Council accepted the newly formed Canadian branch's affiliation with itself, pledged its support and cooperation, and invited this first-ever colonial branch to submit occasional reports of any actions taken.[48] The Canadian Red Cross Society was born.

✝

The idea of the Red Cross migrated to Canada long before any official organizing efforts were undertaken and made itself felt in subtle ways: costume choices at fancy dress balls, flags cobbled together on fields of battle, and a corps of volunteers privately raised to help treat the sick and wounded. The drive to create an actual Red Cross organization, when it appeared, emerged from within a close-knit male community interested in reforming the medical provisions of the Canadian militia. Tradition has attributed to George Sterling Ryerson the responsibility for the establishment of the Canadian Red Cross Society, and he is undoubtedly central to the story. However, Ryerson by no means acted alone. The soldier-surgeon with a penchant for associational life and a high opinion of his own place in the social hierarchy was part of an intricate social, political, and professional network which shared, at least to some extent, his concern with military medical reform. From this complex network of military and medical men came the AMOMC, the SJAA, and eventually, the Canadian Red Cross Society.

The creation of the CRCS as an organization had little, if anything, to do with humanitarianism in the abstract and everything to do with the desire of certain individuals to reform Canadian military medicine. When a reform effort from within the military initially failed, George Sterling Ryerson and his like-minded peers turned to voluntary aid associations as an alternative. But as they would soon find out, the CRCS was formed too late to serve the purpose for which it was intended. The year 1896 saw not only the birth of the CRCS but also the appointment of a new minister of militia and defence, Frederick Borden. Borden would soon spearhead a reform of the militia from within that would leave the newly formed CRCS with precious little to do.

2

TO SOUTH AFRICA AND BACK,
1896–1914

On 5 November 1900, the streets of downtown Toronto were bedecked in red, white, and blue bunting as more than 100,000 men, women, and children lined the sidewalks to wave handkerchiefs and cheer on a procession of 10,000 military men. The marchers were mostly locals: veterans of the Fenian Raids (1866–70) and the 1885 Northwest Uprising, members of Toronto militia regiments, and – the highlight of the parade – newly returned South African War troops just off the train. Toronto's ornate stone City Hall was brightly illuminated for the occasion, while the words "Heroes of Paardeberg, Welcome Home" were spelled in lights just beyond the green expanse of Queen's Park. As the massive parade proceeded north along wide University Avenue toward the provincial legislature, it passed under the third great centre of attraction that day: the enormous castle-like Red Cross Arch which temporarily spanned the avenue displaying Red Cross flags, the Union Jack, and a portrait of Queen Victoria.[1] Dreamed up by the Toronto Ladies' Branch Red Cross and adorned with imperial symbols, Toronto's Red Cross Arch neatly symbolized the strengths of the early Canadian Red Cross Society: the organization owed its brief period of dramatic growth and public favour during the South African War to English-Canadian imperial patriotism, wartime enthusiasm, and women's voluntary labour, rather than to any spontaneous wellspring of disinterested humanitarianism. For this reason, success, like the arch itself, was short lived and ephemeral for the earliest incarnation of the Canadian Red Cross Society.

Active in war, and more or less dormant in peace: this was the Red Cross envisioned by its international founders. The wartime mandate of the British Red Cross directly influenced the establishment of its Cana-

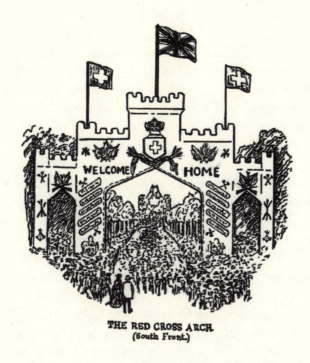

THE RED CROSS ARCH
(South Front.)

Figure 2.1
This sketch from the *Globe* conveys both the impressive scale of
Toronto's Red Cross Arch and the festive pomp of the day's celebrations.
Queen's Park is visible in the distance.

dian branch, which saw in the Red Cross a potential solution to the perceived failings of late-nineteenth-century Canadian military medical provision. The same wartime mandate would fuel the new Canadian Red Cross Society's dramatic growth during the South African War. However, Canadian Red Cross supporters quickly discovered that there were inherent limitations to their organization's wartime mandate in a country most often at peace. After it was officially established in 1896, the Red Cross in Canada fought an uphill battle to establish a permanent foothold in the Canadian charitable landscape. The South African War and the women it brought to the Red Cross fold represented bright spots in this period, but more often it was rough going for the Canadian Red Cross Society in these early years. This was the Red Cross as originally intended.

Slow Start: The Spanish-American War

Having successfully organized themselves and received official recognition from their British parent society in August 1896, the military medical men who made up the membership of the new Canadian Red Cross Society sought out objects worthy of their attention. They found very few. At the first organizational meeting of the CRCS "there was a feeling that the activities of the Society might fairly be extended to other works of mercy in times of peace," CRCS secretary Charles Hodgetts reported to BNAS secretary J.G. Vokes, but "in deference to the expressed wishes of [BNAS president] Lord Wantage" no resolution of this nature was adopted and no action taken.[2] This adherence to a comparatively narrow British view of what was appropriate Red Cross work (as opposed to the more expansive view being taken by some European countries) would have important consequences for the CRCS over the coming years; its impact was also felt immediately. For instance, CRCS members initially considered lobbying the Council of the College of Physicians and Surgeons of Ontario in favour of a standard examination for hospital nurses, but having decided to follow the path marked out by the BNAS, the CRCS instead sat in idleness for a year and a half.[3]

Not until the outbreak of the Spanish-American War in the spring of 1898 did the CRCS have an opportunity to act. True to the instructions it had received from the BNAS regarding the appropriateness of offering medical assistance to other countries at war, in early May the Canadian Red Cross Society issued a call through Toronto newspapers for donations to aid the sick and wounded of the conflict. In order to drum up interest in the campaign and educate the public on the Spanish-American War more generally, Dr Ryerson presided over a lecture at Toronto's Massey Hall arranged by the CRCS, in which the first secretary of a Spanish dignitary spoke on the "Cuban Question."[4] The Massey Hall lecture was well attended, but in terms of public enthusiasm and donation volume, this first-ever CRCS appeal met with a lacklustre response. Furthermore, the American National Red Cross (ANRC) declined the share of the proceeds it was offered, so the CRCS gave the small amount of money it had collected to the Spanish Red Cross alone.

This underwhelming response highlights several challenges facing the society early in its existence. The absence of a substantial Red Cross presence outside Toronto certainly hindered fundraising efforts, and at this early date the CRCS meant very little to Canadians: it was largely unknown, barely established, and completely untested. The lukewarm response also points to the fact that on its own, this humanitarian appeal on behalf of sick and wounded foreign soldiers lacked the power to mobilize the population. Torontonians' humanitarian impulses failed to overcome their general apathy in relation to the Spanish-American War because the competing imperial ambitions of Spain and the United States in Cuba had little relevance for most Canadians. Nor did the CRCS pursue its fundraising efforts for the sick and wounded of the Spanish-American War with the zeal or energy it would use in later conflicts involving Canadian military personnel. All in all, it was an inauspicious but instructive beginning to official Canadian Red Cross work in Canada.

Patriotic, Loyal, Active: The CRCS and the South African War

Not until October 1899 did the Canadian Red Cross Society experience its first real burst of activity and success, when Britain's "last great expansionist imperial war" also became the first time Canada formally sent troops overseas.[5] The outbreak of war in South Africa and the Canadian government's reluctant decision to send a Canadian volunteer force overseas constituted a stroke of particular good fortune for the CRCS: from 1899 to 1902 it had the opportunity to thoroughly undertake the purpose for which it existed. By tapping into English-Canadian imperialism, enlisting women's help, and working closely with the Central British Red Cross Committee, the CRCS was able to provide much-needed supplementary hospital supplies and comforts to sick and wounded soldiers in South Africa.

The emotionally charged Canadian response to the war in South Africa had little to do with South Africa itself. Men like Cecil Rhodes in Britain's Cape Colony coveted the riches of the Transvaal Republic for themselves and its territory for Britain, and spent years badgering the Transvaal into issuing an ultimatum that provided an excuse for Britain to legitimately go to war in South Africa.[6] The issues held little relevance for Canadians (and were poorly understood at best), but as scholars have noted, the South African War "was many wars, depending upon the differing roles and objectives of its participants."[7] There was plenty of room for Canadians to adopt this war as their own, and many did. Prime Minister Wilfrid Laurier thus found himself faced with, on the one hand, strong opposition to participation in the war among French Canadians, and on the other hand a wave of patriotic English-Canadian war enthusiasm (similar to that sweeping the British dominions of Australia and New Zealand).[8] Political expediency led to a classic Canadian political compromise: the Canadian government would equip and transport a volunteer force for which the British government would assume responsibility once it reached South Africa.[9] Both Britain and its white settler colonies attached great symbolic importance to the participation of colonial contingents in this "defence" of the British Empire,[10] a fact that would significantly shape the role played in the conflict by the Canadian Red Cross Society.

English-Canadian pride and war enthusiasm disproportionately exceeded the actual Canadian contribution to the imperial war effort, and produced an explosion of voluntary activity for the benefit of Canadian soldiers. This enthusiasm echoed, on a smaller scale, the "flood of gifts" Britons sent to South Africa through a variety of voluntary agencies.[11] The Canadian Red Cross Society was among the Canadian organizations that responded quickly, opening a Red Cross Fund within days of the federal government's announcement that it would send a volunteer force to South Africa. The first contributors announced in the pages of Toronto's *Globe* newspaper included Governor General Lord Minto ($100), the Ontario government ($500), millionaire meatpacking entrepreneur J.W. Flavelle ($100), and Dr and Mrs Ryerson ($25 each). Each of these sizeable donations served as a public declaration of confidence in the untested Canadian Red Cross Society, and set an example others soon followed.[12] As donations began to fill its coffers, the CRCS sought a use for its funds. In the process, it quickly discovered that there would be limits to wartime voluntary aid: the federal government declined both the society's offer to provide two nurses for overseas service, and a subsequent offer to provide underclothing and socks for the troops.[13] These limitations were harbingers of things to come.

Its initial offers to help rebuffed, the CRCS Central Council instead sent a large number of supplementary medical comforts with the troops of the First Contingent, the first Canadians sent to South Africa, while hastily organized Red Cross committees in Toronto and Ottawa provided a wealth of games, tobacco, fruit, and preserves for the comfort of the men during their sea-voyage. The four nurses sent by the Militia Department along with the First Contingent also received a handsome cash present from the CRCS.[14] Neither the comforts for troops in transit, nor the cash gifts were, strictly speaking, within the purview of the society's mandate to aid the sick and wounded in war. They did, however, answer a patriotic desire to assist the Canadians heading overseas. It was by no means the last time that the society would serve an unofficial purpose of this kind.

The CRCS was able to take a more measured approach to its wartime efforts once the frantic rush of activity that led up to the First Contingent's departure on 1 November 1899 subsided. The CRCS Central Council continued to accept donations to its own fund, but also began to appeal for subscriptions on behalf of the Central British Red Cross Committee for the provision of special hospital trains and other medical aid. The Central Committee was a British body created upon the outbreak of the South African War to coordinate the activities of the BNAS and other war charities helping the sick and wounded.

Meanwhile, the CRCS expanded over the course of the winter of 1899–1900 from a single, Toronto-based council to an organization with multiple branches in various parts of the country. "Black Week," a series of setbacks suffered by the British forces in December 1899, helped propel the expansion of the CRCS, as did a special appeal to women, and the announcement of a Second Contingent to be sent from Canada.

Wishing to expand the scope of CRCS activity, in January 1900 the men of the CRCS Central Council appealed for help to the women of Canada generally, and in particular to the ladies of the National Council of Women of Canada (NCWC). Thanks in large part to the organizational work of NCWC members, the number of Red Cross branches in Canada increased greatly over a matter of months.[15] In some places, such as St Catharines, Ontario, where twenty-three women gathered to organize a local Red Cross (which they later opened to men as well), entirely new organizations were formed.[16] In other areas pre-existing independent women's groups doing war work became Red Cross branches. Innumerable local and regimentally affiliated organizations had sprung into action when the government announced it would send volunteers to

South Africa, and pursuing their own agendas caused a great deal of confusion and overlapping effort. In the face of charitable chaos and competition, many of these small organizations found that Red Cross affiliation offered advantages over going it alone.

There were several compelling reasons to create, or affiliate with, a branch of the Canadian Red Cross Society. The CRCS was one of the few Canadian wartime voluntary organizations with any claim to be a national body, a fact that gave it visibility, prestige, and reach. It possessed a high profile nucleus of influential and wealthy supporters, and (then as now) money tended to attract other money. But perhaps most importantly, through its connection with the BNAS the CRCS had direct access to the battlefront. These advantages also led the Montreal-based Soldiers' Wives' League to act in conjunction with the CRCS despite remaining independent. In time, the majority of work done in Canada for the sick and wounded of the South African War was carried on in the name of the Canadian Red Cross Society.[17] This surge of growth led the CRCS Central Council in April 1900 to develop official procedures for admitting and organizing local branches, codified for the first time in a formal constitution and by-laws.[18]

By the end of the war, there were fifty-three official Red Cross branches in Canada, all located in urban areas. Ontario's thirty-four branches and New Brunswick's nine led the country in Red Cross activity, while Manitoba, British Columbia, Quebec, Alberta, Nova Scotia, and Prince Edward Island each had between one and three branches. These local Red Cross branches varied in size, composition, and activity, depending on the energy of their members and the generosity of their donors. Some branches were composed exclusively of women, while others had one or two men among their officers. Married women dominated the ranks of branch officers, and although it is difficult to gauge the class composition of the branches solely from the lists of officers (which is the only membership information to have survived), larger branches like Montreal/Westmount, Ottawa, Saint John, and Toronto give the impression of a Canadian Red Cross Society being driven at the branch level by the local female elite.[19] The importance of elite social networks apparent in the story of the founding of the CRCS is mirrored during the South African War by the work of New Brunswick philanthropist Lady Alice Tilley, widowed second wife of Father of Confederation Sir Samuel

Leonard Tilley. Lady Tilley's wealth, status, social network, and organizational skill enabled her to organize and oversee her province's nine very active Red Cross branches. Similarly, Toronto society women used their connections to secure rooms in Toronto City Hall which they opened daily to receive supplies, sell Red Cross pins and buttons, and sew invalid clothing with sewing machines and material donated by the Singer Sewing Co. and T. Eaton Co. respectively.[20]

The scant surviving evidence from the Montreal/Westmount branch indicates a similarly socially well-connected female leadership. Quebec's two active branches (in Quebec City and Montreal/Westmount) appear to have been formed and supported primarily, if not exclusively, by Anglo-Quebecers, with considerable amounts of money and goods being forwarded to the Montreal branch from six communities in the English-speaking Eastern Townships.[21] The absence of discernible support from French-Catholic Quebecers is not entirely surprising, given French Canadians' collective distaste for Canadian participation in the South African War. The humanitarian mission of the Red Cross might have been expected to win some support among the anti-war faction, but the society appears to have made no real effort to cultivate such support among francophones. It also seems to have operated solely in the English language, even in Quebec.

Instead of becoming known for neutral humanitarianism, the South African War-era society became closely identified with a pro-war imperial patriotism. The financial support provided to the society through various channels, including government, strongly suggests the usefulness of a voluntary organization as a means to support a voluntary war. The Ottawa branch reported that attendees at its fundraising concerts included Lady Minto (the governor general's wife), Prime Minister Sir Wilfrid and Lady Zoé Laurier, and "nearly all the cabinet ministers in town" – likely including Minister of Militia and Defence Sir Frederick Borden, a generous Red Cross supporter. Such high profile and well-heeled support must surely be responsible for the $4,476.35 contributed by the Ottawa branch to the national Red Cross coffers – the largest donation of any branch in the country.[22] Meanwhile, the Ontario government gave two donations of $500 directly to the CRCS Central Council. Since the federal government had placed limits on its support for the British war effort in South Africa, perhaps Ontario's provincial govern-

ment saw the Red Cross as a way of offering official support through unofficial channels. A number of municipal governments similarly used the
Red Cross as a channel for their financial support. Other subscribers to
the national CRCS fund included Canadian banks, fraternal organizations, literary societies, and a host of private citizens.[23] All subscribers
to the national fund were listed in regular updates in the Toronto *Globe,*
making such donations a public declaration of support – although
whether that support was for the humanitarian work of the Red Cross,
the British imperial cause, or both, remained open to interpretation.

The humanitarian significance of Canadian Red Cross work during
the South African War was frequently linked with, and often eclipsed
by, its patriotic symbolism. Students at Owen Sound, Ontario's Boyd
Street Public School donated an average of four cents per child for a
total donation of fourteen dollars. The school's Principal Douglas
claimed their contribution showed "in a tangible way the spirit that is
alive in the heart of 'Young Canada' to-day towards everything humane
and patriotic." Adult Red Cross leaders similarly constructed donations
of money and goods provided by the children of Saint John, New
Brunswick, as "a lasting object lesson in patriotism and loyalty to Queen
and Empire."[24] While these examples suggest that a variety of children
contributed to the CRCS during the South African War, the organization
has traditionally considered the St Mary's Maple Leaves to be the first
group of Canadian youth specifically dedicated to Red Cross work – the
earliest incarnation of what would later become the Junior Red Cross.
The Maple Leaves were organized by Miss Adelaide H. Clayton, a
teacher at the Collegiate Institute in St Mary's, Ontario. Clayton recalled
in 1937 that her decision to organize the several dozen girls in her English and Moderns classes into a Red Cross club was a result of her
"British blood" being "aroused" by the South African War: "all my
grandsires were officers in the English army," she explained. A patriotically themed tea and bazaar raised much of the $341 the high school-
aged girls donated to the CRCS between April and June 1900.[25]

The patriotic theme appeared in adult efforts as well, particularly
through "patriotic concerts," one of the most popular war charity fundraising methods of the day. Many CRCS branches mounted these concerts, which generally featured a combination of patriotic songs (both
British and Canadian), an address by a local dignitary, instrumental

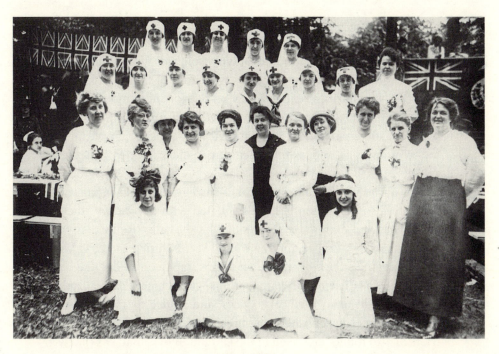

Figure 2.2
The flags, bunting, trestle tables, and backdrop visible behind this group of Montreal Red
Cross volunteers from 1900, as well as the young girls in "Red Cross nurse" costume,
suggest the event may have been a combination picnic and patriotic concert.

music, and poetry recitations. The talent might be provided by local citizens or renowned musicians and elocutionists brought in for the occasion, or both. The result was an enjoyable entertainment that raised money for the chosen organization through ticket sales, while both reflecting and inspiring patriotic sentiments. Above all, the emphasis (as the name implies) was on patriotism: cultivating it, celebrating it, and using it to reap contributions for the cause. The patriotic concert of the St Catharines, Ontario branch of the CRCS featured a military band, a display of drill by local cadets, a number of tableaux presenting military scenes, and an Empire flag drill in which young ladies represented various parts of the British Empire. A large red cross on a shield flanked by Union Jacks surmounted the stage, while a red cross emblem made of lights added a special flair.[26] In these imperially militaristic surroundings, the humanitarian mission of the Red Cross practically disappeared.

This patriotic slant to voluntary work was not unique to the Red Cross, or to Canada. Contemporary newspaper accounts of the South

African War universally ignored or downplayed agony and mess in favour of valour, heroics, and a sanitary version of injury and death in battle,[27] so war charities relied heavily on patriotism to motivate Canadians to contribute. Internationally, this period saw an ever-growing link between wartime patriotism and national Red Cross organizations devoted to aiding sick and wounded citizen-soldiers. John F. Hutchinson has demonstrated that by 1914 national Red Cross societies had become "both an outlet for, and a measure of, a citizen's patriotic enthusiasm," as "devotion to the nation became conflated with devotion to the Red Cross." The most extreme examples of what he calls "Red Cross patriotism" occurred in France and the United States during the First World War, but Japan led the way in the late 1890s. Japan created a Red Cross Society that was the envy of many nations – vast, highly centralized, integrated with the army medical services, and guided by patriotic devotion to the emperor.[28] Without ever reaching such heights, Red Cross patriotism also found fertile soil in the Dominion of Canada as the twentieth century dawned.

The South African War marked Canada's first significant military engagement on the international stage, and many English Canadians strongly identified with the Canadian troops fighting on the South African veldt.[29] The CRCS benefited enormously from English Canadians' collective desire to provide all possible support to the British Empire in its time of need. The patriotism expressed by supporting the CRCS was of the peculiarly English-Canadian variety identified by Carl Berger: it was a love of country, but also a love of empire; an imperialism that was an expansion of nationalism. Although one can imagine French Canadians, farmers, and the working classes, for all of whom imperialism held little or no appeal, finding humanitarian reasons to support the Red Cross, these groups appear to have been for the most part indifferent to the CRCS in this period. By contrast, urban English Canadians for whom the British Empire offered a "sense of power" – and who imagined Canada one day serving as the new centre of the Empire – threw their support behind the CRCS's South African War efforts. By assisting the Canadian soldiers of whom they were so proud, they may have felt they were helping the Empire in Britannia's hour of need.[30] This kind of English-Canadian Red Cross patriotism flourished independently at the grassroots, as the proliferation of patriotic concerts demonstrates, but the society's officials occasionally encouraged Canadians' association of the CRCS with imperial patriotism. In a March 1900 letter, CRCS secretary Charles Hodgetts and acting chairman of the executive committee James Mason appealed "to the loyal and patriotic public of Canada" for their support, which would allow the society "to efficiently fulfil its mission to our brave and gallant fellow-countrymen now upholding, so creditably to themselves and to Canada, the honor and integrity of our beloved Empress Queen and her vast and mighty British Empire."[31] The men of the CRCS Central Council were exactly the kind of middle- and upper-middle-class English Canadians to whom this sort of Red Cross patriotism appealed. Little wonder that it found its way into their organization's publicity materials. Rebecca Gill argues that "Empire, the glory of the British nation, patriotism, and participatory state-citizenship" were central to the South African relief work of British charities as well.[32]

Amid all the patriotic trappings, patriotic concert organizers still worked to remind their audiences of the society's humanitarian mission. No patriotic concert was complete without a few young women dressed as "Red Cross nurses" on hand, serving tea, handing out programs, taking up a collection, and generally adding a festive air to the event. Collections generally took place either during or immediately following a recitation of Rudyard Kipling's poem "The Absent-Minded Beggar." The popular poem urged listeners to "Pass the hat for your credit's sake, / and pay – pay – pay!" in order to support the families and dependents of the average "Tommy Atkins" fighting in South Africa.[33] Audiences seem to have reliably donated significant amounts in response to the poem's sentiment. Costuming became an important element of North American life by the mid-nineteenth century, and by the end of the century it was a ubiquitous element of church and community fundraising events; patriotic concert organizers could turn to a variety of advice books offering instructions for drill formation, dialogues, and costume-making. Even the simplest costumes helped create the sort of festive atmosphere that led audiences to open their wallets cheerfully, and the "dear little Red Cross nurses," as a Toronto society columnist called them, became a fixture at charitable events even when the Red Cross was not receiving any proceeds. Their costumed presence instantly added charm to any ordinary community hall, and teen and pre-teen girls likely enjoyed the embodied pleasure of dressing up "with Geneva crosses on their left arms and pretty little caps coquettishly perched on their heads."[34] The fact that the Canadian Red Cross Society did not yet employ any nurses did not stop Canadians from associating the Red Cross with nursing.

As the "Red Cross nurse" situation indicates, Canadians had a fuzzy conception of what the CRCS did. The Executive Committee issued several pamphlets during the war in an effort to educate Canadians about the Red Cross, but most publicity came from the branch level. Branches had considerable leeway in terms of how they chose to publicize the CRCS. In the absence of a highly centralized propaganda and advertising campaign, as the preceding examples have made clear, the grassroots universally and unequivocally adopted Red Cross work as a patriotic endeavour. The Newmarket, Ontario branch stated bluntly that "every ... patriotic citizen" should "feel it their duty to contribute something," adding that "few nobler objects ever appealed to your liberality."[35] This mingling of the humane and the patriotic helped inspire a flood of donations, but also caused a certain amount of confusion. The society struggled throughout the war to convince Canadians it was not a postal service capable of delivering private parcels to healthy Canadian troops overseas, and in March 1900 the United Empire Loyalist Association wrote to commend Dr Ryerson on travelling overseas as commissioner with the "Red Cross Army Medical Service" – a clear (and erroneous) conflation of the Red Cross and army medical units.[36]

This confusion particularly surrounded the relationship between the Canadian Red Cross Society and the Canadian Patriotic Fund Association (CPFA). The CPFA was formed at the instigation of Governor General Lord Minto in early 1900 in an attempt to organize the chaos of spontaneous donations that accompanied the formation and embarkation of the First Canadian Contingent to South Africa. With high profile support from provincial lieutenants governor and Canadian newspapers, the CPFA quickly became the recipient of the bulk of Canadians' voluntary donations during the South African War. It was specifically intended neither to conflict with local organizations and funds that bought life insurance policies for soldiers, nor to overlap with the mission of the Canadian Red Cross Society. While the CRCS worked for the benefit of sick and wounded combatants only, the Patriotic Fund worked to benefit the wives, children, and other dependents of the troops in South Africa.[37] At the local level communities decided for themselves which organization the proceeds of their subscription lists and patriotic concerts would support, and it was not unusual for the proceeds of a concert to be split between the CRCS and the CPFA. Paris, Ontario created its own Paris Patriotic Society with the express purpose of collecting money for both the CPFA and the CRCS.[38] Although the two organizations' purposes were quite different, the CRCS struggled throughout the war to make it clear that the Canadian Red Cross and the Canadian Patriotic Fund had no connection to one another and had entirely different objects. The language of patriotic giving that surrounded both agencies' work created a connection between them in the minds of the general public that proved difficult to erase.

For modern readers, this patriotic motif may sully (and certainly complicates) what might have been supposed to be a neutral, humanitarian undertaking. But the same national and imperial sensibilities that complicated this work also enabled its humanitarian ends. Whatever their motivation, donors opened their wallets and volunteers gave their time and skills, thereby fuelling an energetic effort to provide sick and wounded soldiers with a wide range of supplementary medical supplies and comforts that they may otherwise have lacked. The government provided medical supplies to its military medical units, but for a variety of reasons these could be insufficient. Sometimes the Boers captured official supplies, or the vagaries of the battlefield held up supply movements. Sometimes official supplies simply ran short before replacements could be secured. Occasionally standard-issue medical supplies did not include some item that medical personnel found to be useful for an unexpected type of illness or injury. Also, government supplies generally did not include less medically necessary "comfort" items that made sick and wounded soldiers' grim convalescence more endurable. The British and Canadian Red Cross societies attempted to fill these gaps, supplementing government medical provisions from supply depots established at several key locations in British-held areas of South Africa.

The wide range of items collected or purchased with funds raised by the CRCS offers a useful glimpse into the state of Western medicine (and particularly battlefield medicine) at the turn of the century. In this period after the discovery of germs but before the creation of antibiotics, keeping patients warm, clean, and nutritiously fed assumed paramount importance, while comforts could make hospitalization less tedious and/or painful.[39] The CRCS therefore focused its efforts on providing items that filled these needs, as a supplement to government-provided supplies. Medically related supplies provided by the society included clothing (shirts and pyjamas in particular), blankets, stretcher frames and mattresses, bandages, soap and sponges, liquors such as wine and brandy (used both to relieve pain and as medicines in their own right, in keeping with common practice at the time), and special "invalid foods" such as beef tea, lime juice, and cocoa. The assortment of comforts sent overseas varied widely as well, encompassing everything from games and books that helped men pass weary hours, to the shorter term indulgences of plum puddings, fruit cakes, and tobacco in all forms.[40]

The work of sewing clothing, packing parcels, and gathering these supplies and comforts for sick and wounded troops fell to the women of the Red Cross, according to a strict, gender-based division of labour prevailing in the CRCS at this time. The men of the Central Council handled relations with the government, the military, and large businesses, while women controlled local Red Cross work. The men of the Central Council played a crucial role in the society's national operations, but it was women's labour and organizational skill that drove both the expansion and the output of the Canadian Red Cross at the branch level. When President J.M. Gibson conveyed the society's hearty thanks to its female volunteers in the society's 1902 report of its war work, he expressed a genuine recognition that women had played a crucial role in the society's success between 1899 and 1902.[41]

Gibson and his male peers could thank not only patriotism but also maternalism for the support the society received from English-Canadian women during the South African War. Early in the history of the international Red Cross movement, women of many Western nations discovered how well the caring mission of the Red Cross fit with existing ideals of women's perceived virtues and societal role as mothers. By 1893 Canadians had grown accustomed to female reformers' "maternalistic activism"[42] in many areas of public life, and it was no great stretch for women who ran missionary societies or campaigned for temperance, social purity, or improved urban housing to extend their maternal mission to caring for the wartime sick and wounded. Red Cross work involved caring, some self-sacrifice, and organizational skill, all qualities that women had long brought to their various types of club work.[43] The hands-on tasks of sewing, knitting, and bandage-rolling combined a personal act of creation with a practical answer to real medical needs in the field. This combination of the practical and the personal made Red Cross work an appealing outlet for women's maternalist impulses.[44] Furthermore, although the CRCS had ties to the military, Red Cross work did not infringe on Canadian society's gender norms any more than the reform work Canadian women had engaged in since the latter part of the nineteenth century. In other words, Red Cross work fit perfectly into the Victorian system of thought in which women were the nurturers and caregivers of society.

The female imperialism demonstrated by middle- and upper-class women throughout the British Empire in organizations like the Girl Guides or the Victoria League also found a ready home in the Canadian Red Cross Society after 1899. While some English-Canadian women channeled their empire-building energies into the January 1900 formation of the Imperial Order Daughters of the Empire (IODE), an organization with which the CRCS would work closely in future wars, others turned to the CRCS. Both bodies benefited from a congenial combination of female imperialism, patriotism, and maternalism that circulated among middle- and upper-middle-class English Canadians of the period.[45] English-Canadian women who may have wished to actively participate in the support and defence of the British Empire found their ability to do so, especially in the context of wartime, severely restricted by Victorian social norms. A few women served directly in South Africa, such as Prince Edward Islander Georgina Fane Pope, superintendent of the First Contingent of Canadian Nursing Sisters. Pope wrote that she and her small group of fellow military nurses felt it "a great privilege to serve the Empire in assisting in caring for the sick and wounded in far away South Africa."[46] Most women did not have such direct opportunities, and sought other avenues of service instead. Red Cross work could easily function as a substitute for more active service, allowing women to serve the British Empire by caring for the sick and wounded

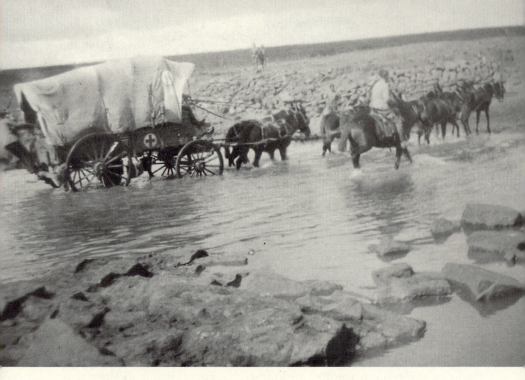

Figure 2.3
Canadian Nursing Sister Georgina Fane Pope photographed this British Red Cross ambulance fording a river near Petermaritzburgh for her own souvenir album. There is no evidence to suggest that Canadians at home ever saw such visual proof of their Red Cross donations at work in the South African War.

through the gift of their time, talents, and money. The CRCS therefore became a logical outlet for English-Canadian women's patriotic, imperial, and maternalist impulses during the South African War.

The Canadian Red Cross would not have been so popular with middle-class English-Canadian women at home, however, without its direct access to soldiers overseas. The two components worked hand-in-hand to make the society a South African War success story. By the end of the war in 1902, the CRCS had processed cash and in-kind donations to a value of $82,379.39 – a small figure compared to the roughly $340,000 Canadians contributed to the Patriotic Fund, or the £178,950 received by the Central British Red Cross Committee from all sources up to May 1901, but equivalent to more than $1.6 million today, and therefore a remarkable figure for a new and relatively little-known organization.[47] The money collected not only provided a wealth of supplementary medical supplies and comforts but also enabled the society to send several CRCS personnel overseas. The first of these was George Sterling Ryerson himself, who sailed with the Second Canadian Contingent in January 1900 to act as Canadian Red Cross Commissioner in South Africa.

Ryerson and the small staff he acquired personally oversaw the distribution of CRCS money and supplies overseas. While countless women and men in Canada continued to organize branches, solicit donations, and collect supplies, Dr Ryerson roamed war-torn South Africa as the overseas embodiment of the Canadian Red Cross Society. It was the kind of hands-on, highly visible public role he delighted in, and the experience became a significant part of his identity, figuring prominently in his memoir written years later.[48] Between February and June 1900, Ryerson spent time in Cape Town, Orange River, Kimberley, Bloemfontein, and smaller places in South Africa, providing supplementary supplies and comforts from Red Cross depots, or paying for supplies purchased in the area. Since the region was too large for one man to cover alone, he appointed assistant CRCS commissioners in several places and left small depots of CRCS supplies with them.

Ryerson and his Canadian staff earned particular praise for their energetic efforts alongside British officials in March and April of 1900, when Ryerson was instrumental in providing desperately needed hospital supplies for British forces newly occupying Bloemfontein. The British troops (including Canadians), already weakened by too little food, fatigue, and exposure, fell victim to an epidemic of enteric fever contracted from the water of the Modder River. The epidemic highlighted weaknesses in the organization of the British campaign, as Desmond Morton explains: "Careful nursing would have cured most of the sufferers, but medical resources had been cut to a minimum to save transport, and now proved hopelessly inadequate to cope." Given the state of medical knowledge and nursing practice at the time, such suffering was not necessary, but the British Army had not fully accepted the "best practices" of civilian medicine. Molly Sutphen's study of the British military response to the 1901 outbreak of plague in Cape Town, for instance, reveals "an Army that did not embrace the talisman of modernity: bacteriology," relying on older, less effective quarantine measures instead of inoculation.[49]

The supplementary supplies Ryerson was able to provide in Bloemfontein led to his appointment, in mid-April, as BNAS assistant commissioner attached to Field Marshal Lord Roberts' army headquarters,
to replace a departing Englishman. The appointment further inflated Ryerson's flourishing sense of self-importance, but it also cemented the positive relationship that already existed between the CRCS and its British
parent organization.[50] Sir John Furley of the BNAS wrote in appreciation
of "the friendly connection which has existed between the Canadian
Branch and the Parent Society" during Dr Ryerson's time in South
Africa, and letters of commendation from British commanders Lieu-
tenant-General Lord Methuen and Field Marshal Lord Roberts spoke
approvingly of Ryerson's work in the field.[51] Lieutenant-Colonel J. Lyons
Biggar, who served as one of Ryerson's CRCS assistant commissioners,
took over Ryerson's CRCS work in South Africa when Ryerson left in
June 1900. That same summer, John Small, a CRCS Central Council
member who was travelling to England independently, was charged with
looking after the needs of sick and wounded Canadian soldiers in England as they made their way back home to Canada.[52]

The success of the society's overseas efforts during the South African
War rested heavily on its relationship with the BNAS, and the CRCS freely
acknowledged its place in a larger imperial Red Cross humanitarian undertaking. This type of "imperial internationalism" animated organizations like the Save the Children Fund and Girl Guides well into the
1930s, so it is not surprising to find it active in the turn-of-the-century
CRCS.[53] This relationship mirrored the place of Canadian, Australian,
and New Zealand troops within the Imperial force fighting in South
Africa. In this vein, CRCS secretary Charles Hodgetts wrote to BNAS secretary J.G. Vokes of his conviction that "whilst we as Canadians have
done something for our own Sick and Wounded yet had it not been for
the facilities afforded our Commissioner [by the BRCS] even the humble
efforts put forth by us would have been of little use."[54] Yet amid the
CRCS's imperial enthusiasm glimmered faint suggestions of a specifically
Canadian nationalism. The British Red Cross commissioners in South
Africa (including Dr Ryerson) looked after Britons and colonials alike,
and the wide dispersal of Canadian troops meant Ryerson could not
help Canadians exclusively. Nevertheless, he and his assistant commis-

sioners did their best to divert the bulk of Canadian Red Cross supplies specifically to Canadians. Furthermore, one of Ryerson's few complaints about CRCS operations in South Africa related to the absence of any identifying mark on CRCS supplies. In his experience, soldiers frequently assumed the supplies they received came from official military stores, unaware that the Red Cross, and specifically the *Canadian* Red Cross, had assisted them.[55]

Another issue that surfaced during the war involved the recipients of CRCS aid. Theoretically the Red Cross used its resources to assist the sick and wounded regardless of which side they fought for, but the society did not emphasize this principle of impartiality to the Canadian public. The Newmarket, Ontario branch, for example, informed potential subscribers that funds collected by the CRCS would be used "first, for the benefit of the sick and wounded of the Canadian contingents; second, for the sick and wounded of the Imperial and Colonial troops at the seat of war; and third, should circumstances justify it, for the assistance of British refugees." In his memoir Dr Ryerson claimed to have used CRCS resources to assist "Briton, Boer and Colonial alike," and certainly all who came under Imperial medical care were assisted; still, the CRCS explicitly and primarily intended to help the sick and wounded of the British Imperial forces. The CRCS offered no assistance to the civilian Boer women and children perishing in British concentration camps after 1900, for example – perhaps simply because they *were* civilians, or perhaps because, like Canada's Protestant churches, imperially minded CRCS leaders felt this means of pacifying the Boer population was justified. This example of what Rebecca Gill calls a "segregation of concern" animated the wider British relief effort as well. Despite their professed internationalism, most late nineteenth- and early twentieth-century Western humanitarian organizations understood the concept of shared "humanity" in a way that privileged national and imperial contexts.[56]

The society's overseas efforts during the South African War earned it a prominent place in the charitable landscape of English Canada. The organization and its work received extensive discussion and praise in celebratory works like *Canadians in Khaki, South Africa 1899–1900*, which appeared in 1900, and W. Sandford Evans's 1901 work *The Canadian Contingents and Canadian Imperialism: A Story and a Study*, both of which included the top war charities in their coverage. Along similar lines, in summarizing the CRCS's war work based on the society's comprehensive war report of 1902, the *Globe* pronounced the Canadian Red Cross Society a "valuable adjunct to modern warfare." The summaries and statistics presented in the society's war report probably influenced the *Globe*'s pronouncement, but likely so too did the praise-filled excerpts of letters and reports from overseas military officers, army chaplains, and Nursing Sisters which the society had carefully compiled and included in a special section of its report. Military nursing superintendent Georgina Fane Pope, for example, wrote in her January 1901 report that she considered the Canadian and British Red Cross organizations' work "to have been of inestimable value." W.G. Lane, chaplain with the 1st Canadian Mounted Rifles, who had encountered Dr Ryerson in Bloemfontein, wrote to Ryerson to say that the supplies he had received for the men from the Red Cross were "sound logic for the continuation of the good work of the society, which you represent."[57] The CRCS needed precisely this kind of endorsement early in its existence.

Not everyone was quite so impressed with the society's South African showing. Lieutenant-Colonel Otter, commander of the Canadians in South Africa, publicly expressed his appreciation to the CRCS – and to the Toronto Ladies' Branch Red Cross in particular, of which his wife was a member – for the money and goods they provided for the troops. Privately, he considered Dr Ryerson to be, in the words of historian Carman Miller, "a self-advertising windbag, whose expenditures were open to question." The source of Otter's animosity is unclear: perhaps he disliked having Ryerson flitting about the war zone, and would have preferred that the CRCS give Otter all discretionary funds for the troops, as the Toronto Ladies' Branch had done when the First Contingent set sail. Or perhaps it had nothing to do with the Red Cross itself, and everything to do with the political manoeuvring on Ryerson's part which had resulted in his promotion above more senior militia officers, back in 1895.[58]

However much Otter may have disliked Ryerson, he kept his criticisms out of the public sphere. No such scruples inhibited William Lehman Ashmead Bartlett Burdett-Coutts, the American-born British Conservative politician and husband of philanthropist Baroness Angela

Burdett-Coutts.[59] William Burdett-Coutts gained notoriety in August 1900 when he used the pages of the *Times* of London to publicly allege, based on his own observations, that sick and wounded British troops received scandalous treatment in Bloemfontein hospitals. This allegation directly contradicted Dr Ryerson's testimony before the British government's South African Hospitals Commission. In his capacity as both CRCS and BNAS commissioner in South Africa, Ryerson stopped in London on his way back to Canada in order to appear before this royal commission charged with investigating the efficiency of the Army Medical Service. The *Toronto Telegram* covered the story of Burdett-Coutts's accusations; it was subsequently picked up by the *Globe* and the *Montreal Gazette*, both of which pressed Ryerson for a response. Having returned to Toronto scarcely two weeks earlier, Ryerson indignantly refuted Burdett-Coutts's charges of neglect, paltry Red Cross supply depots, and unnecessary hardship for patients. Upholding his earlier statement that "there may have been some individual cases of hardship but in general everything was admirably done – under the conditions of war," Ryerson stopped just shy of calling Burdett-Coutts a villain and blackguard. Although the debate continued to rage in the pages of the *Times*, the Canadian press let the matter drop.[60]

The Burdett-Coutts affair foreshadowed the kind of criticism that would plague many national Red Cross societies during the major wars of the twentieth century. Despite the fact that Ryerson and many letter-writers to the *Times* indignantly refuted Burdett-Coutts's allegations, the British politician's feeling that the medical side of military arrangements deserved greater attention was not an unreasonable one. "Thousands of anxious hearts, poor and rich alike, who have as yet been spared a greater sorrow, will be glad to know that everything that is possible is being done for those who suffer in their country's cause," wrote Burdett-Coutts. "And if such is not the case the country ought to know." Nor was his suggestion that all was not as it should be (vigorously denied by Ryerson and others) entirely off base. As historians have subsequently shown, the medical situation in South Africa was dreadful. Imperial troops were routinely plagued by dysentery and typhoid fever (which combined to kill more men than did Boer bullets), and despite the efforts of the army medical services, sick and wounded men in hospital often found unsanitary conditions, poor food, and untrained orderlies.

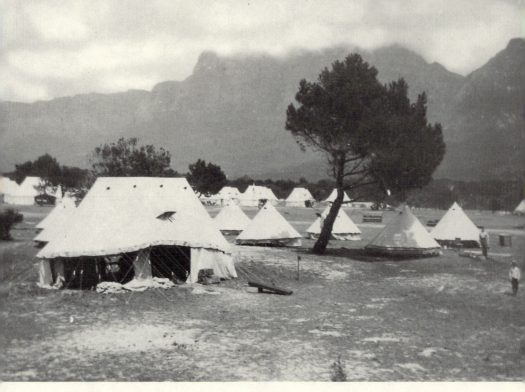

Figure 2.4
Canadian Nursing Sister Georgina Fane Pope extensively photographed the tents
making up the (British) Rondebosch hospital outside Cape Town, shown here.
Dr Ryerson likely visited the hospital as CRCS commissioner.

In some measure this may be attributed to the vagaries of what Dr Ryerson called "the conditions of war," but it also speaks to the fact that medical provision lagged behind other areas of military preparedness within the British Empire. Canadian veterans of the war also recalled the British Army medical service distributing aid "according to rank and title rather than need."[61] This unhappy state of affairs made supplementary efforts like those of the Red Cross a valuable (if insufficient) addition to the medical side of the war.

Red Cross work in Canada benefited from a surge of enthusiastic support when each of the first two Canadian contingents set sail for South Africa, and in November 1900 the CRCS Central Council declared that their work in South Africa would continue "until the last man sails." By that point, however, the height of Canadian Red Cross activity had already passed, having peaked between January and June 1900. After British troops entered Pretoria in June 1900 the war descended into a brutal, drawn-out campaign of guerilla tactics, including farm burnings and the imprisonment of ordinary Boers in concentration camps. Dr Ryerson and Canada's six war correspondents headed home after the capture of Pretoria, and the British Red Cross closed its last supply depot in November 1900, as the war shifted into its new guerilla phase. By the time Canada's Third Contingent set sail in January 1902, charitable fatigue had long since set in, as it had in Britain and elsewhere in the British Empire. CRCS involvement with the Third Contingent was limited to a $500 allotment for the needs of any sick and wounded, and a package of comforts provided by the ladies of St Thomas, Ontario's local Red Cross branch.[62]

The South African War played a crucial role in the history of the Canadian Red Cross Society. As the nineteenth century rolled over into the twentieth this little war allowed the society to expand its membership, saw the CRCS welcome women to its fold for the first time, and gave the organization a chance to prove its usefulness and gain a modest reputation in the process. But as the Third Contingent example demonstrates, the society's growth and success proved transitory. The wave of English-Canadian war patriotism and war enthusiasm which propelled CRCS activity beginning in 1899 receded by the end of 1900, and large-scale CRCS support followed suit. The women whose voluntary labour had fuelled the CRCS's sudden expansion during the early phase of the war quietly returned to their ordinary pursuits.

The Limitations of a Wartime Mandate

When the South African War officially ended in 1902, the CRCS printed a laudatory report recording its accomplishments in that conflict and then fell into a kind of hibernation. The CRCS Executive Committee met irregularly and infrequently, a majority of the branches ceased to exist, and those that initially remained lacked a purpose – enacting a cycle of boom and bust predicted by Henry Dunant in the 1860s. Dunant envisioned national aid societies that, "once formed and their permanent existence assured, would naturally remain inactive in peacetime." But unlike the post-South African War CRCS, he anticipated that "they would be always organized and ready for the possibility of war."[63] The

CRCS followed the lead of the British Red Cross by limiting itself to wartime work, and consequently found it difficult to maintain interest or attract support in peacetime.[64]

The Central British Red Cross Committee's report of its South African War work presented somewhat contradictory lessons drawn from its recent activities when it came to preparing for any future war. On the one hand, the committee felt that "an outburst of popular sympathy with the sufferings caused by war is a matter that may always be relied upon, and should be reckoned with beforehand, so as to render voluntary aid a valuable supplement to the work of the Army Medical Service." The report urged proper integration with the military because the alternative was uncoordinated, delayed, and wasteful voluntary aid which was "a doubtful advantage" and possibly even "detrimental." The committee therefore suggested the creation of peacetime British Red Cross committees in towns, ports, and counties, which would prepare plans for providing hospitals, hospital trains, and hospital ships for any future war. On the other hand, the committee felt an active peacetime Red Cross was "not applicable to the genius and spirit of the British nation" because "it is manifestly impossible that an army that is recruited entirely on voluntary principles should in time of peace excite interest in the homes of the country" and "a Red Cross Society solely for the purpose of preparing for a war which may never come" would not "arouse any great or permanent interest." The British committee supported the coordination of voluntary aid and military arrangements, but saw no point in maintaining an active peacetime Red Cross organization aside from creating the aforementioned plans.[65]

This British perspective was not the only model available to the Canadian Red Cross. The United States, Japan, and European countries with conscripted standing armies, for example, took a very different stance on the role of the Red Cross in peacetime. By the turn of the century, the difficulties of maintaining a well-prepared wartime organization in the absence of war had become abundantly clear, and these countries' Red Cross societies remedied the situation by pursuing peacetime work in the fields of public health and/or disaster relief. Along these lines, in November 1900 Dr Ryerson proposed enlarging the CRCS constitution to allow the society to provide assistance in times of disaster (such as major floods or fires), to provide comforts for healthy Canadian troops as well as the sick and wounded in war, and to work "for other patriotic objects."[66] He probably hoped to capitalize on the Red Cross enthusiasm created by the South African War in order to build a stronger peacetime CRCS. Ryerson's proposal mirrored developments in the broader international Red Cross movement, but did not appeal to his fellow CRCS councillors, who voted against it. The proposed change would have steered the CRCS away from the British model and given it the same mandate as that of the very active American National Red Cross. Instead, after the initial flurry of wartime patriotic enthusiasm died down and even before the official end of the South African War, the majority of Canadian Red Cross activity ceased.

The swift disintegration of the society he had represented so proudly in South Africa must have been particularly disheartening to George Sterling Ryerson. But long before 1902 he recognized that neither St John Ambulance nor the CRCS was the solution he and his peers had sought to Canada's military medical deficiencies. Seemingly convinced that true reform could be achieved only from within the military, Ryerson delivered an address to the Canadian Military Institute in March 1899 (subsequently printed under the title *The Soldier and the Surgeon* and also delivered before a meeting of the revived Association of Medical Officers of the Militia of Canada) in which he echoed now-deceased Surgeon-General Darby Bergin's 1885 recommendation that Canada create a permanent militia medical corps.[67]

As the nineteenth century gave way to the twentieth, the tide finally began to turn for Canadian military medical reform. The appointment of the reform-minded Frederick William Borden as minister of militia and defence in 1896 ushered in an era of significant change. Borden was a progressive Liberal, and an experienced military surgeon whose militia service stretched back to 1869. He was also a well-heeled Nova Scotian who took his civic responsibilities to heart, and a cousin of future Canadian prime minister Robert Borden. The militia and defence portfolio suffered from high turnover and government neglect between 1892 and 1896, lacking both resources and vision in a country wading through economic stagnation and not particularly concerned with military preparedness. Borden's 1896 appointment as minister ushered in a decade and a half of stability and, in time, reform. Four months before the war broke out in 1899, he authorized a Canadian Militia Medical

Department, a trial version of the medical service reformers had been calling for over the past decade. The mad scramble to recruit, organize, equip, and transport the South African War's Canadian contingents was reminiscent of the 1885 Northwest campaign, but Borden experimented with medical equipment, personnel, and training during the conflict. This was how Georgina Fane Pope and her fellow Nursing Sisters ended up in South Africa. After the war, Borden cannily drew on returned South African War soldiers' experience as well as public war enthusiasm to pursue his goal of a more self-sufficient Canadian militia. In Carman Miller's words, the South African war "created a context, impetus, and agenda for Canadian military reform" by bringing Borden, the Department of Militia and Defence, and the Canadian militia to national and imperial prominence. Borden persistently badgered Parliament for more resources (the militia budget increased sevenfold during his time in office), and in 1903 revealed his ambitious plan for a permanent civilian army to replace the regimental system. The following year, a portion of the plan came to fruition in the form of army service, ordnance, engineer, guide, signal, and pay corps, as well as the new Permanent Active Militia Medical Corps.[68] The fledgling medical corps was then reorganized in 1906, a development that likely helped spur the revival in the same year of the AMOMC, this time with the encouragement, subsidization, and participation of the minister of militia himself.[69]

The following year, in 1907, as Germany shattered the British Empire's sense of security by launching an ambitious naval program, the somnolent Central Council of the Canadian Red Cross Society met in Toronto for the first time in five years. The councillors added prominent new members to their number (including the Hon. J.S. Hendrie, Senator G.W. Ross, and Toronto entrepreneur and Casa Loma builder Sir Henry Pellatt) and decided to revive and revamp their organization.[70] No minutes or official records have survived from this early period, but it seems reasonable to assume that the broader reinvigoration of Canada's military and military medical communities helped spur this attempt to resuscitate the CRCS. Desmond Morton calls this period a "moment of Canadian militarism" – a brief window in which the experience of the South African War combined with the growing military rivalry in Europe to create an early twentieth-century Canadian public that engaged with issues of war and peace in a previously unprecedented manner. Parades, pageants, toys, sports competitions, music, and a host of other cultural venues conveyed unparalleled military enthusiasm in English Canada, while a variety of pressure groups ranging from rifle clubs and Boy Scouts to United Empire Loyalists and Military Institutes – precisely the types of organizations and activities already embraced by members of the CRCS Central Council – promoted military preparedness.[71]

Changes within the international Red Cross movement may also have played a part in the Canadian Red Cross revival. In 1906, revisions to the 1864 Geneva Convention recognized national aid societies as auxiliaries to the armed forces, a move that, as John F. Hutchinson demonstrates, both contributed and responded to a "militarization of charity" sweeping the Red Cross world.[72] Change was also afoot within the CRCS's two most obvious models. In the United States the American National Red Cross was reorganized in January 1905 under a new charter as the American Red Cross. The new ARC existed as a national corporation under government supervision, and aging, ailing ANRC founder Clara Barton found herself supplanted by rival Mabel Boardman, who was backed by the weight of the federal government and Wall Street.[73] Across the Atlantic, a lengthy struggle resulted in the July 1905 forced merger of the BNAS and the Central British Red Cross Committee (the South African War creation that united voluntary organizations working for the sick and wounded) as a new British Red Cross Society (BRCS). The revamped BRCS worked under much closer War Office control and received a royal charter confirming the change in 1908. It also deviated from Britain's traditional wartime-only stance toward Red Cross work, moving into the field of active peacetime work through the organization of Voluntary Aid Detachment (VAD) units.[74]

Unlike the British and American Red Cross reorganizations, the rebirth of the Canadian Red Cross Society originated from within rather than from either government or business. Nevertheless, the results for the CRCS resembled those for the BRCS and the ARC: the granting of a charter, and a degree of government supervision for the previously non-governmentally affiliated society. In March 1909 Senator G.W. Ross of Central Council brought forward a petition to the Canadian Parliament for an act of incorporation on behalf of the revitalized Canadian Red Cross Society. The petitioners (who included Dr Ryerson)[75] justified their request on international, imperial, national, and financial grounds. First they explained that a Canadian Red Cross Society already existed in Canada, in affiliation with the British Red Cross Society and in fulfilment of the 1863 Geneva conference recommendation that every country should possess a national society for aid to the sick and wounded in war. Then it reminded Parliament that the CRCS had "greatly aided in diminishing the suffering and loss of the Canadian troops" in the recent South African War. Finally, it argued that incorporation would allow the CRCS to more efficiently and effectively manage Canadians' voluntary donations.[76] Member of Parliament for South Toronto A.C. Macdonell sponsored the bill in the House of Commons, it passed without any recorded debate through all three readings, and on 19 May 1909 the governor general gave royal assent.[77] During this same session, Parliament amended the 1901 Act Incorporating the Canadian Patriotic Fund: clearly the federal government in this period was favourably inclined toward voluntary organizations with the object of aiding soldiers and their dependents. The debate over naval policy that raged in Canada between 1909 and 1911 likely played a role in this regard, by keeping military issues at the forefront.[78]

The 1909 Act of Incorporation set out the purposes and organizational structure of the Canadian Red Cross Society, reserved the use of the red cross emblem in Canada exclusively for the society, allowed the society to hold property up to the value of $50,000, and required the society to provide a financial report to the minister of militia and defence each year. The purpose of the CRCS, according to the act, was "to furnish volunteer aid to the sick and wounded of armies in time of war," in accordance with the spirit and condition of the 1863 Geneva conference and the 1864 Geneva Convention to which Britain adhered; to perform all the duties of a national aid society "in affiliation with the said British Red Cross Society"; and to assume all rights, properties, and duties of the CRCS prior to its incorporation. An eighteen-member, provincially representative governing body (the Central Council) was to organize branches in each province and exercise ultimate control over the organization, while a seven-member Executive Committee it appointed would exercise governing powers when the full council was not in session.[79] With some changes in the number of members and regional representation, this remained the basic governing structure of the Canadian Red Cross Society at a national level for the bulk of the twentieth century.

The swift and uncomplicated nature of the society's incorporation belied its importance. Obtaining a federal charter met one prerequisite for future acknowledgment by the International Committee of the Red Cross as an independent national society. It also advanced the CRCS toward the semi-official position it would come to occupy in Canada. No longer merely a voluntary association with international ties, the CRCS had become a voluntary association whose mandate and role in Canadian society during wartime were enshrined in Canadian law. The charter also recognized the importance of women to the society's past and future success by naming sixteen women (presidents of "local organizations," and in some cases active leaders during the South African War) alongside the thirty-two men incorporated as the Canadian Red Cross Society. These locally respected middle- and upper-class women had carved a small place for themselves in the public sphere through their patriotic and humanitarian efforts for the Red Cross. Their male peers had similarly demonstrated a commitment to the Red Cross through earlier service to, and support of, the CRCS.[80]

The Canadian Red Cross Society's enshrinement in the Canadian statutes coincided with heightened tensions in Europe, and the two factors combined to produce at least the appearance of activity in the society after 1909. Under the patronage of the governor general (Earl Grey in 1910, and the Duke of Connaught after 1911) and the vice-patronage of all nine provincial lieutenants governor, the CRCS once again selected Colonel John M. Gibson, lieutenant governor of Ontario, as its president. The all-male Executive Committee (composed entirely of Toronto residents, including Dr Ryerson) began meeting regularly, if not frequently. The Central Council held its first annual meeting in 1909, drawing together its membership of men who had supported the CRCS since 1896 or earlier (largely Torontonians) plus prominent society ladies Mrs A.E. Gooderham, Mrs Albert Nordheimer, and Mrs Thomas Jaffray Robertson.[81] Beginning in 1910 the society printed slim annual reports detailing the activities and initiatives it had undertaken in the preceding year – reports filled primarily, in the absence of significant activity, by formalities.[82]

Reorganization and incorporation clearly brought renewed energy and enthusiasm to the CRCS faithful at the end of the first decade of the twentieth century, but the society's wartime-only mandate continued to hinder its ability to develop and mature as an organization. The society sent representatives with the BRCS delegation to both the Eighth (London, 1907) and Ninth (Washington, DC, 1912) International Red Cross conferences. But it had to respond to an American Red Cross request for information on CRCS disaster relief efforts in connection with the sinking of the ship *Empress of Ireland* (exactly the kind of activity the ARC would engage in), by stating that "the [Canadian] Society did not engage in such work."[83] Although the BNAS/BRCS moved into peacetime work after its 1905 reorganization, the CRCS continued to adhere closely to the outdated position advocated by long-time BNAS leader Lord Wantage. As John Hutchinson summarizes it, Wantage held that the Red Cross should be "a self-contained and self-perpetuating body of eminent gentlemen who would act as a board of trustees, spending donated funds wisely whenever necessary and prudently saving them when hostilities came to an end."[84] Legitimate Red Cross activity, therefore, proved scarce as long as Canada remained at peace, and CRCS annual reports continued to contain much style but little substance.

Building a truly national organization, responding to correspondence, and monitoring the use of the red cross emblem were three acceptable undertakings for the peacetime society. Supporters in Prince Edward Island organized the first provincial branch of the Canadian Red Cross Society in 1911, and provincial branches were organized in Alberta, Quebec, and Saskatchewan over the next three years.[85] Correspondence from the public made plain Canadians' lingering confusion over what the CRCS actually did: letters occasionally arrived from individuals interested in training as nurses or earning first aid certification.[86]

When the society made half-hearted attempts to move into the fields of amateur nursing and first aid, it failed to gain the necessary momentum. For several years the BRCS encouraged the CRCS to organize and train men and women in small units ready to assist the sick and wounded in time of war, having recently developed its own Voluntary Aid Detachment plan with the British War Office. The CRCS submitted a proposal along these lines to the Department of Militia and Defence, but the militia did not pursue this form of cooperation.[87] Similarly, beginning in 1899 Dr Ryerson publicly advocated the creation of a register of nurses willing to serve in wartime with the Department of Militia and Defence, but the department took no steps in the matter. In April 1912 the CRCS Executive Committee decided to assume the task itself, and took some rudimentary steps over the course of 1912–13 to voluntarily enroll hospital nurses as a Nursing Reserve of the Canadian Red Cross Society. The Executive Committee made enrolling nurses for the reserve a priority in 1913 but had limited success. One reason may have been the concurrent activity of the newly established St John Ambulance Brigade, which was successfully organizing its own nursing divisions and ambulance divisions in various parts of Canada.[88]

The third area of Executive Committee activity, monitoring misuses of the red cross emblem, met with marginally more success. The *Globe*'s editorial page made light of the issue in November 1909, joking that "the name 'Red Cross' cannot be used except under authority of the Geneva Red Cross Society, but hot cross buns are still free from legal embargo."[89] In fact, misuse of the red cross emblem genuinely troubled the CRCS and its fellow Red Cross societies around the world. The Geneva Conventions reserved the red cross emblem exclusively for two uses: first, to protect voluntary and military medical personnel in war by indicating their neutrality in the cause of aiding the sick and wounded; second, to denote the personnel and activities of official voluntary national societies for aid to the sick and wounded. The 1909 Act of Incorporation reserved the red cross emblem in Canada exclusively for the use of the Canadian Red Cross Society, and in 1911 British legislation reserved the use of the emblem for Red Cross societies throughout the British Empire.[90] By 1909, however, the red cross emblem was already in use for a wide variety of purposes across Canada.

A Red Cross brand associated with medical and nursing care had already emerged by this period. The use of the red cross emblem in conjunction with Canadian hospitals, nurses' uniforms, public and private ambulances, certain brands of surgical supplies and drugs, pharmacies, and physicians' offices all testify to its recognizability. In 1912, for example, a Toronto-based organization calling itself the "Red Cross School of Nursing" promised to train nurses by correspondence faster, cheaper, and without the drudgery associated with hospital training.[91] Although improper and illegal, each of these medically related uses at least had a marginal connection to the field of assisting the sick and wounded. More imaginative and inappropriate uses of the red cross emblem documented by the CRCS included appearances on dairies, real estate firms, steamship lines, alcohol, paint, cleaning products, and hairnets. "Is it fitting that such an emblem should be employed to promote the sale of whiskey, gin, stout, chewing gum, or lavatory supplies?" protested the indignant members of the Central Council. A desire to be associated in the consumer's mind with good health, purity, and an absence of germs might explain the dairy, hair net, and cleaning product usage. Since doctors still regularly used alcohol for medicinal purposes, the same might also apply to Red Cross Whiskey and its fellows. The usefulness of the Red Cross brand for real estate or steamships is more elusive. Surely one would not want passengers to associate natural disasters, rescue, or medical treatment with buying a home or ocean travel. Perhaps these businesses simply coveted the visually distinctive and memorable emblem.

In each documented case of infringement, the CRCS Executive Committee took steps to educate the offender on the protocol surrounding use of the red cross emblem and politely requested they desist in its misuse. Many offenders voluntarily agreed to stop using the emblem, but others claimed to have secured the symbol as a trademark prior to the society's 1909 incorporation.[92] Given that the society itself put its emblem to little use in Canada at the time, enterprising Canadians could hardly be condemned for taking advantage of its power.

When Toronto-area South African War troops marched up University Avenue toward Queen's Park along with local veterans and militia members on the fifth day of November 1900, the enormous Red Cross Arch that spanned the street greeted them with the heartfelt message, "Welcome Home." The Toronto Ladies' Branch of the Canadian Red Cross Society had done its part to make the soldiers' return memorable, lobbying the mayor for a public holiday and requesting reduced rates and special trains from the railway companies to encourage out-of-town visitors. The branch paid for its magnificent Red Cross Arch by selling fifty-cent tickets to branch members. The tickets entitled buyers (who included prominent Toronto families and Red Cross supporters like the

Denisons, Gooderhams, and Boultons) to seats on the special specta-
tors' stand adjacent to the arch. Venetian masts (tall poles decorated
with greenery and bearing heraldic shields, including the red cross
emblem) lined University Avenue and added to the festive ambiance. The
downtown celebrations, complete with firecrackers, lights, and a carni-
valesque atmosphere, lasted well into the evening. Several days later, the
Toronto Ladies' Branch in conjunction with Toronto City Council
hosted a welcome evening at Massey Hall, featuring a musical program
and the presentation of souvenir city medals to the returned soldiers. All
proceeds from the evening went toward a "permanent arch fund," since
the ladies planned to memorialize "the part taken by Canadians in
upholding the British flag in South Africa" – a part in which their own
efforts through the CRCS played a role. But the permanent arch never
came to fruition. Like the wartime growth of the Canadian Red Cross
Society, this particular dream proved transitory.[93]

The society's work in the South African War affirmed what the unofficial 1885 Red Cross corps had suggested: that a Canadian voluntary
agency could successfully capture enough public interest and support to
provide useful supplementary aid to the army medical service. The society's South African War involvement helped it establish a connection
with English Canadians, and more importantly with the vast army of
middle-class female volunteers in Canada, while learning useful lessons
about organizing wartime aid and successfully working with the British
Red Cross overseas. Aside from the South African War effort, however,
the society's early decades were marked by false starts, lacklustre results,
and inactivity – failures and struggles that foreshadowed the necessity of
a major peacetime reinvention after 1918.

Although Dr Ryerson became an early Canadian convert to the
broader American Red Cross-style vision of Red Cross peacetime work,
his fellow central councillors proved unwilling to move the CRCS in this
direction. Their strict adherence to the original 1864 concept of the Red
Cross as a wartime-only auxiliary to the army medical services seriously
hindered the early development of the Canadian Red Cross. This form
of the Red Cross as-originally-intended had serious limitations when it
came to maintaining an active, vital, well-prepared organization. By June
1914 the CRCS remained a small Toronto-based body with aspirations

to greater things, whose brief period of moderately high-profile activity at the turn of the century was becoming a distant memory. The first eighteen years of official Canadian Red Cross activity had been respectable, and even admirable, but not exactly overwhelming. Important seeds were sown between 1896 and 1914, especially during the years of the South African War, but the years 1914 to 1918 would do more to shape the Canadian Red Cross's place in Canadian society than all of the previous twenty-nine.

3

A SOCIETY TRANSFORMED BY WAR,
1914–1918

In August of 1915, a full year into what was becoming known as the "Great War," the enterprising members of the Canadian Red Cross Society's Vancouver Branch came up with the idea of selling small, patriotically themed woollen figures to raise money for Red Cross food parcels destined for Canadian prisoners of war (POWs) in Germany. The five centimetre tall handmade mascots, affectionately known as "Woolies" – twenty-six types in all – ranged in price and personage from a ten-cent soldier or twenty-cent nurse, to a one-dollar King George or Lord Kitchener on a white horse. Many Vancouverites gamely sported one or more on their coat lapels, and sales of the Woolies contributed $2,000 (more than $39,000 today) to Red Cross coffers after only seven months.[1] Meanwhile, 1915 brought sorrow to CRCS founder George Sterling Ryerson. The spring battle of St Julien left his eldest son George dead and another son, Arthur, wounded. Shortly thereafter, his wife, Mary, and daughter Laura were torpedoed while crossing the Atlantic aboard the *Lusitania*. Laura survived, but her mother did not. In December Ryerson was asked to relinquish his presidency of the CRCS.[2] It was a difficult year.

These two examples offer glimpses of the enormous impact of the First World War on both the people and the organization of the Canadian Red Cross Society. From near non-existence in the first decade of the twentieth century, the society dramatically expanded in the second, gaining new members, becoming more administratively complex, and outgrowing its founder. The mobilization of volunteer citizen-soldiers from across the country meant that war – and the sickness, wounds, and imprisonment it entailed – was now a concern for a larger proportion of the Canadian population than ever before. The scope and scale of the Great War, the destructiveness of its tactics and technologies, and its reach into the homes and communities of Canadians in all parts of the country transformed the Canadian Red Cross Society and its place in Canadian society. The years from 1914 to 1918 were a watershed in the history of the CRCS, creating the organization as twentieth-century Canadians would know it, and – as Canadians used the Red Cross for their own patriotic, caring, maternal, and social purposes – placing it on a metaphorical pedestal as Canada's leading humanitarian organization.

Organizational Growth and Change, 1914–18

The First World War made the CRCS a national institution. When war broke out in August 1914, the society was ill equipped for what lay ahead, but the surge of patriotism and war enthusiasm that character-ized the first months of the war in Canada brought a surge of money, volunteers, and popular support to the CRCS at the local level. At the provincial and national levels the society welcomed new and capable leaders, and the national Executive Committee did its best to direct supporters' energy and enthusiasm into what it considered appropri-ate channels. This dynamic combination of national direction and spontaneous grassroots initiative rapidly transformed the CRCS from an unprepossessing Toronto-based body into Canada's largest human-itarian organization.

The CRCS sprang into action as soon as war was declared, but its swift response belied its state of unpreparedness. All existing Red Cross branches across Canada received a telegram on 7 August instructing them to immediately begin collecting money for the relief of Canadian and British sick and wounded, but the executive committee that sent the telegrams lacked even a physical office. Although the director-general of medical services for the Canadian military, Colonel Guy Carleton Jones, made the entirely reasonable suggestion that the CRCS establish its na-tional headquarters in Ottawa, the Torontonians of the Executive Com-mittee quickly rejected the idea and instead took up residence in a small brick office building on Toronto's King Street, made available rent-free by the Anglican Synod. The honorary secretary was an overworked medical student, the president and the chairman of the executive shared a single table with the stenographer, and until late August there was no other office furniture and no telephone.[3]

By September, National Headquarters and its few personnel were swamped by responses to the call for local branch mobilization, as well as to the society's first public appeal of the war. The CRCS had $10,000 on hand on 7 August 1914, carefully husbanded since the South African War, and anticipated needing much more. An ad hoc publicity committee quickly launched a poster and newspaper campaign which urged Canadians, "For Humanity's Sake Help the Red Cross." At the same time, the society worked hard to publicize its history, mission, and sound financial practices, in order to establish its trustworthiness in the public mind.[4] Such credentials mattered: with so many different war charities seeking funds, opportunities abounded for shady characters to take advantage of Canadians' generosity in order to make a quick profit. By 1917 the federal government felt obliged to legislate the field with a War Charities Act in order to minimize instances of fraud and poor money management, but it exempted Canada's two premier war charities – the CRCS and the Canadian Patriotic Fund (CPF) – from the act's requirements around issuing permits to fundraise.[5]

The initial appeal was a success: by the end of 1914, the CRCS had raised $275,000, of which it immediately donated $50,000 to its British parent society, the BRCS. The money came from bazaars, bake sales, concerts, door-to-door canvassing, and corporate fundraising by volunteers across the country, clearly indicating that the declaration of war roused public interest in a way the pre-war Executive Committee had been unable to do. New branches were formed and old ones reactivated, so that by the end of 1914, 180 officially recognized local branches of the Red Cross existed in nine provinces: five or fewer in each of British Columbia, Nova Scotia, and Prince Edward Island; fourteen in Quebec, largely in the predominantly anglophone Eastern Townships; and twenty-six or more in each of Alberta, Saskatchewan, Manitoba, New Brunswick, and Ontario. New Brunswick led the pack with forty-seven branches, possibly building on its strong South African War tradition, and almost certainly thanks to the leadership and organizational skill of philanthropist Lady Alice Tilley. By 1918 the ever-expanding society encompassed 1,150 chartered branches across the country, in locales ranging in size and prominence from cosmopolitan Montreal to tiny Eyebrow, Saskatchewan. Keeping in mind that the society's last pre-war annual report (1912) listed, in addition to the national-level officers, only four provincial Red Cross organizations and not a single local branch across the country, it was an astonishing transformation.[6]

In theory, the CRCS was a highly centralized organization during the Great War, with all branches authorized and supervised by National Headquarters. This system was most evident in Toronto, where the national Executive Committee filled the role of an Ontario provincial branch and kept a close eye on the newly formed Toronto branch. More frequently, however, the geographical realities of a vast and sparsely populated country gave local and provincial branches significant latitude and independence of action. This was particularly true in 1914, as National Headquarters found itself with only a general idea of Canadian military hospital needs and next to no idea of what the BRCS might require. In this initial absence of extensive direction from the national level, local branches shaped their work by drawing on South African War experience, National Headquarters' request for money, and their own ideas of what the Red Cross should do. The results varied widely, and National Headquarters found itself deluged by items sent to the Toronto office by well-meaning Canadians who seemed to think the organization was some kind of nationwide yard sale. It took several months to establish clear parameters for branch activity and to clear out the broken gramophones, raincoats, and other detritus. Meanwhile, the personnel and premises of National Headquarters expanded quickly in order to deal with the snowballing volume of (useful) supplies being received and sent out, and the amount of correspondence passing through the office. Soon the King Street offices were filled with unpaid Red Cross officers, paid stenographers, and a growing army of volunteer secretaries, sorters, and packers. In time, headquarters' work also moved to off-site sterilizing, information, and fruit departments, and shipping warehouses in eastern ports. Additionally, it soon became obvious that the CRCS needed a representative in Britain to deal directly with the British War Office and Red Cross authorities there. By the end of September 1914 the CRCS had appointed its first commissioner for England and France.[7]

Although improvisation and experimentation would continue to feature in CRCS work throughout the war, the barely organized chaos of the early war months had subsided by the time the society held its annual general meeting on 22 January 1915. In its place arose a more measured and confident approach, something Dr Ryerson, as president, tried to impress on the assembled delegates and dignitaries. The society had adopted "a system of making careful enquiries" before taking action, he said, adding that "the people of Canada may rest assured that whatever we do will be done after due thought and consideration and thorough investigation." Only five months into the war, the CRCS showed signs of the increasing professionalization that would be among the war's principal long-term impacts on the society. However, professionalization was an ongoing process. Although National Headquarters kept regular monthly accounts of its income and expenses, the Executive Committee did not begin to estimate its monthly expenses and commitments – "so that it might be decided in what manner the Society's resources might best be made use of" – until May 1916. Financial planning became increasingly important as the war dragged on.[8]

The society's South African War experience demonstrated the usefulness of an on-site CRCS commissioner, but offered no meaningful guidelines for coordinating an overseas operation the size of that which soon developed in England and France. The early chaos of National Headquarters was therefore mirrored, if not amplified, when the CRCS attempted to set up operations in Britain in November 1914. The natural but inauspicious (and unrelated) deaths, almost immediately upon arrival, of Colonel Jeffrey Burland (commissioner) and shortly thereafter of Lieutenant E.W. Parker (assistant commissioner) certainly did not help matters. Lieutenant-Colonel Charles A. Hodgetts, a long-time CRCS supporter and former honorary secretary, was dispatched in Burland's place. He was joined early in 1915 by two assistant commissioners, one of whom remained in London with Hodgetts while the other set up operations in Paris and Boulogne. While the London commissioners faced a gruelling workload, the French assignment added an element of personal danger: it involved constant travel from one part of the Western Front to another, often under fire, establishing and supplying advanced stores and liaising with hospitals.[9]

CRCS president Dr Ryerson, no doubt remembering the thrill of his South African adventures, made it known in February 1915 that he wished "to proceed to Europe immediately" as the CRCS commissioner in France. The Executive Committee demurred, and only allowed the fifty-nine-year old Ryerson to travel to France as a CRCS observer with no executive authority.[10] But even if Ryerson had achieved his goal, he would have found that CRCS commissioners during the Great War lacked the wide freedom he had enjoyed in South Africa. The Executive Committee now placed limits on the commissioner's activities and spending, in an attempt to maintain centralized control of all operations. A further check on the commissioner's independence was instituted by January 1917 when, in response to some questionable decisions by Hodgetts, National Headquarters created an advisory, watchdog body known as the London War Committee. Its members – long-time CRCS supporters and Canadian businessmen in London – were empowered to act on any changes they felt needed to take place with regard to the society's overseas operations.

Safeguards such as the London War Committee were vital as the CRCS's overseas activities expanded in volume and importance. During the four years of the war, the commissioner and assistant commissioners were responsible for coordinating the receipt and distribution of 341,325 large packing cases full of supplies sent from Canada and purchasing further supplies in Britain, the total value of which has been estimated to be around $14,000,000.[11] They also supervised the work of various departments, as the overseas operations expanded from a single warehouse and six offices in one building, to six warehouses and more than forty offices in England, with further offices and storage in France, all staffed by a variety of superintendents of supply depots, heads of departments, and legions of British and Canadian volunteers. This overseas work was conveyed to Canadians back home through another wartime development: *Bulletin,* a monthly periodical which debuted in April 1915 as a means of communicating with Red Cross workers, combatting rumours, and encouraging continued effort as charitable fatigue set in. From its earliest incarnation as a slim booklet, *Bulletin* expanded to a thick compendium of information and anecdotes with a monthly circulation of 60,000 by February 1918. Reports from the overseas departments, letters expressing gratitude to the CRCS, and photos of Red

Cross work overseas offered proof to Canadians back home that their Red Cross work mattered.[12]

In the meantime, Ryerson's disappointed hopes for a new commissionership were followed in December 1915 by the Executive Committee's decision not to renew his presidency of the society. Following the British and Australian Red Cross examples, they wished to have "someone high in station" instead, and deputized Ryerson to offer his job to the Duchess of Connaught, wife of Canada's governor general. When the duchess accepted, Ryerson found himself effectively sidelined from the organization he had founded, just at the height of its achievement. He remained a member of the Executive Committee, but felt the loss of the presidency "keenly."[13] The presidential change symbolized a wider transformation in the organization, as the old guard of Red Cross leaders (largely military and medical men) was joined by new faces drawn from a wide array of professions. New CRCS leaders who were volunteers but not amateurs included shipping coordinator Harry Milburne, loaned as a full-time volunteer by the Canadian National Railway; Jean I. Gunn, trained nurse and lady superintendent at Toronto General Hospital, who supervised the sterilization of hospital supplies; and Hugh Langton, historian and chief librarian at the University of Toronto, who oversaw the Toronto component of the CRCS Information Bureau containing records of sick, wounded, and captured Canadian soldiers.[14]

CRCS volunteers new and old, both at home and overseas, pursued their tasks in a complex context of war charities, civilian relief organizations, national and international Red Cross bodies, government agencies and departments, and public opinion. Much to its advantage, the CRCS entered the Great War with an established relationship to the Canadian militia and with the public support and commendation of Prime Minister Robert Borden. Some municipal and provincial governments voted donations to Red Cross appeals, or, as Saskatchewan did, levied a patriotic tax from which the CRCS benefited. There was still room for conflict, however. As Jonathan Vance has shown, Red Cross-government relations were notoriously strained where POWs were concerned, and the CRCS vigorously protested Minister of Militia and Defence Sam Hughes's November 1914 attempt to extend his influence to the voluntary sector by appointing – unasked – three Canadian women to the staff of the society's London headquarters.[15] The mixed social economy of wartime could benefit both sides of the state-civil society partnership, but could just as easily create friction between the two parties.

The society's overseas work brought it into more meaningful contact with the broader Red Cross movement than ever before. Red Cross societies from throughout the British Empire sometimes pooled their labour and resources, and because troops ended up in whichever hospital was closest to hand, they helped care for one another's convalescing soldiers – a fact that offered "the assurance that our Red Cross work is Imperial," Commissioner Hodgetts reported in May 1915. When the United States joined the war in 1917, the CRCS also got its first real exposure to American-style Red Cross work. Although the CRCS considered many responsibilities assumed by the ARC to be outside the proper sphere of Red Cross work, it viewed the ARC's mammoth publicity machine and fundraising success with something akin to envy. Meanwhile, the CRCS's only real interaction with the Geneva-based ICRC came through the neutral Swiss body's distribution of CRCS food parcels for Canadian POWs in Germany. As Caroline Moorehead explains, the ICRC "was oddly detached from the work carried out in its name" in this period, its relationship with national Red Cross societies "ill-defined and compliant." When the Canadian society sought direction or guidance it looked not to the ICRC but to the BRCS – of which it was still officially considered a branch.[16]

Throughout the war the CRCS worked in conjunction with, or relied heavily on, the BRCS in its the overseas operations. The British society had the advantages of greater experience, physical proximity to the Western Front, a larger organization, and a bigger budget. There is little sign in the surviving records of a relationship between the CRCS and the French Red Cross, an omission that seems strange given that so much of the fighting took place in France. It may be a result of the language barrier, but more likely stems from the fact that, as a colonial Red Cross branch, the CRCS had no legal rights except through the BRCS. From the very first CRCS commissioner's arrival in London, all commissioners were instructed to conform to "the custom and practice of the parent Society," aided by attendance at BRCS Executive Committee meetings. Despite such close relations, the CRCS alone was responsible for the direction and scope of its First World War activities, and relied less on BRCS direction as the conflict wore on. By the time it composed its report to the 1921 International Red Cross conference in Geneva, the CRCS emphasized (as it had in its own publications by 1918) that "the Canadian Red Cross Society is not a Branch of the British Red Cross." Of course technically it *was*, for as long as Canada remained a British colony. A statement in the first draft of this same 1921 report explained that the CRCS "was the first *colonial* Branch incorporated in the British Empire," but, in a telling change, was subsequently altered to read "first *overseas* Branch" [italics added]. The CRCS's altered sense of its relationship to the BRCS by war's end reflected Canada's own subtly shifting sense of identity in this period.[17]

Just as important as relations with governments and other Red Cross bodies were the society's relations with other Canadian voluntary and charitable organizations. The society's fellow large national organizations – including the CPF, the IODE, the Women's Institutes, the Salvation Army, the YMCA and YWCA, the National Women's Patriotic Society (NWPS), the Canadian War Contingent Association, the St John Ambulance Association (SJAA), and St John Ambulance Brigade (SJAB) – were potential competitors, but the CRCS established cordial relations with most of them, and avoided major conflict with others, frequently by establishing clearly delineated respective spheres of activity. This was particularly true of the CRCS's greatest potential competitors, the SJAA and SJAB. A plan adopted by the Canadian Militia Council in March 1914 explicitly authorized any of the SJAA, SJAB, or CRCS to organize Voluntary Aid Detachments in Canada's various military districts, a situation that made wasteful competition and overlapping a real possibility. Therefore, at a 14 August 1914 meeting convened by the governor general (patron of both the CRCS and the SJAA), representatives of the three organizations formed a National Relief Committee on the pattern of Britain's new Joint War Committee of the British Red Cross Society and Order of St John of Jerusalem, and agreed on their respective jurisdictions of activity for the duration of the war. The SJAA would train and organize Voluntary Aid Detachments, while the SJAB would provide personnel for the VADs and the Army Medical Corps. The CRCS would undertake all fundraising and provide grants to support the SJAA and SJAB work, as well as funding its own work for the sick and wounded and POWs. Although occasionally inclined to downplay St John's financial needs, the CRCS came through with the necessary funds, and the three groups seem to have functioned smoothly in their respective spheres throughout the war. No doubt this relative harmony was aided by the participation of a handful of military medical men in the upper echelons of both groups.[18]

As important as the Red Cross-St John agreement was, women's involvement was even more crucial to the success of the CRCS wartime program. When Canadians went to fight in South Africa in 1899, the CRCS Executive Committee went looking for women, appealing to the National Council of Women of Canada (NCWC) for help. In contrast, when Canada went to war in August 1914, Canadian women came looking for their Red Cross Society. By early September, groups like the Women's Institutes were writing to National Headquarters offering their assistance and seeking direction for their war work. A Mrs Plumptre of Toronto wrote on her own behalf, "regarding the enrolement [sic] of ladies on the council of the Red Cross Society, also about assistance which the ladies were desirous of giving."[19] This simple inquiry began a decades-long relationship between the CRCS and Mrs Plumptre, who became a highly influential Red Cross leader.

The South African War had given the men of the Executive Committee an idea of how useful women could be to their work, but Mrs Plumptre's insistence on female representation on the body that governed the society's day-to-day affairs was something else entirely. They wisely accepted the expertise on offer and added Mrs Plumptre and national IODE president and CRCS Central Council member Mrs A.E. Gooderham as "associate members" of the executive.[20] Plumptre in particular brilliantly embodied the ways by which maternal feminism could be used to create a powerful, public, activist role for women in this era. When she approached the CRCS in 1914, Adelaide Plumptre was an Oxford-educated forty-three-year old mother of two young children and wife of Henry Pemberton Plumptre, rector of Toronto's prestigious St James' Anglican Cathedral. She had previously taught at Toronto's Havergal College private school for girls, and took an active part in the Girl Guides, the YWCA, the NCWC, the CPF, and the Toronto Women's Patriotic League. Contemporaries described her as "a born organizer" possessed of "unlimited energy and plenty of ability," and a keen-minded "executive genius."[21]

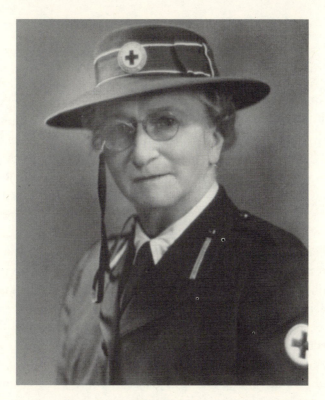

Figure 3.1
Adelaide (Mrs H.P.) Plumptre, in uniform as president of the
Ontario Division CRCS in the 1920s. She began reshaping
the national society in 1914, and continued to do so for the
next thirty years.

At the very first Executive Committee meeting she attended, Adelaide Plumptre submitted a pamphlet of sewing and knitting instructions which were printed, updated, and reissued quarterly for the duration of the war. At her second meeting, Plumptre was appointed superintendent of supplies, and proceeded to institute a thorough system of record keeping at the society's warehouses, as well as production quotas for provincial and local branches. Her arrival heralded the advent of a rationalized outwork production system for Red Cross supplies the likes of which had never before been seen in Canada. In creating these systems Plumptre likely drew on two contemporary approaches influential from the late-nineteenth century until well after the Great War: first, the Progressive reformers' belief in the power of efficient bureaucratic methods and the right of charities to intervene for the greater good; second, the manufacturing sector's

embrace of scientific management as a means to increase both the quality and quantity of production.[22] In 1915 she was made CRCS honorary
secretary, becoming the first female voting member of the national Executive Committee, which was the true centre of power in the CRCS.

Despite the presence of Plumptre and Gooderham, the CRCS national
executive remained a male stronghold, as did many provincial Red Cross
executives. Men oversaw corporate fundraising efforts, held all but one
of the overseas commissioner positions, and contributed large amounts
of money to Red Cross appeals. Some older men and young boys also
knitted socks; other men worked in CRCS warehouses. Yet women were
the heart and soul of the organization, holding dominion over branch-
and auxiliary-level activity. It was they who organized bake sales, knitted garments, sewed and rolled bandages, held benefit concerts and afternoon teas, and canvassed their neighbourhoods and churches. Overseas
it was women who visited soldiers in hospital, brought them treats and
took them for drives, sat by their bedsides, and traced the missing and
wounded. Women's tangible, caring work for the CRCS encouraged a
clear gender-based division of labour: as several Calgarians pointed out,
it was only fair that since women were doing the hands-on work, men
should finance it.[23] The importance of women's work for the CRCS during the war, likely combined with some behind-the-scenes pressure from
Adelaide Plumptre and others, resulted in an increased female presence
on the CRCS Central Council. By 1917 the council included six women
as general members and seven others as provincial representatives – a
small but significant change.[24]

Of course, not all women chose to work for the Red Cross. Many middle-class women directed their efforts toward other war charities; some
chose not to volunteer at all. Although the society attracted support from
all classes, and from both rural and urban Canadians, working-class men
and women were probably proportionally under-represented among volunteers. Volunteering required leisure time, or the means to pay someone
else to look after one's domestic responsibilities, so many working-class
Canadians would have lacked the time or means to volunteer. Paid labour
may have attracted some of these Canadians instead.[25]

After women, the CRCS counted Canadian children among its most
prolific volunteers, and the Great War marked the unofficial beginning of

a sustained Junior Red Cross in Canada, perhaps influenced by the war work of Boy Scouts and Girl Guides across the country. In September 1914 Montreal artist and handicrafts advocate May Phillips created a children's Red Cross group in the town of Greenfield Park, Quebec, and by 9 October 1914 some Ontario children were similarly organized into local age-specific auxiliaries of the Red Cross. A school group in Northgate, Saskatchewan is often cited by the CRCS as the first officially recognized "junior" Red Cross branch in the world because it received its own separate charter (just like an adult branch) in 1915. The Northgate Juniors' founder, trained nurse Emily Holmes-Orr, recalled in 1938 that "the older people" in the hamlet believed Red Cross work would train schoolchildren "no matter how tiny they were, to help bear the burden their country was bearing." By the end of the war the Saskatchewan provincial branch was receiving donations from 221 school-based or independent "Junior Red Cross" groups. May Phillips's earlier work with Greenfield Park children was honoured in the 1920s and 30s by both the Canadian and American Red Cross organizations for founding what later became the Junior Red Cross, but children's documented Great War work in Ontario and Saskatchewan, as well as the earlier South African War work of the St Mary's Maple Leaves, makes it clear that young Canadians were independently drawn into Red Cross work in many parts of the country.

Children's Red Cross work mirrored their elders': the Greenfield Park children's group, for example, made more than 1,400 garments in its first year, packed fifty special parcels at Christmas and sixty-eight at Easter, and sent relief cheques to the Belgian queen, the Prisoners of War Fund, and the Serbian and Montenegrin Red Cross Societies.[26] The most extensive contemporary discussion of young people's Canadian Red Cross war work appears in Lucy Maud Montgomery's *Rilla of Ingleside*, a fictional account of the war years in Prince Edward Island that draws heavily on the author's own wartime experience in Ontario. Anne Shirley Blythe (formerly of Green Gables) encourages her teenaged daughter Rilla to form a junior Red Cross auxiliary among the local girls on the grounds that "they would like it better and do better work by themselves than if mixed up with the older people." The subsequent activities of the "Junior Reds" bring out Rilla's hitherto undiscovered executive

ability and form an important part of her transition from girl to woman
over the course of the book – a coming of age Montgomery uses to symbolize Canada's growth to maturity through the crucible of war.[27]

Numerous narratives produced during and after the war celebrate the
universal support the CRCS received during the war. Mary Macleod
Moore, a Canadian journalist overseas, wrote in 1919, "The appeal of
the Red Cross was comprehensive. You read of the people formerly
called the Doukhobors making large donations to the Red Cross Campaign Fund, and you heard of Indians and Esquimaux raising money to
be sent to the Red Cross ... Old French women knitted socks to be put
in the Red Cross boxes, and the little girls in schools all over Canada
worked hard for the soldiers that they might send Christmas greetings
to hospitals."[28] The contributions of aboriginal Canadians in the West
were particularly celebrated, as were those from other ethnic minorities
such as the 106 men and two women of Lethbridge, Alberta's Chinese
community.[29] But as Robert Rutherdale points out, efforts by war charities to applaud contributions from ethnic minorities during the war
often reveal the presence, rather than the absence, of barriers to these
groups' participation in the upper levels of the organization.[30] On a national scale the CRCS embraced the individual contributions of a diverse
population divided by gender, class, language, and ethnicity: socks from
the File Hills aboriginal community in Saskatchewan were as welcome
as those from the (white) Toronto Women's Patriotic League, provided
they were knitted to the proper specifications. At the local, provincial,
and national executive levels, however, the divisions and hierarchies of
the pre-war social order remained substantially intact. The CRCS was
run by white, middle-class, largely anglophone, and frequently Protestant, Canadians.

These inclusive narratives of CRCS support mask another notable absence: evidence is scarce, but French-speaking Quebecers do not seem
to have embraced the society and its work to the same extent as other
Canadians. Moreover, there was a marked absence of discussion on the
subject at the time. Some francophone Quebecers did work for the
CRCS, but the groundswell of wartime grassroots support evident in
other provinces seems to have been lacking in many Quebec communities, and much of the society's support in Quebec appears to have
come from its anglophone population. By 1918 Saskatchewan had

more than 300 local branches reporting to the provincial branch, while Quebec had fifty-one – four of them actually in neighbouring parts of Ontario. Montreal and Quebec City possessed large, thriving branches, and in predominantly francophone Trois-Rivières French- and English-speaking women worked together for the local Red Cross, but Robert Rutherdale notes that compared to other war charities in the city the branch was small and its work lacked prominence.[31]

The reason for lower levels of francophone support is unclear. Perhaps the society's attractiveness was diminished by its close ties to its British parent organization, or its often imperially tinged appeals; after all, many francophone Quebecers were at best ambivalent about Canadian participation in the war, and at worst outright opposed to it. Likely the almost exclusively anglophone composition of the Quebec provincial executive did not help, nor did the absence of any substantial CRCS ties with the French Red Cross. The national society's failure to make a concerted effort to attract – or even simply to accommodate – unilingual francophones almost certainly hindered greater francophone support. The simple matter of translating CRCS materials into French – first raised in October 1914 in a letter to Ottawa newspaper Le Droit, and inter-mittently revisited thereafter – was repeatedly deflected by National Headquarters and left to the discretion of the Quebec provincial branch, which similarly did nothing. Given this trend, the 1917 joint CPF-CRCS campaign in Montreal that deliberately courted francophones probably owed its success to CPF influence rather than CRCS initiative. Since the CRCS quite literally did not speak their language, it is not surprising that francophones appear to have been less eager to support the society than their anglophone compatriots.[32]

From a financial standpoint Ontario and the Western provinces were the bastions of CRCS support, although the Maritimes provided massive amounts of voluntary labour, and wealthy Montreal helped make Quebec's cash contribution a substantial one. Between 7 August 1914 and 31 December 1919, cash contributions from Ontario made up 41 percent of the total $9,073,485.56 received, while the four Western provinces, led by Saskatchewan, contributed a further 40 percent. Quebec and the three Maritime provinces collectively provided 11 percent, with the remaining 8 percent contributed by the Yukon territory, the United States, Cuba, and "other."[33] The significant financial role played by the Western

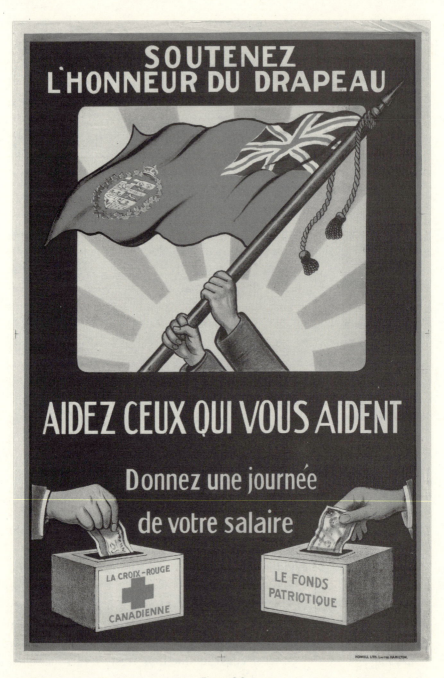

Figure 3.2

Red Cross patriotism is on display in this poster from a joint CRCS-CPF appeal that urges readers to uphold the honour of Canada's flag by donating a day's pay. "Help those who help you," it adds, emphasizing a reciprocal relationship of care and protection between home front and front lines.

provinces led them to protest the composition of the society's Ontario-dominated governing bodies. The massive nationwide growth of the CRCS since 1914 had rendered the Executive Committee and Central Council unrepresentative of the organization's membership, and in 1916 the CRCS Act of Incorporation was amended in Parliament in order to increase the membership of both bodies. The changes made official space for Mrs Plumptre and Mrs Gooderham on the executive committee and added provincial representatives (both female and male) to the council.[34]

The society rang in 1914 as a small committee of military and medical men in Ontario with loose ties to a handful of inactive branches elsewhere; by 1918 it had grown into an active, accomplished, and truly national organization. What began as a disorganized system steadily improved in efficiency and professionalism to become a remarkably well-oiled machine by war's end. In short, from an organizational perspective, the First World War was a fundamentally transformative period for the CRCS.

Transatlantic Caring: The CRCS Overseas

The organizational transformation of the CRCS between 1914 and 1918 took place – and mattered – because it enabled the society to fulfill its *raison d'être*: providing aid and comfort to sick and wounded soldiers and prisoners of war. Although the existence of the Canadian Army Medical Corps (CAMC) limited the potential role of the CRCS (civilian volunteers were not allowed near the actual battlefields, for instance), there was still ample room for voluntary aid. Many Canadians accordingly took pride in helping their sick, wounded, and captured countrymen through the Red Cross.

Thanks to the ubiquity of the red cross emblem (prominently worn by medical service personnel of all the combatant nations), the term "Red Cross" came to be freely associated in Canada with all aspects of battlefield medicine. Toronto's *Globe* newspaper, for example, used "Red Cross" to refer to army medical services of all nations, often mislabelling the doctors and nurses of the CAMC as "Red Cross surgeons" and "Red Cross nurses." A popular patriotic song of 1918 extolled the virtues of wartime nurses by claiming "Mid the war's great curse / Stands the Red

Cross Nurse / She's the rose of No Man's Land." The term "Red Cross work" similarly became convenient shorthand for civilians' (and especially women's) work for a wide variety of war charities. As Adelaide Plumptre put it, "only a very small section of the public understands or cares about the proper legal sphere of Red Cross work. To the average person, 'Red Cross' stands for 'war relief' of all kinds."[35]

Some countries used Red Cross Society personnel within their military medical services, but Canada did not. By this time military medical reform had succeeded to the point where it was assumed from the outset that the CAMC would provide its own doctors and surgeons, but the question of nurses was less clear. The CRCS proudly selected and dispatched a contingent of twenty nurses in the first year of the war and paid for several dozen more selected by the SJAA, but these nurses never worked as a unit and were not allowed to work in Canadian military hospitals overseas, the latter a privilege CAMC Matron-in-Chief Margaret Macdonald jealously guarded for CAMC Nursing Sisters. The CRCS nurses were instead deployed in British hospitals by the BRCS or taken on by the British War Office. More than half of them subsequently transferred to the CAMC (which offered military rank and higher pay) or the Queen Alexandra's Imperial Military Nursing Service. The CRCS more successfully engaged nurses to work in a Red Cross convalescent home for soldiers in Ogden, Alberta between 1915 and 1916, until the home was transferred to the government's Military Hospitals Commission. In 1918–19 a small group of CRCS-employed nurses in Canada assisted soldiers' wives and children at eastern seaports and on trains. One was Saint John, New Brunswick native Bertha Gregory, a trained nurse who travelled from New Brunswick to British Columbia in 1919 on a train filled with Canadian veterans' wives and children. Gregory continued her Red Cross work with immigrating families after the war as a nurse with the CRCS Port Nursery at Saint John, from 1920 to 1922.[36]

Despite the small number of actual nurses employed by the CRCS during the war and the limited nature of their work, the popular image of the "Red Cross nurse" prevailed. The confusion may have stemmed in part from the visibility of VADs – partially trained, overwhelmingly female volunteers used to supplement trained nurses in hospitals at home and overseas. Canadian VADs were indirectly funded by the CRCS (through the 1914 Red Cross-St John agreement) but wholly recruited, trained, and deployed by the SJAA. The VAD uniform (including skirt and blouse, white apron, and long veil) resembled the CAMC Nursing Sisters' uniform and sometimes sported a prominent red cross emblem on the apron bib. Of the 2000 Canadian VADS enlisted by November 1918, 500 worked overseas, either in British military hospitals or in assorted other roles such as driving CRCS ambulances in France, working in CRCS recreation huts, or staffing the CRCS rest home for nurses in Boulogne.[37] Thus, Canadians can hardly be blamed if they mistakenly assumed VADS were "Red Cross nurses."

The ambulances driven by Canadian VADS were among the 120 modern motor vehicles purchased by the CRCS and sent overseas by January 1916. Ambulances were a popular item for Canadians to donate through the CRCS because their role transporting patients offered a tangible opportunity for donors to help rescue the sick and wounded. Driven by Canadian VADS, BRCS volunteers, and others, CRCS ambulance convoys were eventually stationed in Paris, Étaples, and London, with individual vehicles also dispersed throughout England.[38] Each vehicle had the name of the CRCS emblazoned on its side, making it a moving billboard proclaiming Canadians' desire to reach across the Atlantic and care for their troops.

The CRCS mission to comfort and aid the sick and wounded led the society to equip or provide special equipment for canteens, games rooms, recreation huts, rehabilitative workshops, and/or nurses' quarters at most of the Canadian hospitals in England and France.[39] It also prompted the society to equip or construct its own general hospitals, convalescent hospitals, and rest homes overseas – facilities that a serviceman would reach only after passing through a regimental aid post, several dressing stations, and a casualty clearing station, as he was moved progressively further back from the trenches of the Western Front.[40] By the end of the war the CRCS had equipped or built five hospitals and two rest homes in England, as well as a large hospital in France: the King's Canadian Red Cross Convalescent Hospital at Bushey Park; Princess Patricia's Canadian Red Cross Convalescent Home in Ramsgate; the Canadian Red Cross Special Hospital at Buxton (specializing in rheumatic patients); the Officers' Hospital in the Petrograd Hotel, London; the Duchess of Connaught's Canadian Red Cross Hospital near Taplow; Canadian officers' rest homes in Sidmouth and Bexhill; and a state-of-the-art 520-bed hospital at Joinville-le-Pont, France. Through sheer persistence Matron-in-Chief Margaret Macdonald persuaded Colonel Hodgetts in 1915 to add rest homes for Canadian military nurses to the roster, and by the end of the war four were in operation: two in London, one on the English coast at Margate, and one in Boulogne. Most of these facilities were conversions of buildings on loan from wealthy Britons, but others included purpose-built pavilion-style wards known as "hut hospitals" or "hutments." By the end of the war the society had provided some 3,700 hospital beds in its various facilities.[41]

The Duchess of Connaught's Canadian Red Cross Hospital (also known as Taplow or Cliveden) was the society's first hospital overseas and remained the society's showpiece throughout the war, welcoming 24,000 patients by war's end. It grew from 110 beds in a converted indoor tennis court to 1,040 beds in numerous hutments, and received lavish praise for its efficiency, comfort, and overall superiority. Jeffrey Reznick convincingly argues that such praise for wartime hospitals (common in Britain) was calculated to boost morale and dull the horrors of war. Even so, there seems to have been something special about this particular hospital, possibly deriving from the beauty of the Astor family's Cliveden estate, on which it was situated. It was a popular posting for medical personnel and a coveted location for convalescing soldiers. "My days at Taplow were the happiest I spent overseas," recalled Canadian Nursing Sister Anne Ross, years later.[42]

The society's pride inclined it to boastfulness where its hospitals were concerned, so the criticism it received from Special Inspector-General Herbert Bruce in Bruce's politically charged 1916 critique of the CAMC came as a rude shock. Bruce charged that the CRCS's new special hospital at Buxton was poorly situated and served no useful purpose; in the midst of arguing that the entire CAMC needed reorganization he also singled out for criticism the Cliveden hospital and "special arrangements" it had received. It cost more to operate hospitals jointly run by the CRCS and the Department of Militia and Defence, he argued, than it did to run those solely controlled by the department. Around the same time, concerns arose that Colonel Hodgetts was mismanaging the society's overseas affairs, particularly Cliveden. This collective onslaught of criticism led the CRCS to establish its advisory London War Committee in late 1916. As a result of the committee's investigations, and in line with

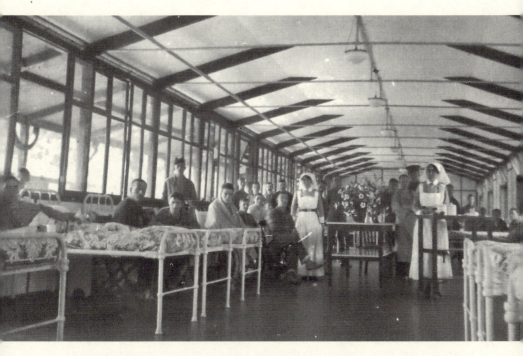

Figure 3.3

Inside a purpose-built "hut" ward at the Duchess of Connaught's Canadian Red
Cross Hospital on the Cliveden estate at Taplow, England. The long pavilion style
and large windows reflected contemporary understandings of the curative value
of fresh air and sunshine.

Bruce's recommendations, in 1917 the society turned over the management of its four major hospitals in England (Cliveden, Bushey Park,
Buxton, and Ramsgate) to the Department of Militia and Defence to be
run like any other Canadian military hospital. However, the CRCS retained responsibility for the buildings and equipment and continued to
provide comforts, supplementary supplies, and special equipment.[43]

Another option would have been for the society to simply tighten its
inspections and administrative practices, rather than turning over its
hospitals to the state. This raises the possibility that CRCS leaders themselves saw the logic of state-run health services, and/or were weary of
these administrative responsibilities and preferred to focus their energies elsewhere. This was certainly the case when, decades later, the advent of Medicare made it possible for the society to turn its outpost

hospitals over to local or provincial governments. More broadly, although it may have seemed at the time to be the product of a unique wartime context, this extension of state control over medical facilities provided by the voluntary sector, undertaken in the name of efficiency, merely anticipated by a couple of decades the Rowell-Sirois Commission's 1940 recommendation that greater state intervention would be required if civilian health care provision in Canada was ever to approach equitable access for all citizens.

Some of the society's most meaningful work overseas took place through the CRCS Information Bureau and its Prisoners of War Department. Both were innovations of the First World War, because providing aid to POWs and tracing the sick and wounded had only been added to national Red Cross societies' purview as of 1912. The high casualty rates on the Western Front soon rendered the task of keeping track of Canadian sick, wounded, and deaths in hospital too vast and complex for the CRCS commissioner to undertake alone, while simultaneously reinforcing the importance of the task. A single soldier could easily be lost, his friends and family left in agonizing uncertainty. In early February 1915, prominent Montreal philanthropist Lady Julia Drummond was authorized to establish an information bureau which would provide a personal touch for the sick and wounded, and bridge the gap between soldiers and their distant loved ones. Lady Drummond was the twice-widowed second wife of senator and Bank of Montreal president Sir George Alexander Drummond, Montreal's leading pre-war elite female reformer, and a suffragist. Her only surviving son, Captain Guy Melfort Drummond, was killed in action in 1915, leading Drummond to throw herself (and a substantial portion of her own wealth) into Red Cross work to aid and comfort other mothers' boys.[44] A year and a half after the creation of the Information Bureau, Mrs Plumptre believed, "nothing has more entirely convinced the public of the value and efficiency of the Society's work than the system of gifts to wounded men, of visitors for Canadian patients and of information for their relatives on both sides of the sea."[45]

The Information Bureau began with Lady Drummond and two other women labouring away in two rooms, but quickly expanded to fill twenty-five rooms and occupy hundreds of volunteers (both British women and Canadian officers' wives who came to England during the

war) in five departments: Enquiry, Parcels, Newspapers, Drives and Entertainments, and Prisoners of War. The Enquiry Department contained
a further eight subsections of its own, and by December 1917 each day
the department had thirty-seven people recording casualties in the files
and twenty women writing to families with updates on their loved ones'
conditions. They sent an average of 1,800 letters per week, and based
their updates on weekly reports sent in by nearly 1,000 Canadian and
British women who worked as CRCS hospital visitors in England's 900
hospitals. When tracing specific soldiers reported missing, or the circumstances surrounding an individual's death, the CRCS relied on the
BRCS Missing and Wounded Enquiry Bureau's volunteer searchers, who
scoured rest homes, base depots, ambulance trains, and hospitals in
France and England, and talked with men in the same battalion as the
missing individual.[46]

The POW Department became a special unit of the Information Bureau after the Second Battle of Ypres in May 1915, when the number of
Canadians in enemy hands noticeably increased. The BRCS had by this
time established a dominant role for the Red Cross in the provision of
aid to POWs, and the ICRC had set up a massive card index in Geneva
to track the growing numbers of POWs on both sides of the conflict.[47]
The POW Department benefited from the capable direction of Evelyn
Rivers-Bulkeley, a former lady-in-waiting to the Duchess of Connaught.
Like her colleague Lady Drummond, Rivers-Bulkeley assuaged her
personal grief – in this case, from the loss of her husband, who was
killed in October 1914 – through voluntary work. The CRCS Information Bureau's POW Department collated lists of captured Canadians
(which reached the British Foreign Office through neutral governments)
and used them to compile a card index of Canadians in captivity. Du-
plicates were held in Canada by the CRCS National Headquarters and
also the Department of Militia and Defence.[48]

The POW Department also assumed the role of relief agency for Canadian POWs, using volunteers to pack standard CRCS food parcels that
were distributed to Canadian prisoners via the neutral ICRC. The parcels
contained tinned and other non-perishable food items intended to supplement the meagre prison camp diet, which generally consisted of some
variation on soup, bread, and coffee. Food quickly became a preoccupation for bored prisoners, and the parcels served a morale-boosting

function as well as a nutritional one. An unnamed Canadian prisoner wrote in 1915 that the parcels showed "some one did not forget us Canadians," while T.R. Richard, who spent twenty-five months in a camp in Westphalia during the Great War, insisted in 1943, "had I not received Red Cross parcels I would not be living today." Many POWs felt the same. The society seized on this idea of CRCS food parcels as the only thing standing between captured Canadians and death in enemy hands, making the most of POW symbolism in CRCS publicity and public appeals as the war progressed.[49]

Approximately 3,800 Canadians were captured during the First World War, and although the CRCS was not the only organization involved in Canada's POW relief effort, it was arguably the most important. Yet, as Jonathan Vance demonstrates, a climate of "mutual suspicion" characterized relations between the CRCS and the federal government where POW relief was concerned. The mixed social economy of wartime was anything but conducive to service-provision, in this instance. The CRCS often acted without consulting Ottawa, while Ottawa was reluctant to admit the society's value as a partner. Despite numerous attempts to streamline and improve the system, the CRCS POW Department and various ministries in the federal government worked independently and sometimes at cross-purposes throughout the war, with no single, central office to which Canadians could turn with their inquiries. Unlike other areas of more cordial cooperation, in this realm voluntary aid and government initiatives existed in uneasy and inefficient tension. Fortunately the various antagonisms did not keep the resulting relief effort from benefiting POWs themselves.[50]

POW relief was not the only new area of humanitarian work undertaken by the CRCS overseas: in October 1918 the society entered the field of civilian relief as well. The idea of providing direct, non-hospital-based relief to French civilians was raised earlier in the war, but the CRCS executive committee hesitated to act beyond the provisions of the Geneva Conventions. The CRCS finally entered this field when, in October 1918, Sir Frederick Treves of the BRCS "expressed his opinion that aid to non-combatants suffering from the consequences of war was legitimate work under the Society's Constitution." Now, as the Allies pushed Germany out of Belgium and France in the final months of the war, CRCS workers followed behind the advancing front, working closely with the Canadian Expeditionary Force (CEF), the CAMC, and local citizens' committees to distribute clothing, food, hospital supplies, and comforts to refugees and destitute citizens.[51]

The society's largesse also extended beyond its own work during the war. Tens of thousands of cases of CRCS supplies flowed into French hospitals, while the society provided substantial grants to a range of medically related causes, including the Scottish Women's Hospitals, the French Wounded Emergency Fund, and the IODE Hospital for Officers, as well as the (non-health-related) Maple Leaf Clubs for Canadian soldiers on leave in London. Fellow Red Cross societies also received both money and supplies, with such transfers viewed as demonstrations of practical support for Canada's allies. Donations to a sister society were not as overtly partisan as offering supplies or money to a government, but they still made a political statement: the CRCS aided the British, French, Serbian, Belgian, and Montenegrin Red Cross organizations, but not the German or Austrian Red Cross societies. Only when Italy switched sides and joined the Allies did the CRCS begin forwarding supplies to the Italian Red Cross.[52]

If You Cannot Give a Life: Red Cross Work on the Homefront

The CRCS could not have accomplished its important overseas work without its close associations with the BRCS and the CAMC, or the assistance of the ICRC (where POWs were concerned) – but it was the CRCS supporters and volunteers back home in Canada who truly enabled the society to do its work overseas. Their experience of Red Cross work was unglamourous and often tedious, largely limited to fundraising and/or making comforts and hospital supplies. The money they raised paid for CRCS ambulances, hospitals, and POW parcels. The garments, supplies, and treats they prepared found their way to sick and wounded soldiers from the entire British Empire and Canada's other allies.

Different parts of the country could and did do different types of Red Cross work: port cities could assist disembarking soldiers, sailors, and war brides, while sphagnum moss (used in bandages) could be found only in certain provinces; rural Canadians often contributed produce instead of cash, while urban citizens could more easily undertake door-to-door canvasses. Local interests, economies, and personalities influenced the activities of each branch or auxiliary. Yet overall, Red Cross work across Canada was directed into a limited number of channels approved by National Headquarters. One of the key lessons the society had learned from its South African War effort was that, being more flexible and portable, money was always preferable to material and supplies.[53] CRCS leaders therefore initially hoped to limit branch activity to fundraising, but it proved impossible to uphold the "money, not goods" principle. Canadian women and children wanted to do something tactile and concrete for soldiers, and the CRCS quickly realized it would be wiser to guide this impulse into useful channels than to lose support by trying to quell it. Hands-on work and fundraising, therefore, came to occupy most CRCS volunteers in Canada during the war.

Canadians were determined fundraisers, using superfluities shops, dogs bearing collection boxes, patriotic crafts, bazaars, teas, flag days, door-to-door canvasses, and anything else they could think of to raise money for the Red Cross. Their efforts garnered more than $9,000,000 in cash for the CRCS during the four years of war (equivalent to over $171,000,000 today) and more than $6,000,000 for the BRCS.[54] Prominent CRCS supporters within the business community, such as CRCS Executive Committee chairman Noel Marshall, brought hundreds of thousands of dollars' worth of donations in cash and kind to the CRCS by making the most of their corporate contacts. Patriotic concerts – that favourite technique of South African War fundraisers – remained popular, perhaps because they entertained while they opened pocketbooks. Also in the tradition of the previous war, although now on a grander scale, many local branches of the CRCS and the CPF cooperated in fundraising. Canadians were now clear on the two funds' different objects, but organizers no doubt hoped that when Canada's top two war charities combined forces the double appeal to Canadians' patriotic and humanitarian impulses would result in increased contributions, as well as eliminating competition between the two organizations. Many volunteers worked for both the CRCS and the CPF, and young girls in "Red Cross nurse" costume occasionally appeared at CPF fundraising events.[55]

Fundraising and publicity went hand-in-hand. Provincial branches sent travelling Red Cross speakers to small communities and outlying districts across Canada to encourage local volunteers, drum up support, and publicize the society's work overseas. Some communities heard Red Cross speakers in tandem with military recruiters, as L.M. Montgomery did on 10 December 1916, when she attended "a Red Cross lecture in the church – an illustrated lantern affair." She noted in her journal that "several soldiers were present and after the lecture they made recruiting speeches." There were probably exceptions, but by and large Canadians seem not to have felt the two causes – recruiting men for the trenches, and caring for sick and wounded servicemen – conflicted, and may instead have believed they were compatible. Both drew heavily on Canadians' patriotism and sense of duty, and at least one CRCS poster from the period explicitly linked enlistment and Red Cross support. In stark bold letters it exclaimed: "If you cannot GIVE A LIFE you can SAVE A LIFE by helping the Canadian Red Cross." Discussion of Red Cross efforts may have aided recruiting by making the war seem more survivable, or by reassuring potential recruits they would be looked after. The paradoxical notion of making war more humane was one of the reasons some observers had objected to the Geneva Conventions back in the 1860s, and it created a tension in the early Red Cross movement between those who saw the conventions as progress toward a more civilized world and those who perceived how useful Red Cross societies could be to nations at war.[56]

Further fundraising and publicity crossover existed between the CRCS and its sister Red Cross organizations. The most prominent examples were the massive and hugely successful 1915 and 1916 "Our Day" campaigns to raise money in Canada for the BRCS. The nationwide Our Day campaigns (spearheaded by the provincial lieutenants governor) were promoted as an opportunity for all citizens to show their support for the British Empire at war. The CRCS supported the campaigns and benefited from all of the Red Cross publicity they generated, but came to resent this incursion into what the society considered its own territory. The 1915 campaign earned nearly $1,500,000 from Ontario alone, money in which the CRCS had no share. Subsequent requests for a CRCS-led "France's Day" and for a Montenegro Red Cross campaign were

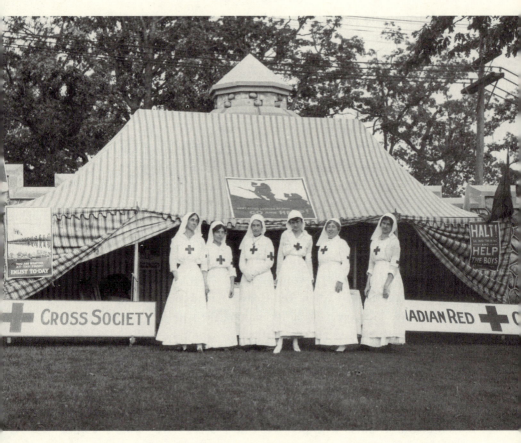

Figure 3.4
Military recruiting posters inside and outside of this Red Cross tent at Toronto's Casa
Loma emphasize the connection some Canadians made between enlistment and Red
Cross care. The female volunteers in front of the tent seem to range in age from twenty
to fifty, showing the wide appeal of dressing up in "Red Cross nurse" costume.

put off, then made optional at each province's discretion. In a context of
taxes, government loan appeals, and competition from other war charities, CRCS leaders agreed by 1918 that these appeals simply required too
much time and energy, and they were discontinued.[57]

Even a straightforward transfer of money or goods from one national
Red Cross to another served an important symbolic purpose, as the
American Red Cross in particular was well aware. Early in 1918 the ARC
War Council made a well-publicized $500,000 donation to the CRCS for

use in France, as a public expression of support between allies. In thanking the ARC, CRCS leaders directly linked Red Cross cooperation to national wartime cooperation, suggesting that the Red Cross bond further strengthened the two countries' ties as neighbours and allies.[58]

Once the United States joined the Allies in 1917, the CRCS benefited from the advertising finesse of ARC campaigns, as newspapers and word of mouth brought ARC publicity north of the border. Government and business came together on the ARC War Council and turned the organization into a powerful patriotic propaganda tool. John Hutchinson writes that after America's entry into the war, "contributing money and time to the Red Cross became a kind of patriotic obsession, which brought out the best and the worst in the American genius for publicity and hoopla."[59] There is no evidence to suggest CRCS leaders resented the Americans' late and self-congratulatory entry into the war, although they might justifiably have done so. Instead, the American involvement seems to have provided a timely boost. Canadians already linked the Red Cross to patriotism, but the onslaught of brash ARC win-the-war propaganda helped renew Red Cross enthusiasm among some war weary Canadians. Albertans attributed a sudden surge in southern Alberta Red Cross growth in June 1918 to "people whose friends had told them of what was being done in the United States."[60] The influence was far from one-sided: in February 1918 Dr Ryerson was invited to speak about the society's wartime experience at ARC chapters along the Pacific coast, from Seattle to Los Angeles. "There were three ways of getting subscriptions for the Red Cross," he told his audiences: "first, an appeal to sympathy; second, an appeal to self-interest (for the people had sons and brothers in the service); and third, an appeal to patriotism." All three approaches would be staples of CRCS (and other Red Cross societies') appeals throughout the twentieth century. To this day both sympathy and self-interest remain central to humanitarian fundraising more broadly.

Aside from fundraising, CRCS volunteers in Canada engaged in a range of more concrete work for the sick and wounded. This work included preparing hospital foods for shipment overseas as a supplement to those the society purchased in Britain. The CRCS Fruit Kitchen in Hamilton, Ontario used professional equipment and a volunteer workforce from 1916 onward to produce "invalid foods" and special treats: tomato soup, canned chicken, pickles, jam, and jelly.[61] Beginning in

1916, volunteers waded through bogs in British Columbia and the Maritimes to collect sphagnum (also called peat) moss while others graded and sterilized the collected moss and assembled it into bandages. As the war progressed the remarkable absorbency of this moss made it an important resource in the face of an absorbent cotton shortage. By November 1918 CRCS volunteers were producing approximately 200,000 to 300,000 finished sphagnum dressings each month for the British Army. Natalie Riegler estimates that this level of output would have required 500,000 women to give four hours of voluntary labour each day, not including those collecting the moss in peat bogs.[62]

Another group of Red Cross volunteers worked with ex-soldiers: the Halifax branch cooperated with other organizations to meet and entertain Canadian troops disembarking in Halifax, while volunteers across the country visited veterans in local hospitals and convalescent homes, providing them with the same comforts as those convalescing overseas. During the summer of 1918, the Department of Militia and Defence agreed to the society's plan to continue providing comforts and visitors after the war and to construct, operate, and maintain "Red Cross Lodges" in connection with military hospitals. The lodges were intended as a homey, comfortable meeting place for hospital patients and their relatives. These plans ensured that the society's work would continue after war's end, and indicated a sense of long-term responsibility for the care of veterans not seen in the South African War-era CRCS.[63]

Although the CRCS was involved in this wide range of homefront activity, one area of endeavour came to symbolize not only Red Cross work as a whole but also women's special contributions to the war effort: the making of supplementary clothing, comforts, and hospital supplies – and above all, sock-knitting. CRCS leaders may have preferred cash contributions, but by September 1914 they recognized that "women's work making garments ... ha[d] cash value, and serve[d] to keep up interest in Red Cross." Mrs Elaine Nelson of Toronto (a young singer whose Great War contributions included Red Cross work, farming, munitions work, and entertaining the troops) recalled that, at least in urban areas, before the war "there was no reason for anybody to knit" because store-bought goods were available. The war years produced a veritable knitting revival, she remembered, as older women taught the skill to a new generation, specifically for the purposes of war work.[64] Hand-knit socks became the stereotype of women's work, but Red Cross volunteers throughout the British Empire also produced multiple varieties of bandages and dressings, towels and bedding, garments for hospital patients (such as pyjamas, slippers, or bed jackets), and comfort bags containing such items as a toothbrush, toothpaste, comb, writing paper, and envelopes.[65] These were sent from local branches to provincial and national Red Cross headquarters, shipped overseas to Britain, divided between CRCS warehouses in London, Shorncliffe, Paris, and Boulogne, and finally distributed to hospitals as required. They therefore constituted a tangible link between Canadians at home and Canadian troops overseas, and the resulting sense of connection probably accounts for the popularity of this work among volunteers.

The field of caring for Canada's fighting men was crowded, and it was once again thanks to clearly delineated roles and inter-agency cooperation that the CRCS was able to function effectively. The Salvation Army and the YMCA focused on entertainment, recreation, and spiritual guidance for combatant soldiers, while the National Women's Patriotic Service Committee and Canadian War Contingent Association provided field comforts to combatant troops. This left the field of comforts for sick and wounded soldiers to the Red Cross, which undertook this responsibility with the crucial support and participation of the women of the IODE and the Women's Institutes. The result was the aforementioned resurgence in the popularity of knitting, such that in November 1914 widely read Canadian women's magazine *Everywoman's World* lightheartedly reported hearing needles "going clickity-clack from coast to coast." Not all Red Cross sewing or knitting was done by hand or for free – some large requests from the BRCS were filled through CRCS purchases of manufactured goods, while the Toronto Women's Patriotic League combined war charity and aid to the impoverished by paying a number of unemployed working-class women to do Red Cross sewing each day. At the same time, the voluntary effort continued, with women plying their needles in living rooms, church basements, and concert halls, and on front porches, streetcars, and university campuses.[66]

Socks became a joke in some quarters, as critics questioned the usefulness of the millions of pairs sent overseas each year. The fact that they were coming at soldiers from all directions – from the CRCS, IODE, Canadian War Contingent Association, regimental associations, and individual relatives – probably did constitute overkill, but the wet, cold trench conditions and the seriousness of the ailment called Trench Foot made keeping one's feet warm and dry an issue of genuine concern. Not every willing volunteer was equipped to meet the standards set by Mrs Plumptre, however. British VAD Vera Brittain's confession that she found "even the simplest bed-socks and sleeping helmets" well beyond her abilities would no doubt have resonated with some Canadian women. Plumptre urged volunteers to remember that garments that did not meet CRCS specifications or were badly knitted were "really useless," and chided them with the message that "the object of the Red Cross is not to provide materials for working parties and to occupy the time of the workers, but to provide garments which are really suitable for men to wear."[67]

The Nova Scotia provincial branch took determined steps to avoid shoddy workmanship by standardizing and rationalizing women's voluntary production as much as possible. Although it still accepted articles made elsewhere across the province, the branch centralized production in its Red Cross workroom at the Halifax Technical College. Under the supervision of Nova Scotia branch vice president May Sexton the work was carried on "as in a factory, each group doing a certain thing," with a regular schedule for producing specific items each day. Various women's organizations supplied shifts of workers, and their work on the sewing and knitting machines was supervised and inspected. This model of scientific management was financed by monthly contributions from five hundred Halifax businessmen.[68] Yet, whether produced in a farmhouse or a factory-style setting, CRCS comforts were intended to introduce something familiar, homelike, and personal – the equivalent of a hug, bedtime story, or special blanket – into the austere and regulated existence of recuperating soldiers. Private Samuel Porter of Toronto both clarified and underscored the importance of comforts in a letter of thanks to the Red Cross branch in Patterson Settlement, New Brunswick: "Now I don't want you to think that the Army don't [sic] supply us with socks, for they do, but they are not like the socks that Mother makes."[69] Such reassurance must have encouraged knitters to keep their needles clicking.

To accommodate advances in medical and surgical techniques, the money CRCS volunteers raised now sometimes paid for specialized items of medical and surgical equipment, but in other respects most of the items the society sent overseas would have been familiar to a South African War convalescent: bandages, crutch pads, towels, and other ancillary items, as well as the comforts laboured over and collected by volunteers back home – not just socks, but also jam, games, books, special Christmas stockings, and maple sugar. Overseas CAMC Nursing Sister Sophie Hoerner observed that the men in her hospital seemed to appreciate any little comforts or attentions directed their way, but that they were especially mad for cigarettes. Many Canadian funds and organizations made sure they got them, but the CRCS was one of Canada's biggest providers of tobacco, distributing nearly 37,000,000 cigarettes and 82,000 lbs of loose tobacco by February 1918.[70]

Hoerner praised the comforts and hospital supplies provided by the CRCS, writing from Étaples in August 1915 that supplementary Red Cross supplies were crucial to her work. In her own words, "The work of the Red Cross is keeping us going. We couldn't do without that. It's a superb work and the boxes are wonderful. It's our reserve when we run short and we need all and everything they send, the patients getting many comforts that they would have to do without."[71] Naturally, not all convalescing soldiers were so keen. Some disliked the standard bandage, which restricted their movement; others resented gramophones and evening concerts in the hospital wards because they could not choose *not* to listen.[72] Some Canadians at home also may have disliked the fact that their donations to the society could not be directed to a specific regiment, individual soldier, or combatant troops. Despite such dissatisfactions, CRCS comforts and supplies appear to have accomplished the society's goals of supplementing CAMC medical supplies, temporarily comforting or distracting convalescing men, and reassuring soldiers they were not forgotten by the people at home. "Good people, your parcels are helping to win this war," Lieutenant Allen Otty assured his family members back in New Brunswick, in March 1917.[73]

The positive overseas results of the society's homefront work did not mean its war effort was free of challenges. Despite attempts to regulate women's work through a combination of patriotic appeals and scientific

management, women retained ultimate control over their voluntary
labour. National Headquarters intermittently received word of poorly attended meetings, a general lack of enthusiasm, or women who would not
"settle down to work." CRCS officials chastised women for failing their
men and their country, while local branches strove to revive enthusiasm
through efforts such as deliberately combining sewing and socializing
into one evening program.[74] Some volunteers responded to these tactics,
but the fact remained that labour voluntarily given could always be voluntarily withdrawn.

The relative invisibility of the society's overseas work, to those in
Canada, produced another serious problem: recurrent rumours of sock-
selling from 1915 onward. Canadians naturally wondered if the comforts
they sent actually reached soldiers, and in a context where war profi-
teering was considered an unforgivable crime, the ubiquitous socks took
on a new symbolic importance. The possibility that gifts freely given by
Canadians might be sold to soldiers for someone's profit angered Canadians, as did an accompanying rumour that Red Cross supplies sat in
warehouses unused, while soldiers went without (a rumour that, as Margot Duley shows, similarly plagued the Women's Patriotic Association of
Newfoundland). A separate rumour insinuated that provincial and national CRCS officials were paid large salaries at the expense of aid to soldiers.[75] Sociologist Ari Adut points out that scandal can be exacerbated
when the perceived transgressor has high status, and also when the scandal appears to demonstrate "a deficiency of internal control within the
transgressor's group."[76] Both the society's place as a leading Canadian
war charity and the accusations of moral laxity among some CRCS workers, therefore, served to increase the impact of the rumours.

In the pages of *Bulletin* and newspapers across the country, the society attempted to combat these rumours by refuting their charges and
explaining the actual situation: the CRCS did not sell socks, hospitals
had only to request supplies in order to receive them, and with the exception of the overseas commissioners and a handful of bookkeepers
and stenographers, the society's many officers paid their own expenses
and provided their services free of charge. Colonel Hodgetts was asked
to investigate the operations of the CRCS depots overseas, just in case,
but discovered none of the rumoured problems. Mrs Plumptre's attempts

to trace those who had bought Red Cross socks turned up an endless chain of hearsay and no identifiable purchasers.[77]

In 1916 Alberta branch president R.B. Bennett attributed the "slanders and words of mistrust" to enemy attempts to undermine Canada's war effort; in 1919 journalist Mary Macleod Moore similarly called the persistent rumours "a 'Made in Germany' story."[78] The rumours never completely died, but seem to have peaked in 1916 – the same year CRCS leaders observed a decline in supplies received – and slowly declined thereafter. The rumours may have constituted a form of backlash against the ubiquity of the Red Cross in wartime Canada. They may also have sprung from confusion overseas: so many organizations provided comforts – including a variety of national Red Cross societies – with different policies attached, and so many comforts and supplies changed hands in so many places that it was probably difficult to distinguish who was doing what.[79] Marc Bloch writes that "false news is probably born of imprecise individual observations or imperfect eyewitness accounts," at which point "the error propagates itself, grows, and ultimately survives only on one condition – that it finds a favorable cultural broth in the society where it is spreading."[80] No doubt someone, somewhere, did sell socks: perhaps unscrupulous Red Cross volunteers, black marketeers, or soldiers. Back in Canada, the rumours themselves – these magnified misperceptions – were the problem.

Ultimately, the long duration of the war had the greatest impact on the donations and labour Canadians gave to the Red Cross. Financial contributions remained high throughout and women produced comforts and supplies in abundance. Yet the war took its toll. By 1917 permanently maimed and disabled soldiers were returning to Canada in large numbers, presumably leading some women to channel their energies away from volunteering and toward caring for their loved ones at home. At the same time the increased demand for women in paid labour likely also removed some women from the voluntary sector. Income tax, inflation, and Victory Loan campaigns ate into Canadians' disposable incomes. War weariness and charitable fatigue sapped citizens' enthusiasm and energy. CRCS documents do not allude to it, but the same labour shortages that prompted the federal government to introduce military conscription in 1917 surely had some impact on the voluntary workforce as well: there simply were not enough Canadians to do all the jobs that needed doing in a country embroiled in a bloody, industrialized "total war." The combination of all these factors meant that women's production flagged noticeably, and cash contributions flowed less freely. H.B. Dawley of Courtney, British Columbia wearily observed in 1916 that "a person is called on two or three times every week to give some money to one of these funds and then they have all kinds of red cross entertainments or something of that kind."[81] And although seeing the physical results of modern warfare in returning soldiers might lead some Canadians to redouble their efforts for the Red Cross, it might just as easily convince others of the futility of jam and balaclavas in the face of machine guns and mustard gas.

War weariness, charitable fatigue, rumours, criticism, and competition for Canadians' time and money made it more difficult for the CRCS to undertake its war work, but the society carried on regardless. It was able to do so because Canadians, taken as a whole, did not waver in their support. Mrs Plumptre was justified in her belief, expressed at the height of the sock-selling rumours, that people would not lose interest in the Red Cross "until they lose interest in their own wounded and captured boys."[82]

Canadian Love-Gifts: The Many Meanings of the Wartime CRCS

Given the plethora of other war charities in Canada, the negative rumours in circulation, and the increasing levels of war weariness and charitable fatigue felt by Canadians as the conflict wore on, Canadians' extraordinary commitment to their Red Cross appears at first glance remarkable. The source of this commitment lay in the range of positive meanings with which both CRCS officials and ordinary Canadians endowed the organization and its work – meanings that proved more powerful than weariness, criticism, and competition. The CRCS publicity committee and CRCS leaders like Mrs Plumptre advanced certain perspectives on Red Cross work, but ordinary Canadians also contributed to the creation of meaning through the ways they used the Red Cross locally, supported it, talked or wrote about it, and associated it with various aspects of the war effort. Among the most prevalent reasons Canadians supported the CRCS during the Great War were Christian conviction, patriotic belief in the war's military purpose, emotional attachment to the troops, the energy and enthusiasm of youth, and the desire to build a public life for women.

By 1914 the international Red Cross movement was already steeped in a heady mix of humanitarian and charitable values, summarized by one Alberta newspaper as a belief in universal charity "regardless of creed, color [sic] or race."[83] The question of CRCS neutrality could have been a sticky one in wartime Canada, but the society never denied its international links or claimed not to aid any enemy soldiers that might fall into British hands. That this did not become a problem may be a result of the pro-British slant of most individual CRCS volunteers. It may also reflect the fact that the "humanity" Canadians were asked to help through the society was vague enough to encompass the enemy if necessary but seems to have been generally understood as being Canadian, British, imperial, and Belgian/French, in that order. No one mentioned the German women knitting for their own soldiers, or the work of the German Red Cross. In Francis Marion Beynon's loosely autobiographical wartime novel *Aleta Dey*, otherwise "very mild and reasonable" women in Aleta's Red Cross sewing circle voice anti-German sentiment as strong as any official propaganda. This suggests that at the local level, the degree to which the Red Cross lived up to its humanitarian ideals was determined by individual members' inclinations rather than national or international Red Cross policy. For this reason, pacifists like the fictional Aleta or real-life Francis might feel more at home in some branches or auxiliaries than others.[84]

Although the CRCS was deliberately non-sectarian and never officially affiliated with any particular religious faith or denomination, many Canadians supported the CRCS out of Christian conviction. Lady Drummond referred to her Information Bureau as a "ministry" to wounded soldiers and their next-of-kin, while New Brunswick branch secretary Elsey Clements described the meaning of the Red Cross with religiously tinged phrases like "the healing of both body and spirit" and the "call to service." This Christian element may have been one factor that led many Mennonite and Quaker women to feel comfortable working for war charities like the CRCS, as they attempted to walk what Marlene Epp describes as the "fine line between patriotism and pacifism." Reformer Nellie McClung suggested in 1917 that the red cross emblem would be a fitting sign for women to wear as they pieced civilization back together after the war, the red symbolizing God's creation of all people and the blood they shared, and the cross serving as a reminder of Jesus Christ and his mission to save and minister to others.[85]

These individual inclinations to understand Red Cross work through a Christian lens (generally not a feature of official CRCS publicity) were reinforced through the use of so-called "high diction" – the language of Service, Sacrifice, Honour, and Duty – in remarks about Red Cross work. One way for Canadians to grapple with the appalling inhumanity of the Great War, Jonathan Vance points out, was to derive solace from the idea of "redemption through sacrifice," drawing parallels between Christ's sacrifice on the cross and their own sacrifices during the war.[86] Being separated from friends and loved ones who enlisted, sometimes for many years, was of course a sacrifice in itself. But the language of sacrifice went beyond these partings. Canadians could speak of doing their duty or serving and sacrificing for the nation in the context of financial donations or tedious bandage-rolling sessions as easily as they could speak of enlisting in the CEF or dying in the trenches in this way. The actual activities were not at all comparable, but the language that surrounded them could be the same.

The ideas of service and sacrifice similarly informed Canadians' association of Red Cross work with their patriotic support of the nation and empire at war. During the Great War, Red Cross patriotism returned to Canada after lying dormant since the end of the South African War. Contributions to war charities like the CRCS were considered indications of a community's patriotism, and Red Cross branches large and small proudly published detailed figures of how many comforts they had sent to National Headquarters, and how much money they had raised. A March 1915 newspaper report of Medicine Hat's outstanding contributions, which ended with an appeal urging Calgarians to equal or greater efforts, was typical of the way civic pride and competition were used to tap into this patriotic spirit.[87]

Mrs Plumptre claimed that in the early days of the war, "Red Cross work (in its widest significance) ... afforded almost the only outlet for [women's] desire to serve and save." Since women could not risk their lives in defence of their country, she wrote, "they turned the torrent of patriotism into the channels of lowly service." The Canadian government stood to benefit from encouraging or at least not undermining this Red Cross patriotism because, as Jeffrey Reznick argues, the resulting "culture of caregiving" helped sustain both manpower needs and civilian morale: voluntary aid to sick and wounded troops meant more soldiers returning to the trenches and civilians who felt good about their contribution to the war effort.[88] The voluntary aspect of this work, however, was sometimes questionable. Red Cross work was frequently framed as a duty owed in return for the service and sacrifices of Canadian soldiers. From the Toronto *Globe*'s editorial call for civilians to "discharge their obligation to those at the front" by subscribing to the CRCS fund, to the tiny Bradford, Ontario branch's assertion that with five local boys at the front the branch "expects to have everybody knitting who stays at home," Canadians made it clear to one another that those who could not or would not fight must contribute in a different way. By extension, failing to contribute to the war effort in any form was not an option. The idea of Red Cross work as service to the nation – as a way for those barred from military service by age, gender, or health to "fight" at home – appeared in all the combatant nations. John Hutchinson argues that this fight-or-knit idea helped legitimize the modern concept of total war in which civilians may play a role nearly as crucial to victory as that of the military.[89]

The patriotism expressed in relation to the CRCS and its work was flexible, conveying pride, love, and support for a variety of objects ranging from local recruits to the entire British Empire. Although the patriotic aspect of CRCS work frequently took the guise of imperial sentiment, as the war progressed it became important to distinguish the *Canadian* contribution to the relief of the sick and wounded, echoing the growing Canadian nationalism frequently cited by historians as forged in the crucible of the war. The badge worn by CRCS hospital visitors in England – a small red cross superimposed on a maple leaf – subtly asserted the distinctiveness of the *Canadian* Red Cross contribution to the British imperial war effort.[90] The society was by no means a nationalist organization by 1918, but it had come a long way from the "British National Aid Society for the Sick and Wounded – Canadian Branch" of the South African War.

The concept of "love-gifts" – elaborated by Adelaide Plumptre in 1917 – combined this patriotic meaning of Red Cross work with another important lens through which Canadians viewed the CRCS: that of caring. Plumptre wrote that "the aim of the Red Cross is to provide an outlet for the love and gratitude of a people towards its protectors." In her view bandages and hand-knit socks were "love-gifts" from the nation, a tangible demonstration of Canada's care for its sick and wounded. This love was directed at soldiers both individually and collectively, and since Canadians viewed Canadian soldiers overseas as "Canada personified" – "the embodiment of all its aspirations and potential" – caring for the bodies of sick and wounded Canadians also meant caring for the nation itself.[91] However, while love-gifts might spring from a spontaneous burst of love and concern, the CRCS considered itself a middleman charged with ensuring that ordinary Canadians' caring was properly organized and rationally applied.[92] Hence the importance of commissioners, quotas, and standardized knitting instructions.

The caring aspect of Red Cross work touched many Canadians on a deeply personal level. The term "comforts" neatly expresses both the purpose and the effect of much Red Cross work. While items such as socks and cigarettes did not determine a soldier's likelihood of survival or recuperation, they were intended to comfort and cheer him at a vulnerable moment. At the same time, providing the items (even from an ocean away) brought comfort to volunteers themselves. The physical labour of making comforts acted in the same way. L.M. Montgomery's fictional Rilla Blythe observes in March 1917 that "we all find we cannot do any work that requires concentration of thought. So we all knit furiously, because we can do that mechanically." Knitting and sewing were concrete, controllable responses to tragic and terrifying situations beyond women's control. Engaging in them in the company of other women brought a further comfort to women experiencing difficult separations from, and losses of, loved ones. For this reason Bruce Scates calls women's wartime voluntary work "emotional labour," noting that both the work and the company helped mediate women's loss and bereavement.[93]

Many Canadians responded positively to the CRCS Information Bureau's work of tracking down the missing and caring for the wounded when distant loved ones could not. Letters of appreciation poured into the society's Toronto and London headquarters, conveying the relief and gratitude family members felt at receiving details of a soldier's whereabouts and condition, and offering support for the society's work. One family in Ontario wrote, "Our pain for the Boys at the front are [sic] largely overcome when we know that if they get hurt that their own friends are there to receive them" – a statement which says a great deal about why Canadians supported the CRCS in the First World War. Modern mass media made it clear that the members of the CEF were in danger, and that illness, wounds, and capture were real possibilities, but geographical distance and practical considerations made it impossible for most Canadians to provide hands-on assistance. The CRCS stood in overseas as "their own friends," caring for the vulnerable.[94]

"I appreciated more than words can convey," a British Columbia woman wrote in regard to her husband, "the first news I received relating to his poisoning from shrapnel, for no other authentic news reached me and I knew I was receiving an unbiased report from you and that was the greatest comfort and assurance to me with all that distance between us." As Eric Schneider has argued in the British case, Red Cross work tracing the missing, wounded, and circumstances of death for both officers and ordinary soldiers constituted "a rare case of truth-telling" during the war, augmenting the brusque and undetailed official notifications provided by military authorities. Jay Winter suggests that this branch of Red Cross work not only linked soldiers and their families but created a kinship bond in which the Red Cross itself became an extension of family. Such kinship bonds are evident in statements such as that of a Quebec woman who wrote to the Information Bureau about her son, saying "I noe you have a mother's love and I will say good bye and god Bless your good work [sic]." Families hungered for information, no matter how grim, and for this reason the work of the Information Bureau was among the most meaningful of the society's many Great War activities.[95]

The care and comfort motifs running through wartime CRCS work often found expression in a discourse of "mothering." Since it stood in for wives and mothers on the other side of the Atlantic who were "too far away to pet their boys," Mary Macleod Moore dubbed the Information Bureau the "Mothering Bureau," and asserted that whether young, old, married, or single, women Red Cross volunteers were engaged in acts of mothering. CRCS advertising and contemporary tributes to women's wartime voluntary work frequently emphasized the connection between mothering and the wartime Red Cross. This international trend found its ultimate expression in artist A.E. Foringer's poster for the American Red Cross of a *pietà*-style Red Cross nurse cradling a wounded soldier, entitled "The Greatest Mother in the World" – included in the introductory chapter of this book.[96] The First World War proved to be the high water mark for the discourse of mothering in the CRCS, but it remained a prominent part of the society for many more decades.

The CRCS attracted such widespread support in part because it put a new patriotic and humanitarian spin on traditionally "feminine" activities. This made it appealing and unthreatening to conservatives like staunch anti-feminist Sir Andrew Macphail who praised the CRCS for bringing "a touch of the larger humanity, an element of the feminine" into the austere lives of soldiers. At the same time it became an outlet for the patriotic energies of maternal suffragists like Nellie McClung in rural Alberta and Agnes Dennis in Halifax (where the pre-war Halifax Local Council of Women converted itself into the Nova Scotia provincial branch Red Cross when war broke out).[97] Like nineteenth- and early twentieth-century reform movements and women's organizations before it, the CRCS offered women a means of extending the domestic sphere and blurring the distinction between private and public. Some Canadians shifted their opinions on suffrage during the war, considering women's work for the CRCS and other war charities as demonstrating their worthiness for full citizenship. In the words of a *New Glasgow Enterprise* reporter, women had proved that theirs was "no longer the weaker sex, but one that in a great emergency prove[d] itself strong and true."[98]

On many levels wartime CRCS work was social: it was undertaken in the society of others, it offered an opportunity to socialize, it was subject to social surveillance and social pressures, and it reflected the pre-

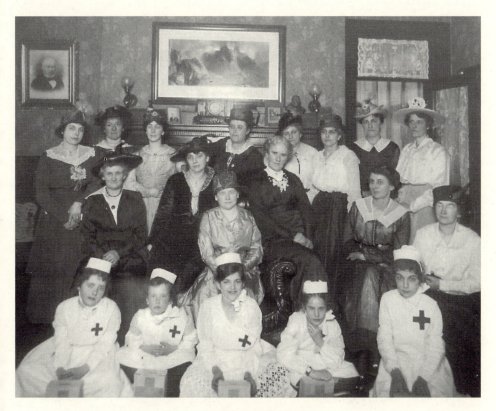

Figure 3.5
Members of the North Branch CRCS in Montreal gathered for a fundraising event one afternoon in 1917 and recorded the occasion with this formal photograph, framed and preserved for posterity. Unlike most volunteers in historical CRCS images, these women are named. Back row, left to right: Mrs M.C. Hopkins, Mrs Sayer, Mrs Frazer, Mrs F. Read, Mrs Owen, Mrs Lewthwaite, Mrs Finlayson, Mrs Aikinson. Middle row: Mrs Barber (secretary), Mrs Ramsay, Mrs Scott (assistant treasurer). Front row: Mrs Cleveland (president), Mrs Munro (hostess), Mrs McKenzie. The girls in costume (with collection boxes) are identified as possibly being the daughters of (left to right) Hopkins, Sayer, Ramsay, Aikinson, and Munro.

war social hierarchy. Fundraising events provided a guilt-free opportunity to dance, play cards, or attend concerts. Dull and repetitive tasks like bandage-rolling were often undertaken in the social space of a CRCS branch or auxiliary where socializing with others helped keep volunteers at their tasks once the initial novelty and patriotic fervour wore off. This social side of CRCS work was clearly displayed in a 1916 anecdote in the *Bulletin*, which humorously relayed the story of a visitor to National Headquarters. The woman explained that her fellow local volunteers did not like to make shirts and pyjamas because the sound of the sewing machines drowned out their conversation.[99]

Social surveillance was similarly in evidence throughout the war. The "fight or pay" / "fight or knit" mentality cultivated by war charities like the CPF and the CRCS meant that Canadians kept tabs on one another's charitable war work and donations. Newspaper acknowledgments of individual knitting and sewing output, for example, helped women monitor one another in rural British Columbia communities, producing peer pressure to contribute. No doubt some CRCS branches experienced scenes such as those Vera Brittain witnessed in the British context, where being *seen* to contribute was as important as the contribution itself. The well-to-do ladies of Buxton, England, Brittain recalled, "wasted so much material in the amateur cutting-out of monstrous shirts and pyjamas that in the end a humble local dressmaker … had to be called in to do the real work, while the polite female society of Buxton stalked up and down the hotel rooms, rolled a few bandages, and talked about the inspiration of helping one's country to win the war." The existing social hierarchy also influenced branch and auxiliary leadership: L.M. Montgomery's literary fame and position as minister's wife led to her appointment as president of the Leaskdale, Ontario CRCS branch, a position she did not want but felt duty-bound to accept when invited. Other volunteers found their social authority increased through their association with the CRCS, as they organized time, resources, and labour under the banner of the red cross emblem.[100] Thanks to a combination of secular humanitarianism, religious conviction, emotional attachment to the troops, patriotism, feminism, anti-feminism, and social pressures, the Red Cross was an integral part of life in wartime Canada.

Postscript: Halifax and Siberia

While the First World War consumed the bulk of the society's energy, two other events also claimed a share of its attention in this period. The Halifax Explosion (1917) and Canada's Siberian Expedition (1918–19) each diverted resources from the CRCS war effort and heralded, in different ways, further developments in the ongoing evolution of the Canadian Red Cross.

A tragic and unexpected chapter of the society's work in Canada during the Great War opened with the collision of the steamships *Mont Blanc* and *Imo* in Halifax Harbour on the morning of 6 December 1917. The resulting explosion and ensuing tidal wave destroyed homes and buildings, killed nearly 2,000 people, wounded many more, and left 10,000 Haligonians homeless.[101] Upon hearing of the disaster, the American Red Cross, with more than forty years of domestic and overseas disaster relief experience, immediately sent supplies and relief workers from nearby Boston. The CRCS, by contrast, had no history of disaster relief activities before 1917, and (many years earlier) had explicitly voted down Dr Ryerson's proposal that the society enter that field. However, the gravity of the situation quickly overrode any concerns about official mandate, and local and provincial branches rushed into the breach. Supplies in Saint John, New Brunswick intended for France were diverted to Halifax, and the Nova Scotia branch brought in a trainload of doctors and nurses from elsewhere in the province.[102]

Both the immediate emergency response and longer term relief and rehabilitation efforts were coordinated by the experienced ARC team, but the CRCS played an important role as well. Nova Scotia branch vice-president May Sexton (who happened to ride on the same train to Halifax as the Bostonians) shared with the ARC team her vast and personal knowledge of Halifax, its civic and philanthropic organizations, and its most influential citizens. Mrs Sexton and the ARC team jointly agreed on priorities for the relief mission, and members of the ARC team later singled her out for praise.[103]

When the ARC team later met with Halifax civic leaders to discuss reorganizing the relief effort, it was at May Sexton's urging that thirty-four volunteers and ten soldiers seconded from the CEF were organized into a special Medical Supply Committee, chaired by CRCS shipping agent Harry Milburne, and vice-chaired by Sexton herself. Although the committee fell under the umbrella of the city's newly reorganized relief effort, in practice it became largely a CRCS undertaking. In the Red Cross workroom at the Halifax Technical School, some 300 women met to sew bandages for five days straight, and volunteers handled the receipt of donated food, clothing, footwear, hospital supplies, and money, as well as its distribution to area hospitals and dressing stations. On 15 January 1918 the ARC offices in Halifax officially closed, and by March

1918 the CRCS had re-stocked its storeroom on a rehabilitated Pier 2 and resumed its work in Halifax for sick and wounded soldiers in local military hospitals.[104]

The CRCS contribution to relief and rehabilitation after the disaster was overshadowed by that of the ARC, which was more important, better organized, more visible, and more symbolically powerful (its work representing Allied friendship and long ties between Nova Scotia and New England). Nonetheless, the CRCS played an integral part in the overall relief effort. The Halifax Explosion thus became the first instance of the society undertaking domestic disaster relief, inaugurating what would come to be a central pillar of Red Cross work in Canada.

As opposed to the Halifax Explosion, which took the society in a new direction, the Siberian Expedition more closely approximated the kind of aid to sick and wounded soldiers with which the CRCS was familiar. In August 1918 the Canadian government promised to contribute 4,000 troops for an Allied military intervention in Siberia, in aid of the anti-Bolshevist White Russians then battling the Red Army for control of Russia in the wake of the 1917 revolution. When Canadian soldiers travelled to Vladivostok, the CRCS followed close behind.[105] Once it decided to send CRCS aid to Siberia with the CEF, the Executive Committee diverted comforts and hospital supplies produced in the four Western provinces for use there. It also chose Colonel John Stoughton Dennis Jr as a new CRCS commissioner in Siberia, and authorized the opening of a Vancouver warehouse. Canadian military personnel arrived in Siberia in October 1918, and by December the CRCS had established itself in Siberia as well. The Siberian mission had barely begun when the Great War came to an end, but the military intervention continued. For reasons of economy and efficiency in this far-flung locale, the CRCS departed from previously accepted policy: it distributed comforts provided by the Canadian War Contingent Association to combatant soldiers, in addition to providing comforts to the sick and wounded who were the society's special province.[106]

The Siberian mission was an extension of the CRCS's work in England and France, where the society worked closely with the military and other Allied Red Cross societies and provided comfort and a morale boost to Canadian soldiers far from home. However, it also closely resembled Dr Ryerson's time as CRCS commissioner in South Africa. The small Siberian mission lacked the complex bureaucracy that grew up around CRCS operations in England and France, the society worked as closely with the BRCS in Siberia as it had in South Africa, and Colonel Dennis had more opportunity for hands-on involvement in the tradition of Dr Ryerson than did the CRCS commissioners in Europe. It also eventually (and somewhat reluctantly) incorporated the new turn toward public health work and civilian relief taken by the entire international Red Cross movement in the aftermath of the Great War. In the absence of combat injuries on a Great War scale among Allied troops in Siberia, much CRCS aid went toward anti-venereal disease and anti-typhus measures. After the 1919 withdrawal of the Canadian troops, CRCS workers in Vladivostok stayed on, providing medical aid and relief supplies to White Russian refugees, railway workers, the poor, and sick and wounded White Russian soldiers, until 1921. This CRCS aid was a mere drop in the bucket of need, but it marked a clear departure from earlier policy and was more in line with the new public health turn of the 1920s.[107] As such, the small CRCS mission to Siberia bridged the periods of war and peace both temporally and substantively. It barely registered on the radar of most CRCS supporters, but symbolically it was the product of things past and a harbinger of things to come.

✚

For the overwhelming majority of Canadians, their experience of the CRCS during the Great War was profoundly local, and their "hometown horizons" (in Robert Rutherdale's phrase) shaped the work they did and how they understood it. But through the CRCS Canadians also became part of an "imagined community" of Red Cross volunteers, in the now-famous words of Benedict Anderson.[108] The provincial, national, imperial, and international tiers of Red Cross activity magnified and extended the efforts of individual Canadians and their communities: through the CRCS's international affiliation Canadians could even reach behind enemy lines, sending parcels to Canadian POWs in Germany. Few (if any) other organizations could boast the same reach. Furthermore, the wide variety of activities that fell under the umbrella of CRCS work, and the many and varied meanings that Canadians could attach to them, contributed to the society's broad appeal. The Canadian Red Cross Society spoke in the languages of Christianity, patriotism, feminism, caring, and social expectation – although apparently not in French. No wonder, then, that a broad spectrum of Canadians embraced their Red Cross Society and placed it on a pedestal during the war.

The CRCS emerged from the war transformed: no longer largely the preserve of men, of Ontarians, or of elites, the CRCS of 1918 was a coast-to-coast voluntary and charitable behemoth that had successfully harnessed the grassroots desire of the masses to aid their suffering fellow citizens, and administratively evolved in order to coordinate the provision of a staggering amount of tangible aid to the sick, wounded, and captured. No one cared that the society had not provided the direct battlefield assistance Henry Dunant originally envisioned, or reformed Canadian military medicine, as G.S. Ryerson once desired. Serving as a link between citizens on the home front and citizen-soldiers overseas was enough – and perhaps even better than those founding goals – in the context of twentieth-century total war. The society therefore ended the Great War as a force to be reckoned with. The November 1918 Armistice, however, introduced a disturbing existential question for this bigger, better Canadian Red Cross: *what now?*

4

THE BATTLEFIELDS OF PEACE,
1919–1939

In the spring of 1939, two dozen children, students of all ages from Joannes School No. 2 in Farmborough, Quebec, laboriously pulled rotting tree stumps from a quarter acre of their schoolyard and created a gravel walk from the dirt highway to the door of their log cabin-style schoolhouse. The children of this new settlement area – part of a colonization scheme in which the provincial government gave unemployed urban men and their families tracts of unsettled land in remote parts of the province – took turns sweeping the schoolroom floor after school each day. They assigned the roles of "doctor," "nurse," "policeman," and "fireman" among themselves on a weekly basis, in order to monitor their collective cleanliness, keep the younger children off the highway, cut kindling, and keep the fire going during school hours. These efforts to improve their own health and beautify their schoolyard were undertaken as a chartered branch of the Junior Red Cross – a fact the girls and boys proudly related, along with details of their activities and a photo of their group, in a letter to Jean Browne, the national director of the Canadian Junior Red Cross in Toronto.[1] Somehow, between November 1918 and April 1939, the Canadian Red Cross Society had shifted its focus from sick and wounded soldiers in European military hospitals to pioneer children in a log schoolhouse in outpost Quebec. What happened?

Having established itself by 1918 as the country's undisputed leader among wartime humanitarian aid organizations, the CRCS spent the ensuing two decades renegotiating its place in the Canadian voluntary sector, its relationships with other Red Cross bodies, and its appeal to Canadians themselves. What is known among historians of the voluntary/

charitable sector as "mission drift" – a gradual movement away from an organization's original mandate or mission – was, for the Canadian Red Cross during the 1920s and 1930s, not so much a drift as a sharp yank on the rudder, both deliberate and dramatic. In a move that was part war memorial and part pragmatism, interwar Red Cross leaders strove to redefine their mission and broaden the scope of their work in order to build a better Canada one healthy citizen at a time and keep their organization vital and prominent in the process. The society took on this new work confident that it could simply redirect the resources and volunteer labour that it had commanded in wartime in order to achieve the same degree of success in the public health field. Instead, it met with conflict and competition from other public health agencies, declining public interest, and dwindling funds. Despite these challenges, the interwar years were a pivotal period for Canada's leading wartime humanitarian aid organization. The Canadian Red Cross Society's decision after the First World War to stray from its original mandate and move into peacetime public health work – a self-reinvention it promoted as a form of nation building – proved to be a pragmatic response to postwar social conditions. It also pointed the organization in the direction it would travel for the next ninety years.

The Many Transformations of Peacetime

When the armistice ending the Great War took effect on 11 November 1918, the Canadian Red Cross Society's first task was to wrap up its overseas operations. In a gesture toward all soldiers of the CEF, CRCS nurses met soldiers' wives and children at eastern Canadian ports when they arrived from Britain and accompanied them across the country by train.[2] In the absence of any clear direction from its parent British Red Cross Society, the CRCS also decided, on its own initiative, to stray ever so slightly from previously accepted policy limiting it to work for sick, wounded, or captured soldiers in order to undertake relief work for civilian refugees returning to devastated areas of Europe. The care of wounded and permanently disabled soldiers who required assistance remained paramount,[3] but the society eventually provided some $300,000 in cash, plus clothing and hospital supplies, for refugees in France, Belgium, Romania, and Serbia. Leftover wartime hospital supplies and equipment were either shipped home and distributed to provincial and local CRCS branches or sold overseas. The CRCS hospital facilities at Bushey Park were presented to the London County Council as a home for delicate children; the hospital huts at Cliveden were given to the City of Birmingham as a hospital for crippled and tubercular children.

This could easily have been the end for the Canadian Red Cross Society. Having disposed of its surplus wartime medical supplies, the society might have quietly upheld its promise to assist sick and wounded veterans by maintaining a small body of hospital visitors to offer the usual comforts and company, and otherwise demobilized until such time as another war (heaven forbid!) required it to once again spring into action. Many Canadians imagined that this would be the case, and at war's end eagerly laid down their knitting needles or set aside their collection boxes. Many branches and most auxiliaries closed their books.[4] However, the overwhelming success and strength of the wartime organization led other Red Cross supporters to envision a future in which the society had a significant role not only in wartime but in peacetime as well.

The idea of peacetime Red Cross work had circulated within the international Red Cross movement for some time. Delegates to the 1912 Ninth International Red Cross Conference in Washington, DC (including CRCS representatives Mrs A.E. Gooderham and Dr Ryerson), for example, overwhelmingly voted to extend Red Cross work around the world into peacetime projects, "as without it the work would die of inanition and lack of public interest in time of war." The difficulty of maintaining a viable wartime relief organization in the absence of war weighed heavily on the minds of many national societies' leaders.[5] Yet the Canadian Red Cross, still following the wartime-only mandate laid out by its British parent, took no steps in this direction prior to the Great War. Not until 1916 did the CRCS Executive Committee begin thinking, even vaguely, about peacetime. In June of that year it opened the Duchess of Connaught's Canadian Red Cross Endowment Fund. Leading lights in the society feared a repeat of the "great difficulties" the CRCS had faced between the end of the South African War and the beginning of the Great War, and the endowment fund was intended to provide a base of financial support for future work.[6] But although CRCS leaders hoped to "maintain the organization and the interest in the work" after the end of the Great War (whenever it might come), not until 1918 did the society begin to seriously consider an enlarged mandate.

By 1918 the society had assembled a massive, well-respected organization from coast to coast, and many supporters were loath to see it disappear. Surely, they argued, it would be a shame to let such a vast army of volunteers, so much public goodwill, and such well-filled coffers simply sit idle once the war ended. Some Red Cross leaders were probably also reluctant to lose the status and power they gained through their Red Cross roles. On many levels, it felt good to be involved with this organization. Why allow it to disappear? This line of reasoning allowed George Sterling Ryerson to make his last major mark on the organization he founded and championed through long years in the charitable wilderness. At the February 1918 Central Council meeting he once again proposed that the CRCS move into the field of peacetime work; this time Central Council agreed. Ryerson considered this to be the capstone on his work of founding the society.[7] If he had not proposed the move, someone else in the organization would likely have done so eventually, but it seems fitting that the society's founder also officially set it onto the path of peacetime work that would so substantially influence its place in Canadian society. The following day the Duke of Devonshire (doing triple duty as governor general, patron of the society, and husband of the society's president) urged the CRCS not to disband when the war came to its eventual conclusion, stating that making the society a permanent fixture in Canadian life would be "one of the greatest steps which could be taken."[8] This ringing vice-regal endorsement was a welcome support, but the Great War continued to demand the full attention of Red Cross leaders until the end of 1918, and the CRCS took no immediate steps to develop a peacetime program.

Although pragmatism undoubtedly played a role in the society's decision to pursue peacetime activity, the CRCS had more than its own continued existence in mind when it decided to take on public health work. In the face of the appalling standards of health revealed by medical examinations of military recruits during the Great War and the millions of deaths around the world during the conflict and the subsequent Spanish Influenza epidemic, public health took on new significance in the postwar world. In addition, it became increasingly evident that large numbers of ordinary Canadians in rural, northern, and new settlement areas lacked access to basic health care services. The society's move into public health was a strategic manoeuvre, but it was also rooted in genuine national health concerns.

Likewise, the decision to expand the CRCS's mandate took place in an international context of concern over public health in which charitable organizations were urged to tackle the problem. The CRCS was only one of many national Red Cross societies whose leaders were eager to venture into new fields and build on their wartime successes rather than subside into inactivity. As political leaders met at the Paris peace conference of 1919 to remake the world in what American president Woodrow Wilson and other idealists hoped would be a kinder, gentler fashion, a simultaneous movement was taking shape among the leading national Red Cross societies: one that aimed to remake the world along healthier lines. Henry Davison, president of the American Red Cross War Council, conceived the idea of a League of Red Cross Societies (LRCS) that would coordinate and advise the national societies in public health and disaster relief work, along the lines of the peacetime work undertaken by the American Red Cross for decades prior to the First World War. The League of Red Cross Societies, as its name implied, was to be a non-governmental version of the new League of Nations, and Davison envisioned it making a similarly important contribution to sympathy and brotherhood among nations.[9] The International Committee of the Red Cross was displeased by the plan, viewing the LRCS as a competitor for leadership of the Red Cross movement, but the "Big Five" Red Cross societies – British, French, Italian, Japanese, and American – became founding members of the LRCS regardless.[10]

The new LRCS immediately convened a gathering of international medical experts in Cannes, France. The April 1919 Cannes conference produced a series of recommendations meant to direct national Red Cross societies around the world toward those aspects of public health that could most benefit from their help. Venereal disease, tuberculosis, typhus, child welfare, malaria, preventive medicine, and public health nursing emerged as the areas of most pressing need.[11] Armed with this broad mandate from leading international health experts, the LRCS opened its membership to Red Cross societies other than the Big Five, and thanks to Henry Davison's influence with Woodrow Wilson, support for the Red Cross movement was written into the League of Nations Covenant.

Article 25 of the covenant pledged member nations to support the work of their Red Cross societies in "the improvement of health, the prevention of disease, and the mitigation of suffering" during both peace and war.[12] National Red Cross societies eagerly adopted this three-point mission statement and convinced their respective governments to integrate it into their official charters. Now enshrined in both international and national law, the new three-point mission statement was used for leverage as Red Cross societies carved out new peacetime territory for themselves, sometimes treading heavily on the toes of both voluntary and government organizations in the process.

Since Canadian Red Cross Society leaders and supporters played no role in the development of the LRCS idea and organization, they were not content to be patient (as the BRCS advised) and wait for events to unfold on the international stage. Instead, as the CRCS wrapped up its wartime work, CRCS leaders began mulling over amendments to their constitution and pondering potential uses for leftover war funds.[13] These discussions were halted by the BRCS in January 1919, in order to await the results of an upcoming International Red Cross conference which would sort out the legal implications of extending Red Cross activity outside the bounds of its original mandate under the Geneva Conventions.[14] The delay proved highly influential. The CRCS had been thinking on a rather small scale, and the results of the Cannes conference opened its eyes to a grander project: public health as the new frontier.

Four days after the conclusion of the Cannes conference, CRCS honorary solicitor Norman Sommerville wrote to acting prime minister Sir Thomas White and asked him to introduce a government bill to amend the society's Act of Incorporation so as to extend the society's purposes in Canada to include "prevention and alleviation of human ills and suffering" during peacetime.[15] By mid-May 1919 the Canadian government's initial reservations were overcome by the British government's intention to grant the BRCS a similar charter, and the fact that Article 25 of the League of Nations Covenant called upon signatory governments to support national peacetime Red Cross work.[16] The CRCS modified its requested amendment to reflect the three-point statement found in Article 25, and the bill passed quickly through Parliament.

No longer fettered by its wartime mandate, the society was now empowered "in time of peace or war to carry on and assist in work for the improvement of health, the prevention of disease and the mitigation of suffering through the world."[17] As what would today be termed an organizational mission statement, it had a grand, noble ring to it, in keeping with the idealism of the day. Being enshrined in Canadian law, it also gave the CRCS carte blanche to involve itself in as many varieties of health and welfare work as it chose. The language of both the statement originally submitted to Parliament and the LRCS version eventually adopted was deliberately broad, inclusive, and widely empowering. Over the course of the twentieth century it would help the society to justify its involvement in a range of activities, from outpost nursing stations to blood donor recruitment, from water safety training to the distribution of clothing and butter to Canadians suffering the effects of the Great Depression.

Propelled by the momentum of the entire Red Cross movement's entry into peacetime public health work, in 1919 the CRCS barrelled enthusiastically into the field armed with a national mandate to improve health, prevent disease, and mitigate suffering. After consultation with a variety of professionals – notably North American public health experts like C.-E.A. Winslow[18] – the society formulated its own national plan. The task of drawing up the society's first peacetime program fell to Adelaide Plumptre, a key figure in the more business-like second generation of CRCS leadership which had emerged during the Great War. Mrs Plumptre's remarkable record of voluntary service both within and outside the society made her a natural choice to draft the plan that would guide the society in coming years.[19]

The CRCS National Peace Policy drawn up by Mrs Plumptre in 1919 and adopted by Central Council set out a clearly defined series of relationships and duties to guide future work by the society at all levels. War work came first, and the wartime agreement with the St John Ambulance Association and Brigade would be upheld until all war work was finished. In terms of new peacetime work, the most striking change related to the role of the provinces. Within national guidelines, the work of the society would henceforth be directed by largely autonomous provincial branches, which through a variety of means would guide local branches in promoting child welfare, good hygiene, and proper sanitation in their communities. National Headquarters would ensure that the CRCS remained in line with developments in the international Red Cross

movement, but would take a hands-off approach to provincial and local
activity. The national Executive Committee would liaise with the federal government and national voluntary organizations, coordinate aid to
any provincial branch that requested it, and serve as a channel of communication among provincial branches, national, and international Red
Cross bodies. The society as a whole would act as an auxiliary of the
new federal Department of Health, in addition to its role as an auxiliary
of the medical branch of the Department of Militia and Defence. Specific
tasks that Plumptre set out for the society across Canada included form-
ing a national medical and nursing service, encouraging universities to
establish nursing departments, promoting St John Ambulance Association courses in first aid and home nursing, keeping national and provincial reserve funds and lists of medical personnel for use in emergencies,
and generally cooperating with governments and other agencies working toward similar public health goals.[20] It was an ambitious plan for an
organization with next to no prior experience in peacetime work, but it
bore the confident stamp of the society's wartime experience.

The provincial branches of the CRCS found themselves with a much
greater role in program development and delivery after 1918, because a
single health program for all of Canada would not have been politically
feasible, expedient, or appropriate. The 1867 British North America Act
assigned responsibility for health and education to the provinces rather
than to the federal government, and the First World War had inadvertently strengthened the provincial branches of the Red Cross, while
health care needs and standards across the country varied widely. The
CRCS National Peace Policy therefore offered a broad national vision
statement and practical direction on who was responsible for what, but
left the details up to each province.

This latitude produced an array of Canadian Red Cross public health
activities, which differed from community to community, as local initiative and provincial direction dictated. In Nova Scotia, for example,
the National Peace Policy became the basis for the provincial branch's
"Ten Point Program" which set out specific practical objectives and
programs the Nova Scotia Red Cross intended to carry out. In Prince
Edward Island, the Red Cross became the leading organization engaged
in public health work, and over the interwar period it directly influenced the creation and shape of the provincial Department of Health.

The Quebec provincial branch resisted civilian public health work for years and instead focused on the care of unemployed and sick veterans and their families; British Columbia similarly held out against public health work for some time. By contrast, Alberta's provincial Red Cross became a whirlwind of activity, its efforts embracing such dissimilar work as aid for drought-ridden farmers in the south of the province during the 1920s, a Crippled Children's Hospital, and the "Red Cross Lady" radio program.[21]

A global influenza (or "Spanish Flu") epidemic ravaged Canada during the late autumn and winter of 1918–19, ultimately killing an estimated 55,000 Canadians (and likely more than 30 million people worldwide). Among its many legacies, the epidemic provided an early, unwitting example of how the Canadian Red Cross would pursue its public health goals during the interwar period. In spite of the severity of the epidemic, the CRCS did not mobilize to combat it in any nationally coordinated fashion.[22] Provincial branches were given permission to help, and on their own initiative many provincial and local branches turned their energies and resources toward assisting those in their communities stricken with Spanish Flu. Alberta's provincial branch assisted ninety-four communities by issuing supplies worth more than $13,000, cooperated with the local boards of health, and used Calgary and Edmonton supply depots to get medical supplies to branches in outlying districts. Nova Scotia and New Brunswick organized similar province-wide responses. Elsewhere, some individual local branches tackled independent relief work. One example was Border Branch in Windsor, Ontario, which facilitated the provision of nursing care, hot meals, drugs, bedding, and medical supplies to more than two hundred local families on a pay-as-you-can basis after the Essex Health Association approached them for help in January 1919.[23] A coordinated national response to the epidemic would have offered a more consistent standard of care and relief, but the localized responses were much more characteristic of the approach the Red Cross would take to public health work over the coming decades.

The provincial autonomy spelled out in the CRCS National Peace Policy and demonstrated during the Spanish Flu epidemic was evident in other important ways. At the end of August 1919 the society finally completed its national organization by creating provincial branches for

Ontario and British Columbia. In a symbolic recognition of the expanded role they would play in peacetime work, provincial branches were renamed provincial "divisions" in 1920. Provincial autonomy marked a fundamental shift away from the previous relationship between national and provincial levels of the CRCS. During the Great War, National Headquarters controlled most provincially and locally raised funds, set quotas and standards for sewn and knitted goods, and conducted all relations with other governments and Red Cross bodies. This all changed with the inauguration of peacetime work. Provincial divisions developed their own activities and relationships with federal and provincial government departments, while local branches did likewise with municipal governments.[24] Meanwhile, wartime expansion outside previous Red Cross strongholds in Ontario, New Brunswick, and Anglo-Quebec resulted in broader provincial representation on Central Council, the society's legislative body. However, the day-to-day affairs of the national society continued to be run by the Ontario-based members of the Executive Council, as a result of the society's decision to remain headquartered in Toronto.[25]

Despite losing much of the control it had exerted during the war, National Headquarters was determined to maintain a permanent role in the work of the society. To this end, it established a permanent national office at 410 Sherbourne Street in Toronto, from which it initiated a number of its own programs. Home nursing classes, the Junior Red Cross, and the Red Cross Seaport Nurseries at Halifax, Saint John, and Quebec City were nationally coordinated, although provincially administered.[26] By carrying on the society's relations with the ICRC, the LRCS, and other national Red Cross societies, the national office contributed significantly to the overall functioning of the society during this period. Nonetheless, its role had been diminished since 1918.

National-provincial Red Cross relationships were not the only site of upheaval during the interwar years: the society's international status also underwent important changes. During the Great War the CRCS had taken major strides toward both behaving and viewing itself as an independent Red Cross organization rather than as a branch of the British Red Cross Society. The Canadian society's pride in its leading role coordinating CRCS and BRCS relief operations in Siberia attested to this, as did the certificate of recognition issued by National Headquarters to all organized groups which assisted the society in its Great War work: there was nary an imperial symbol to be found amid the maple leaves, beavers, provincial flags, and red crosses which adorned the certificate.[27] Yet despite such evidence of movement toward a distinctly *Canadian* Red Cross identity, the CRCS remained firmly attached to the BRCS. The CRCS had been keen to work with the BRCS and make use of the British society's greater resources and clout during the war, and the Canadian society's hesitance to embrace full independence mirrored Canada's own uncertain and tentative slide into national independence from Britain during this period. As Margaret Macmillan notes, "full independence was not something to be undertaken lightly"[28] – membership in the British world had its privileges. Convenience and longstanding ties of affection kept the CRCS within the imperial Red Cross fold.

International recognition of the Canadian Red Cross Society as a fully independent, national Red Cross society, therefore, came as a result of postwar changes in Canada's relationship to Great Britain rather than any move to attain full independence from within the CRCS itself. The 1926 British Empire Conference, which informally defined the status of Great Britain and its dominions as autonomous entities free to deal independently with both internal and external affairs (later formally codified in the 1931 Statute of Westminster), brought the changing political status of the British Empire to the notice of the ICRC. When the ICRC requested clarification, the BRCS politely informed the Swiss committee that the Red Cross societies of Canada, Australia, New Zealand, South Africa, and India were no longer branches of the BRCS but autonomous societies which should be recognized as parties to the rights and obligations of the Geneva Conventions. Having neither sought nor particularly desired a change in its status, the Canadian Red Cross thus found complete independence from the British Red Cross unceremoniously thrust upon it. On 15 November 1927 ICRC president Gustave Ador officially welcomed the Canadian Red Cross Society to independent status as a national Red Cross Society, but this change in the CRCS's international status initially proved more symbolic than tangible. The October 1928 IRC conference in The Hague offered the CRCS its first chance to attend as an independent society, but Central Council let the opportunity slip by. Instead, the society asked a BRCS delegate to do double duty and represent the CRCS as well.[29] The enduring strength of the bonds of

Empire in this period were further demonstrated by the sole exception to the low CRCS attendance at international Red Cross gatherings in the interwar years: the large Canadian delegation at a special 1930 British Empire Red Cross conference. In contrast, a BRCS stand-in for the CRCS was considered sufficient for the IRC conference in Belgium the following year.[30] The CRCS's priorities and affinities beyond its own Canadian borders were clearly still imperial rather than international or North American through the 1920s.

Justifying, Promoting, and Resisting Mission Drift

As the CRCS embarked on its new work in the 1920s, it deployed a particularly vague definition of health. Nineteenth-century public health initiatives principally addressed issues such as combatting epidemics and regulating water, sewage, and food production.[31] In contrast, the society's interwar conception of public health revolved primarily around a broad sense of the public good or the health of the nation rather than around an individualized notion of health as the opposite of sickness, injury, or disability. This flexible conception of health allowed the society to create programs that addressed both "real" bodily states like dental cavities, malformed limbs, and maternal death, and what might be termed "perceived" bodily states – non-biological conditions of being, such as citizenship and Canadian-ness. During the interwar period the CRCS also focused its efforts largely on improving the health of rural Canadians, a definite shift away from nineteenth-century public health approaches which had concentrated on urban health reforms. The poor health of many Canadian military recruits revealed after 1914 forcibly demonstrated that rural Canada was not fostering the good health many Canadians had long assumed it to be producing. Rural and outpost Canada no longer appeared to be the haven of fresh air, clean water, and natural good health assumed by nineteenth-century reformers.[32] Instead, organizations like the CRCS viewed it as lacking in the knowledge and services essential to good health, and worked during the interwar years to rectify the situation. The society's flexible conception of health helped it justify its engagement in a variety of projects throughout the interwar years.

As it moved into peacetime work, the CRCS attempted to impress on the public its fitness to lead a postwar Canadian public health crusade. In this it echoed the efforts of the international Red Cross movement as a whole. At the international level, figures like American public health expert and director of the LRCS Department of Public Health Dr C.-E.A. Winslow cited the movement's non-political and non-partisan character, its possession of public confidence born of the war, and its worldwide membership as proof that "the Red Cross, and the Red Cross alone" could mobilize popular feeling to the degree "which is necessary to make the control of preventable disease a solid reality."[33]

To achieve this mobilization within Canada, the CRCS produced a torrent of literature promoting both health and the Red Cross. Some of this material had a purely practical purpose, such as instructing mothers in the care of infants or setting out the guidelines of good nutrition, but much of it attempted to rally readers to the Red Cross cause using words and images that could be categorized under the umbrella of nation building. One 1922 CRCS campaign pamphlet went so far as to blatantly ask on its cover, "Nation Builders. Are You One?"[34] The nation building imagined through Red Cross work could be physical, as when Central Council chairman James W. Robertson argued in 1928 that "the physical vigor of this nation could be greatly improved in two generations" if Canadian children could be taught to follow the rules of good health and hygiene. It could also be less tangible, such as CRCS national commissioner Dr F.W. Routley's assertion to a 1927 radio audience that the CRCS outpost hospital service would help Canada reach "its true greatness" by bringing medical help and comfort to men and women in new settlement areas and thereby encouraging others to follow these pioneers' example and populate unsettled areas of Canada.[35] The society neatly summarized its interwar nation-building focus in the materials it prepared for its first nationwide financial appeal since the First World War, which – significantly – took place from Empire Day to Dominion Day in 1927. "The Red Cross is helping to build Canada, to give to the people a better quality of life," promotional pamphlets asserted. The task of ensuring good health for all Canadians would produce far-reaching and long-lasting results, the society concluded: "a people made strong and vigorous," and "young lives inspired and trained to true citizenship and service."[36]

The idea of nation building had particular significance for Canadians after 1918. The Great War not only influenced CRCS leaders' desire to undertake peacetime work but also quickly gave that work a meaning and purpose beyond mere physical health. The deaths of so many men, the loss of so much youthful promise, had to be redeemed through a better postwar world. The society explicitly linked its current efforts to the recent war, in materials such as the mid-1920s booklet entitled "Still Serving" which asked Canadians, "You gave generously to the Red Cross during the destructive war years. Will you not give equally generously for the constructive work now being done for the upbuilding of our nation?"[37] Wartime references abounded in early interwar Canadian Red Cross health propaganda, and militaristic language and imagery permeated international Red Cross peacetime discourse as well. The LRCS circulated material (sometimes directly quoted by the CRCS) that referred to the "Battlefields of Peace" and "the war against disease." The informal naming of the Canadian Red Cross's peacetime work as the "Crusade for Good Health," and the use of Joan of Arc images, drew on Christian-soldier and medieval warrior references which combined nation building, war, Christianity, and health in a mixture every bit as potent as the one produced by the CRCS during the Great War. It also echoed crusader imagery widely used in stained-glass windows commissioned and installed as Great War memorials.[38] These references to battle and war drew on Canadians' positive wartime relationships with the Red Cross to try to mobilize continued support. Shirley Tillotson's study of Community Chest appeals in Vancouver during this period suggests that military allusions may also have been deployed to undermine the association of charitable fundraising with femininity – as exemplified by the traditional charity teas, bazaars, and balls – in hopes of recruiting more male volunteers.[39]

Like crusader imagery, the ideas of service and sacrifice woven through much interwar CRCS publicity literature linked the organization to both war and Christianity. Throughout this period the most explicitly Christian aspects of the CRCS's language and imagery echoed the Social Gospel movement's pre-war emphasis on social reform as a type of practical Christianity. For instance, the Great Depression prompted the Ottawa branch of the Red Cross to pair the image of a white-garbed Red Cross nurse with the well-known words of Jesus in the Gospels:

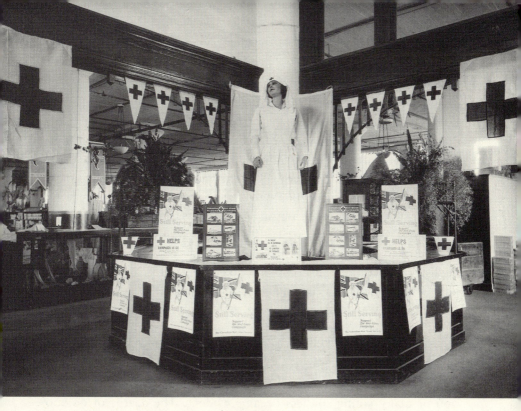

Figure 4.1
This early 1920s Saskatchewan Division display in a department store shows the
connections made between CRCS wartime service and peacetime public health needs.
Joining the familiar red cross emblem and "Red Cross nurse," posters on the counter
highlight the province's eight outpost hospitals, orthopaedic surgery for children,
and assistance to Great War veterans, united by the nationwide campaign slogan
"Still Serving."

"For I was hungered, and ye gave me meat: I was thirsty, and ye gave
me drink, I was a stranger and ye took me in, Naked and ye clothed me,
I was sick, and ye visited me."[40] The connection also went beyond publicity materials. Child welfare and immigration, two important interwar
Red Cross priorities, had long been on the agenda of many Social Gospel
adherents. Although the Social Gospel had lost some of its momentum
by 1918, its legacy clearly animated organizations like the CRCS, in
both their activities and the way they positioned their work in a Christian context.[41]

The influence of the Great War is further evident in the fact that many
Red Cross leaders in Canada saw their peacetime work as a war memorial. Journalist and long-time Alberta Red Cross leader Mary Waagen
told an audience in her home province, "I always visualise that the best

monument we can raise here in Canada to the men who fell in the war
is the building up of these better [public health] conditions."[42] The entire Canadian myth and memory of the war reassured Canadians that
the war dead willingly gave their lives to provide Canada with "a future
of greatness built on the sacrifices of the war years." In order to truly
keep faith with the dead, Jonathan Vance argues, Canadians believed
they must "start at home by putting their efforts towards building a better nation."[43] In this vein, a 1926 Red Cross radio talk in Nova Scotia
alluded to Colonel John McCrae's already famous war poem by assur-
ing listeners that the Red Cross "has taken up 'the torch' and will 'keep
faith' with those who sleep on Flanders Fields."[44]

The Great War further influenced the CRCS's interwar public health
work by infusing it with fears of "race degeneration." As Mariana
Valverde notes, such fears circulated among the Anglo-Saxon ruling
classes in Canada, the United States, and England beginning around the
turn of the twentieth century and increased as the poor physical condition of many young soldiers became evident. The deaths of 60,000
Canadians in the Great War, swiftly followed by a nearly equivalent
number of deaths from Spanish Flu, made the health of the nation an
issue of grave concern and breathed new life into the public health movement. Reformers specifically directed their attention toward mothers and
children. Canadian children were national assets, and their health was
therefore an issue of national significance.[45] James W. Robertson of the
CRCS asserted in 1921 that poor health was a feature of "backward
civilizations," and concluded, "It ought not to be so in Canada." This
concern over the quantity and quality of the population – known as
eugenics – became an international ideology during the interwar years.
As Marouf Hasian Jr argues, "the myths of national degeneration" encouraged citizens to see child-rearing as a national duty, and poor health
as a social problem rather than a purely individual matter.[46] In order to
address this perceived decline in the quality of the population, the CRCS
focused much of its effort in three particular areas: mothers, children,
and citizenship.

In its interwar concern to reach mothers, the Canadian Red Cross
contributed to a wave of early twentieth-century advice, prescriptive
literature, milk depots, and well baby clinics created by a variety of
voluntary and government bodies, all attempting to transform the art of

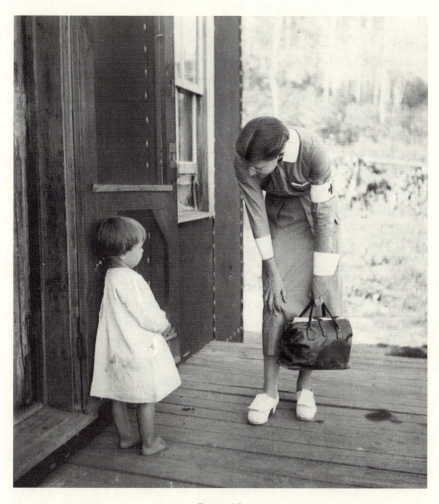

Figure 4.2
Rural children, like this one being visited by a CRCS outpost nurse, were a key
demographic targeted by the society's interwar public health work. Better babies would
make a better Canada, and render the sacrifices of Canada's war-dead worthwhile.

mothering into a precise science and therefore influence the quality of
Canadian children.[47] After 1918, the CRCS, like these other organizations
and government departments, worked to bring the "gospel of health" to
mothers across the country, thus ensuring (they hoped) a healthier future
for Canada, one baby at a time. In addition to the actual work the CRCS
undertook in relation to maternal health and health education, Red Cross
work and workers themselves were cast in a maternal light throughout
the interwar years. The convenor of the Halifax Red Cross Seaport

Nursery, Mrs McManus, wrote that her committee welcomed immi-grants "in the name of that internationally known 'greatest mother of them all' the Red Cross," while she and her committee of ladies were described in the late 1920s in a distinctly mother hen-like role, as they "hover[ed] around, keeping a watchful eye over all."[48] The maternalist aspects of the CRCS's interwar work continued to hold the society in good stead in a Canada where, as Veronica Strong-Boag notes, "proper performance of maternal duties gave women cause for personal pride and public approval."[49]

Children were a cornerstone of interwar CRCS public health efforts. As early as 1915 Canadian feminist (and Red Cross volunteer) Nellie McClung wrote that postwar restoration and rebuilding would require more than a return to the status quo: not *more* children, but *better* chil-dren.[50] The society's new Junior Red Cross wing quickly became one of the most significant of the CRCS's activities because it played a crucial symbolic role as well as offering more practical health benefits for stu-dents. In publicity materials and internal communications, the Junior Red Cross was explicitly set forth as a peacemaking tool – in other words, as a way to redeem the failures of the pre-war and war years. It was also seen as a way to transmit a spirit of giving – one of the few positive as-pects of the war years – to the younger generation.[51]

Concern for the quality of the country's children was not limited to the Canadian-born. George Nasmith, chairman of the national Junior Red Cross committee during the early 1920s, claimed the program was a great Canadianizing force because it brought about "similarity of views of life and service in Canadian children from coast to coast" and helped foreign-born children learn "ideals of citizenship, of cleanliness, of health, of beauty and of service." In Saskatchewan in particular, as Nancy Sheehan has shown, the Junior Red Cross was promoted in rural schools as a convenient means of Canadianizing the province's large for-eign population and improving the standards of rural life more gener-ally.[52] Through its work at East Coast seaports and on the Prairies, the CRCS displayed great confidence in the ability of health information, clothing, and diet to help transform immigrants – not just children, but adults as well – into good Canadian citizens.

The society's hard-sell approach, with its persistent emphasis on Red Cross peacetime public health work as a nation-building endeavour –

whether as war memorial, maternalist enterprise, peacemaking tool, or Canadianizing effort – was a necessary response to the fact that, especially during the early interwar years, many Canadians felt the organization should not be engaged in peacetime work at all. During the February 1920 CRCS annual meeting, Agnes Dennis of Halifax claimed that "the responsibility of the peace-time program of the Canadian Red Cross had been laid upon it, instead of being sought,"[53] an idea that appeared frequently in the society's publications and campaign literature throughout the 1920s. No doubt some ordinary Canadians supported the continued work of the Red Cross after the armistice, but the rapidity with which volunteers dropped out of the organization, the strident protest from certain women's organizations, a limited amount of dissent from the upper echelons of CRCS leadership, and the resistance of the Quebec and British Columbia divisions, indicate that the Canadian population as a whole did not push the society into peacetime work. Former CRCS president Sir John Gibson and a handful of others within the society had opposed the move into peacetime work back in 1918, and two of the society's greatest wartime supporters – the Women's Institutes and the IODE – resented the CRCS's incursion into their peacetime territory. Each group sent resolutions of protest to both the CRCS Executive Committee and the prime minister, proclaiming their desire "to return to their original independent freedom of activity." The CRCS also came into some conflict with the new federal Department of Public Health, created in 1919, and failed throughout the interwar years to create a meaningful working relationship with the Dominion Council of Health. Alberta Division's Mary Waagen later recalled that "every man's hand was against the idea of Red Cross work in peacetime, except those who were active Red Cross members."[54]

The enormous effort the CRCS had to put into convincing the Canadian public, through its campaign literature and publications, that it was right and good for the society to pursue public health work in peacetime, attests to Canadians' ambiguity about this new phase of Red Cross activity. Fear and resentment surrounding the society's new peacetime work increased until the organization was forced to address the issue. In early 1920s publications Canadian Red Cross leaders both acknowledged and attempted to diffuse Canadians' ambiguity and resentment, claiming that suspicions and fears that the CRCS would try to monopolize the field came from those who "did not know the Red Cross Society or its workers."[55] The society missed the point. The problem was that Canadians were all too familiar with the CRCS from the recent war. The degree to which the Red Cross had overshadowed and even swallowed up other worthy war charities and women's groups provided a chilling example of what might lie in store for existing peacetime voluntary health organizations.

In response to such concerns, the society organized a national Red Cross Advisory and Consultative Committee in the spring of 1920, with representatives from the national and provincial branches of the CRCS, plus representatives from a range of Canadian public health agencies and professional associations. Yet as late as 1939, after two decades of CRCS peacetime work, the society's broad mandate still proved controversial. In a telling exchange between Charlotte Whitton, Canadian Welfare Council founder and executive director,[56] and George P. Davidson, director of social welfare for the British Columbia provincial government, Davidson confessed he considered the CRCS "purely opportunistic in its approach," as it tried to be "all things to all men." Both Whitton and Davidson felt that provincial Red Cross divisions – British Columbia and Ontario in particular – spent an unacceptably high proportion of their income on administrative costs, but as Whitton's assistant Marjorie Bradford pointed out, taking the society to task on this issue was difficult when Canada's governor general served as president of the society. Davidson spoke for countless government and voluntary workers when he summarized the root of his animosity toward the CRCS. In his view, Red Cross leaders were convinced that "they have a mission in life," and for this reason "they have reserved to themselves the divine right of doing anything and everything that governments are not doing in a given community."[57] Davidson's assessment was apt, if irate. The "opportunistic" approach and sense of mission, which so irked observers like Whitton, Davidson, and Bradford, were the very things that helped the CRCS survive two long decades of peace.

The occasionally superior and patronizing attitude of certain Red Cross leaders no doubt contributed to other organizations' frustration and bitterness over the society's move into public health work. In 1919 and 1920 CRCS representatives frequently spoke of filling a "big brother" role, advising, encouraging, and coordinating the work of other health agencies in Canada. This was the role the new federal Department of Health intended to fill, which caused some initial friction. So did the new department's focus on health issues related to immigration and the military, which were federal responsibilities and therefore within its constitutional jurisdiction, but were also two areas the CRCS was concerned with. Beyond these small tensions, the society's move into peacetime public health work also presumed an expertise in the field that other agencies justifiably resented. The CRCS had a combined total of six years of wartime health work to its name, while organizations like the IODE, the Victorian Order of Nurses (VON), and the various arms of St John Ambulance possessed decades of experience in peacetime and public health work.

Once More unto the Breach: The Peacetime Red Cross in Action

This, then, was the context of organizational momentum and outside resistance in which the Canadian Red Cross Society attempted to reinvent itself. What the transformation looked like on the ground was something else again. Immediately following the Great War, the CRCS possessed one definite advantage over many other public health organizations in Canada: it had money, and plenty of it. Since the CRCS and CPF had been exempt from the 1917 War Charities Act, no government legislation regulated how their substantial leftover wartime funds must be used. Resentment did not keep other public health organizations from seeking financial help from the CRCS, and, as it had during the Great War, the Red Cross briefly became a sort of peacetime granting agency. The society considered such grants as one way of exercising its stated policy of assisting and cooperating with other organizations engaged in public health work, and by 1921 had provided funds to a range of agencies including the SJAA and SJAB, the Canadian National Council for Combatting Venereal Diseases, the Canadian National Committee for Mental Hygiene, and the Canadian Association for the Prevention of Tuberculosis.[58] Grants relating to mental hygiene and venereal disease represented the society's only real engagement with these two major elements of the interwar public health movement, and may have been spurred by the relevance of these issues to some returned veterans. The third major interwar public health concern, tuberculosis, on the other hand, strongly influenced the society in this period. Between 1918 and 1925 nearly $90,000 of the society's surplus war funds went to support the work of the Canadian Tuberculosis Association (equivalent to three years' worth of all the salaries and staff travel expenses paid by the national society at mid-1920s rates), and the anti-tuberculosis campaign visibly influenced the twelve rules of the Junior Red Cross Health Game, which emphasized fresh air, rest, "proper" nutrition, and limiting the spread of germs through coughing, sneezing, and spitting.[59] The decision to grant funds to the St John Ambulance Association and Brigade sprang from a less benevolent motive. When members of the St John Ambulance in Canada proposed to extend wartime cooperation into a permanent postwar joint committee of the CRCS, the SJAA, and the SJAB, the society (keen to be released from its enforced relationship with St John Ambulance) preferred instead to settle a small portion of its left-over war funds on the two St John groups and cut all "restrictive ties."[60]

Beyond grants, several major types of activity united the diverse provincial Red Cross efforts during the interwar years. The first was work for Canadian veterans of the Great War. Inspired by physical re-habilitation work Dr Ryerson observed in France in 1915, the CRCS es-tablished workshops in major cities across Canada to provide retraining and sheltered employment for disabled veterans. Some provincial divi-sions provided, supported, and staffed Red Cross lodges attached to vet-erans' hospitals, which offered a home-like atmosphere for patients to enjoy on their own or with visiting friends and family. Quebec Division was a leader in providing extensive relief and assistance to ex-soldiers and their families, in response to crop failure, sickness, or maternity needs.[61] Veterans clearly remained a priority.

Although the society valued its work with ex-soldiers, another pro-gram came to vie for pride of place in its peacetime program: the Junior Red Cross. The organization's new youth wing combined the twin themes of the CRCS peacetime program: nation building through health, and keeping the society alive and vibrant in peacetime. Classroom teachers (often with the encouragement of their provincial minister of education or school principal) voluntarily integrated the Junior Red Cross program into their regular curriculum, supported by posters, magazines, lesson ideas, and other resources provided by the Red Cross – resources that supported practical, activity-based, child-centred, progressive educational methods in ways that many school textbooks and curriculum guides then in use did not.[62] As members of a Junior Red Cross branch, children elected officers and conducted their meetings using parliamentary procedure, raised money for a Crippled Children's Fund,[63] performed plays with a health and hygiene theme, and were charged with improving their own health by following the rules of the Health Game. Since most national societies had their own Junior Red Cross programs, Canadian Juniors were also able to participate in pen pal and portfolio exchange programs with students in other countries. In 1922 Junior membership ranged from a low of 250 children in Nova Scotia to 45,000 children in Saskatchewan. By 1939, after two decades of diligent promotion, there were more than 14,000 Junior branches in Canada, with 425,000 paid-up members.[64] The society promoted these figures as a testament to the spread of solid values of health, service, and international understanding. And if the Junior Red Cross raised money, brought young members into the fold, and led them to become adult volunteers, all the better.

Immigrants also attracted widespread interest from Red Cross workers across the country. After the Great War, the CRCS joined the ranks of select church groups and voluntary organizations that the federal government allowed to access newcomers directly at their point of entry, thus becoming one of what Franca Iacovetta calls in a later period the "gatekeepers" of Canadian society.[65] Interwar restrictions on Asian immigration meant that such work centred on the eastern Canadian ports of Halifax, Saint John, and Quebec City, where British and European immigrants landed by the boatload until the Great Depression led Canada to close its doors to further arrivals. The CRCS Seaport Nursery Service used its allotted space in the immigration sheds to bathe, feed, and entertain the babies and children while offering the mothers tea, general assistance, and a respite from childcare responsibilities during the interval between official examinations and the departure of westbound trains. Red Cross volunteers used this brief time with immigrant families to begin the assimilation process, providing a copy of the *Canadian Mother's Book* to mothers with young children, substituting Canadian baby bottles and garments for makeshift or traditional ones, and trying to "teach a little Hygiene and Health to these new Canadians."[66]

On the prairies, CRCS health work also focused heavily on immigrants. In 1925 and 1927, for example, the CRCS received grants (jointly provided by the British Red Cross, the Overseas Settlement Committee of the British government, and the Canadian Department of Immigration) to be used in relieving "distress arising from sickness or suffering" among immigrants who came to Canada under the British Empire Settlement Scheme. The Alberta Division was particularly concerned about the health and hygiene standards of the province's large numbers of Central and Eastern European settlers.[67] While other voluntary organizations and government departments were also engaged in immigrant work, leaders like Alberta Division's Mary Waagen believed the non-governmental status of the Red Cross and its familiar emblem "bearing the badge of humanity and service" gave it an advantage with Eastern Europeans whose homeland experiences had left them wary of state interference.[68]

One of the society's best-known interwar undertakings directly assisted immigrants, veterans, mothers, and children alike. Through the outpost hospital program the CRCS provided small cottage hospitals and nursing stations in remote, under-serviced, and newly settled parts of the country, where physicians and hospitals were scarce or distant. As Linda Kealey and others have argued, "voluntary efforts [like the Red Cross outposts] provided key assistance at a time when publicly supported health care was non-existent or minimal." Women's work as nurses and midwives was particularly crucial to health work in rural and remote areas. Kealey's study of New Brunswick outposts reveals the degree to which the state relied on the voluntary sector to provide vital services during the interwar years. More broadly, the society's interwar provision of outpost hospitals and public health nurses across Canada, as well as its grants to public health departments, allowed the state to shirk what later generations would consider its duty to provide a basic infrastructure of health services outside the largest urban areas.[69]

The Alberta Division pioneered outpost work in the early 1920s when prolonged drought conditions left some communities unable to maintain their small hospitals on their own; the program subsequently spread across the country. Red Cross outpost hospitals and nursing stations eventually existed in locations as diverse as the British Columbia interior, small-town Saskatchewan, Quebec's Magdalen Islands, northern Ontario, and rural Nova Scotia.[70] Outpost nurses dealt with all kinds of

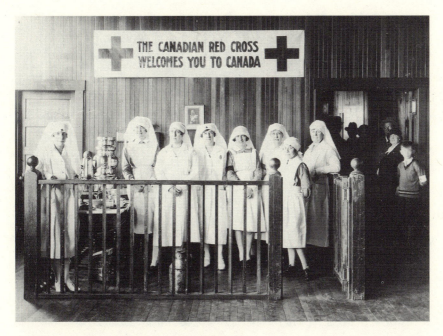

Figure 4.3
Volunteers at the society's port nurseries in Saint John, Halifax, and Quebec City
welcomed new immigrants with tea, coffee, and cookies (visible to right of left-most
volunteer) and the internationally recognized emblem of the Red Cross. Other
volunteers stand in the shadow of the doorway at right, including a young boy wearing
a Red Cross armband.

health needs, many of them normally the province of a physician, from
rheumatism to childbirth to serious injuries requiring first aid. In communities lacking many types of infrastructure and services, outpost
nurses might be called on to perform tasks well outside the bounds of
nursing, such as "writing letters, baptizing infants, and conducting fu-
neral services." They also served as public health educators, attempting
to improve community standards of hygiene and uproot medically un-
sound superstitions and folk practices.[71] Although many patients came
to the outpost, the nurses also paid house calls, braving bad weather and
long distances to reach their patients by foot, horse, dogsled, snowshoe,
or boat. The doctors and senior nurses technically assigned to "supervise" outpost nurses were based too far away to be of immediate help,
so successful outpost nurses needed pluck, ingenuity, and self-confidence

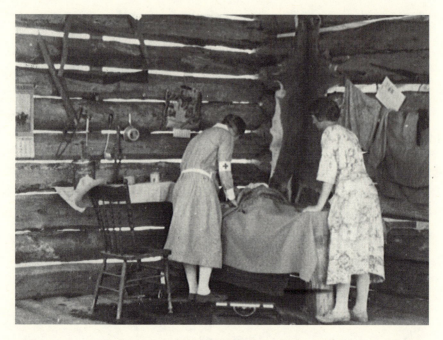

Figure 4.4
The primitive conditions on display in this log cabin, where an outpost nurse is visiting
a bedridden patient (possibly a child), indicate that medical care was not the only basic
necessity in short supply for those living in remote settlement areas of interwar Canada.

in order to succeed in their challenging and largely self-directed work.
Contemporary studies showed that women of childbearing age and their
infants were particularly vulnerable in underserviced rural and remote
areas, a fact the Red Cross, the VON, and others who established outposts kept in mind when establishing nursing stations and cottage hospitals. Unsurprisingly, new mothers and babies constituted a majority
of the outpost nurses' patients.[72]

Across Canada, the CRCS engaged in a wide range of other health-
related activities. A number of provincial divisions helped establish and
finance the first Canadian courses in public health nursing at the universities of British Columbia, Toronto, Western Ontario, McGill, and
Dalhousie. Many divisions offered courses in first aid or home nursing,
either independently or in conjunction with the St John Ambulance
Association. Red Cross nurses visited lighthouses in British Columbia;

Alberta Division established its own Crippled Children's Hospital; Saskatchewan, Manitoba, Quebec, New Brunswick, and Nova Scotia divisions each supported or directly provided travelling clinics which brought medical or dental care to remote areas of their respective provinces. Local and provincial branches also provided relief and emergency supplies to Canadian communities suffering from a variety of disasters, including forest fires, epidemics, mining accidents, a prairie cyclone, and at least one major flood. In connection with its ongoing disaster relief work, the society once again attempted to enrol registered nurses for voluntary service in war or disaster, with limited success.[73]

In pursuing these public health activities across the country, the CRCS saw itself as an auxiliary to government. The responsibility for enacting and administering public health measures rested solely with government, the society affirmed, but as a nationwide voluntary organization, the Red Cross could offer useful assistance to official health authorities. The Cannes conference, the creation of the LRCS, and the inclusion of Article 25 in the League of Nations Covenant (calling on signatory governments to support national peacetime Red Cross work) only reinforced the fact that such was the duty of the Red Cross, CRCS leaders argued. One shining example of positive government-Red Cross cooperation during this period was the Vetcraft program which offered sheltered employment in a workshop setting to disabled ex-soldiers in Victoria, Vancouver, Winnipeg, Montreal, Halifax, and Saint John. Disability, as Morton and Wright observe, "trapped its victims," who faced the possibility of permanent poverty. The government looked to retraining and curative workshops to return veterans to some measure of self-sufficiency. The Department of Soldiers Civil Re-establishment (DSCR) could easily have funded and operated the Vetcraft workshops on its own (as it did in Ontario, where Ontario Division refused to participate for unknown reasons), but instead it provided 85 percent of the funding and the CRCS the remaining 15 percent, while the management was turned over to the CRCS. The DSCR considered Red Cross management desirable in part because of the society's "excellent reputation" with the public, with veterans, and with manufacturers who might otherwise resent such subsidized competition. It also believed that veterans themselves would prefer non-governmental control of the workshops. The Vetcraft program is an example of the state pursuing a partnership with the voluntary sector in order to attain its desired ends through alternate means. In 1927 the new Department of Pensions and National Health took complete control of some of the workshops, but in the meantime the program offered a counterpoint to the interwar trend identified by James Struthers in which voluntary agencies pushed resistant governments to intervene more actively in social conditions. In the Vetcraft case, it was the government that pursued CRCS involvement.[74]

Isolated instances such as the Vetcraft workshops aside, the society's confident self-publicity and trumpeting of its federal peacetime charter masked the fact – retrospectively acknowledged in 1938 – that as the 1920s opened "there was not much enthusiasm shown in the official endorsation of its new activities." Government support had to be won over time.[75] Nor was a lack of government cooperation the only unforeseen problem faced by the CRCS. No amount of new Junior members could make up for a lack of adult voluntary effort and diminished financial giving. Having confidently expected that its vast network of local branches and auxiliaries might be turned to peacetime work with little difficulty, the society instead found that its wartime volunteers deserted in droves. Auxiliaries dissolved or turned their attention back to their original purposes, while most small, rural branches closed their books. In towns and cities devoted volunteers kept a nucleus of support alive, but with some difficulty. Many Canadians were not convinced of what the LRCS's Dr C.-E.A. Winslow called the Red Cross's "logical leadership" in public health, while others had no affinity for public health work. Even when supporters successfully organized new branches, it proved "difficult to get enough people to take an interest in it to carry on any aggressive work," as Trenton, Nova Scotia branch secretary Alice Phelan observed in 1929.[76]

In peacetime the composition of the society's body of supporters changed beyond a simple decline in the number of volunteers. Public health work and the Junior Red Cross brought a new brand of women (and some men) into the Red Cross fold. These Canadians were professionals – primarily nurses and teachers. Some were paid; others (such as the teachers who organized their students into Junior Red Cross branches) applied their professional skills in a voluntary capacity, in a similar fashion to the experts in transportation, textiles, and nursing who had donated their skills to the CRCS as advisers during the war. After 1919 the society's work slowly but surely came to rely on the support of trained professionals – and increasingly it paid them for their services.[77]

Falling Short: Challenges of the Great Depression

As if the changes brought about by the end of the war and a shift to peacetime work were not enough to shake up the society, the decade of the 1930s brought a new set of issues and complications to the table, primarily related to the financial crisis that set in at the end of 1929. For instance, during the mid-1930s the CRCS finally began to take a greater interest in the international Red Cross movement, perhaps in light of the increasingly troubled nature of international relations and the possibility of another war. Ironically, during the early 1920s, when it was flush with cash, the CRCS had not been particularly keen to participate in the wider Red Cross world; now that it began to take a greater interest, the economic crisis of the 1930s left the society with little money to send its own delegates to IRC conferences. By 1938 the selection of representatives became contingent on whether any CRCS members might already be in London during the time of the upcoming conference.[78] Having won a place for itself on the international stage during the Great War, the society spent most of the interwar years hidden in the wings, first from lack of interest and later from lack of funds.

The IRC conference attendance problem symbolized a more general financial difficulty. By the late 1920s it became obvious that the money the society had so freely given to other public health agencies earlier in the decade could not easily be replaced. National fundraising campaigns such as that of 1927 failed to meet their targets, and waning funds at the end of the 1920s gave way to outright financial crisis in some provincial divisions when the Great Depression hit Canada.[79] In 1931, with the support and assistance of long-time Red Cross supporter Prime Minister R.B. Bennett, the CRCS launched a National Emergency Appeal. Much to the surprise and dismay of CRCS leaders, who confidently expected a repeat of the society's oversubscribed wartime appeals, the campaign failed to meet its objectives. The society's ability to ease the suffering caused by the economic crisis and prairie drought was hampered, and provincial divisions had to cut back on their regular public health-related programs as well. At the same time, the disparate impact of the Depression on the various provinces produced tensions and alienation between provincial divisions and National Headquarters.[80]

The Great Depression impeded the society's ability to raise money, but simultaneously introduced unanticipated avenues of activity into the CRCS peacetime program. By 1928 the difficulty of definitively attributing diseases such as tuberculosis, cancer, epilepsy, or diabetes to war service meant that many veterans could not claim aid from the federal government. This in turn led increasing numbers of veterans to seek assistance from the Red Cross when they were unable to work. The problem was only compounded after 1929, as economic depression threw healthy veterans out of work and poverty exacerbated the health problems of others. The Montreal and Toronto branches were among those that consequently operated large hostels for single, homeless, unemployed veterans. By 1933 there were nearly as many ex-soldiers in hospital as in 1920, and Red Cross volunteers across Canada were visiting their bedsides at a rate of over 1,000 visits per day. During the winter of 1930–31, the Department of Pensions and National Health used the CRCS, with its national network of branches, as a distribution agent for bedding and clothing for needy Canadians.[81] The CRCS supplemented the government's efforts by taking a leading role in providing local clothing relief, with large quantities of clothing donated used, purchased new, or knitted in Red Cross workrooms and Junior Red Cross branches across the country. As they were able, provincial and local CRCS branches also provided layettes containing essential baby care items, food vouchers or baskets, small emergency funds, and/or rudimentary care in their respective areas.[82]

Nancy Sheehan argues that the existence and assistance of voluntary agencies like the CRCS allowed governments to delay and limit their acceptance of the responsibility for relief,[83] and while this may have been the case overall, for some CRCS leaders the problem was exactly the opposite. Mary Waagen and D.M. Duggan of the Alberta Division, and Norman Sommerville of the national Executive Committee, each contacted Prime Minister (and long-time fellow Red Cross leader) R.B. Bennett over the course of December 1930 and January 1931, seeking government grants to enable the society to undertake widespread relief work, especially in the West. Duggan confessed that most of the provincial divisions were in debt and the national office could offer no practical assistance. Still, he believed the society had "the skeleton of an organization which could be of real service during these days of distress, but nothing worth while can be accomplished without financial aid from the Federal and Provincial Governments." Sommerville stated that the money was needed to "allay growing unrest," while Waagen's emotionally charged letter invoked Christian duty and wondered why the Red Cross – "the very voice of God in us" – should be "lost to the nation?" Bennett's responses to all three arguments consistently stressed his conviction that "Governments are responsible ... [and] ... must choose their agencies." Inherent in this argument was the fact that the federal government did not choose the CRCS. The prime minister also contended that "People cannot pay taxes to enable the Government to carry on the direct [relief] work, and at the same time be expected to make contributions to ... [voluntary and charitable] agencies."[84] Bennett's federal government, although reluctant to assume the burden of relief itself, would not offload the responsibility onto the Red Cross and other charitable organizations. Lurking behind this dialogue between the prime minister and his erstwhile Red Cross colleagues was the knowledge that American president Herbert Hoover *had* chosen the ARC as the government's channel for providing Depression relief.[85] The ultimate insufficiency of Hoover's voluntarist response and its replacement by President Franklin Roosevelt's state-interventionist New Deal likely kept CRCS leaders from pressing their case with Bennett's 1935 successor as prime minister, Mackenzie King.

Throughout the Depression years the CRCS provided what relief it could in individual localities, and helped many sufferers who did not meet official government criteria for relief. However, the society's lack of money led to the demise of many small branches and limited its effectiveness. CRCS leaders felt they were failing Canadians in need, especially in hard-hit Alberta and Saskatchewan, where average incomes per capita declined 61 and 72 percent respectively between 1928–29 and 1933.[86] However, the Great Depression did not kill the CRCS: in addition to maintaining core programs like the Junior Red Cross and outpost nursing, many local branches took on new responsibilities in providing relief to destitute Canadians. Remarkably, the Ontario Division sailed along in relative prosperity, and was considered by some insiders to be the reason that the entire CRCS stayed afloat at all during the Depression. But the Great Depression undeniably constituted a major blow to the CRCS's ability to effectively function and fulfill its peacetime public health mission. After the Second World War returned the CRCS to its former glory, some supporters who recalled the society of the 1930s were under the impression that it had practically ceased to exist outside Ontario and Quebec.[87]

Through its wide-ranging interwar program of health care education and provision, assistance to veterans, and relief measures during the Great Depression, the CRCS reinforced Canadians' belief that voluntary organizations could provide vital services. In the process, however, it also proved that no voluntary organization, no matter how prestigious or widely supported, could provide comprehensive services in the fields of public health or social welfare. Canadians' early 1920s idealism crumbled in the face of class, ethnic, and regional divisions which reared their heads in ensuing years, and far-reaching social change – including a universal improvement in Canadians' health – remained elusive throughout the 1920s and 1930s. Maternal and infant mortality rates in Canada declined over the course of the interwar years, but as of 1935 the country remained in the bottom third of Western countries for maternal mortality, and came last out of seventeen Western countries for infant mortality.[88] These facts contributed to a growing sense that greater government intervention was required in the areas of delivery, pre-natal, and post-natal care. The CRCS and its fellow charitable organizations accomplished a great deal of good during the interwar years, but they could not do enough to fully meet the needs of a growing country. As the federated charities and Community Chest appeals were discovering during this same period, the more rationalized and businesslike a charity attempted to be, the clearer became the case for making such care and services a public – ie., government – responsibility.[89]

The 1940 report of the Royal Commission on Dominion-Provincial Relations (Rowell-Sirois Report) predicted that "the health activities of governments are only beginning," and considered factors such as the mobility of modern society, urbanization, the growth of wage-earning, and the hazards and occupational diseases of industrialized workplaces,

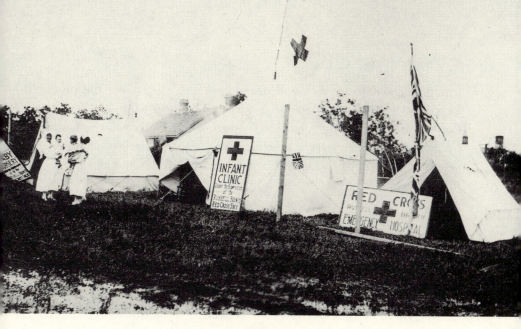

Figure 4.5
Two women in nursing garb (one a volunteer, the other a trained graduate nurse) hold children outside the infant clinic set up in a muddy field by Russell, Ontario's Red Cross branch. Such voluntary efforts offered valuable aid to underserviced areas, but could not fill all the gaps in Canadians' access to health care.

as compelling reasons for all three levels of government to become more involved in the health of Canadian society. The commissioners found a "chaotic situation as regards jurisdiction," but little overlap, stating that they "were impressed by the inadequacy of health services, considering the need, rather than by the existence of duplication."[90] The report on public health that A.E. Grauer submitted to the royal commission paid tribute to the good work of voluntary public health agencies, including the CRCS, but urged greater coordination between the agencies and various levels of government in order to address large gaps. The combined nursing services of the VON and the CRCS, for example, were available to no more than one-third of the population, and many provinces treated health education "as a sparetime activity."[91] In a sense, then, the CRCS's earnest efforts during the interwar years in the public health and social welfare fields inadvertently contributed to the loss of much of that work to government agencies and the new social safety net constructed after the Second World War.

+

The major shifts in policy and international relations that the CRCS experienced between 1919 and 1939 altered the organization's place in Canada and in the wider world. Throughout the interwar years, the Canadian Red Cross worked doggedly to achieve the ambitious and idealistic program put forth in its National Peace Policy. The CRCS peacetime public health program amounted to a grand war memorial project of nation building through health which, although it failed to achieve much that its creators envisioned in 1919, contributed in important ways to the health and welfare of the Canadian population over the two tumultuous decades before 1939. The society ended the second decade of its peacetime existence as an organization that had successfully converted itself from a wartime charity into a peacetime public health agency, financially survived a long decade of economic distress, and moved (at least officially) from being a branch of the British Red Cross Society to being internationally recognized as an independent Canadian society. In spite of these achievements, however, the CRCS was in a relatively sorry state by 1939. It would take a second global war to return the organization to the wealth, power, influence, and widespread support and recognition with which it had entered the interwar years.

Clearly the peacetime program did not allow the CRCS to hold on to its volunteers, its bank balance, or its national prominence at 1918 levels, and yet it did allow the society to maintain a national presence and a skeleton structure during two decades of peace, and bolstered its reputation for doing good works. This in turn would enable the society to swiftly and effectively mobilize in response to the outbreak of a new war in 1939, and – perhaps more importantly in the long run – to return to peacetime work in 1945 and assume responsibility for new initiatives like nation-wide blood collection, without anyone batting an eyelash. Through concrete work in health care and education, and the skilful manipulation of its own image, the Canadian Red Cross Society successfully negotiated an interwar reinvention that was less a "drift" from its original mission than it was a ninety-degree turn.

5

GOLDEN AGE OR TROUBLED TIMES?
1939–1945

"War again! 1939." With these few but evocative words, Lady Julia Drummond autographed a history of her Great War Canadian Red Cross Information Bureau for Norman Sommerville, chairman of the CRCS Central Council. Her simple statement expresses the disappointed resignation many Canadians felt in September 1939, as the Nazi invasion of Poland pulled the British Commonwealth and France into war. Drummond's decision to send Sommerville this small book, and the friendly correspondence about staffing and logistics that ensued, highlights the fact that the CRCS conducted its part in the Second World War (1939–45) with one eye ever on the previous conflict.[1]

The presence of many volunteers and staff who had worked for the CRCS in the Great War (now renamed the First World War) made it easier to reproduce the successes and avoid the missteps of the past. It also enabled the CRCS to mobilize more quickly, effectively, and confidently the second time. By the end of the Second World War more than 2.1 million adults and nearly 900,000 youth – over 28 percent of the Canadian population in both cases – were members of the Canadian Red Cross. They provided an estimated 95 percent of the labour involved in the CRCS war effort, and with other Canadians donated $80 million in cash (approximately $1.13 billion today) by war's end.[2]

The CRCS's Second World War history is in many ways a recapitulation of its First World War history: many of the same kinds of people accomplished many of the same tasks, but on a larger scale. CRCS histories and memoirs of the period reflect these changes, portraying a massive, smoothly functioning organization which, supported by the generosity and goodwill of ordinary Canadians, achieved enormous feats of humanitarian assistance during six dark years of war.[3] In this nostalgic view, the Second World War was the society's finest hour. As historian Jeffrey Keshen has argued of the similarly whitewashed Canadian popular memory of the Second World War as a whole, there is truth in this version, but the full story is more complicated and less flattering. The CRCS *did* shoulder self-appointed tasks of gargantuan proportions and *did* successfully carry them out to widespread praise and approbation. Like Prime Minister Mackenzie King and the Canadian government, the CRCS deliberately strove to avoid the mistakes of the First World War.[4] But behind the scenes, it also engaged in a series of unproductive interagency squabbles, chafed under government restrictions, battled old rumours, and faced new challenges to its ability to help overseas. Although it avoided many of the problems of the previous war, the CRCS found plenty of new ones between 1939 and 1945. As bureaucrats in the federal Ministry of Finance observed in 1942, the CRCS in this period seemed to have "a peculiar aptitude for stirring up trouble."[5]

Same Red Cross, Different Context

The Canadian Red Cross Society entered the Second World War with two great advantages over its First World War self: a national network of branches and volunteers presided over by experienced leaders and a stellar reputation for its work in the previous conflict. In theory, all the CRCS had to do in order to succeed was revert to its wartime footing. In many respects, this approach worked. But the society soon discovered that the national and international contexts in which it now had to work had changed. The society's initial mobilization period and subsequent relationships with the federal government and international relief funds made plain both the benefits and challenges of being the same Red Cross in a different context.

Coverage of Red Cross affairs in the Toronto-based *Globe and Mail* newspaper during the first two weeks of September 1939 – a period covering the separate British and Canadian declarations of war against Germany – conveniently demonstrates many of the ways in which the CRCS's second experience of global war mimicked its first. News items stressed the society's history and relationship to the federal government in order to establish its trustworthiness in the public mind, while the women's pages of the paper recruited women for Red Cross work and noted offers of service from many women's organizations and church groups. Prominent local citizens took on leadership roles in a host of new wartime branches, and reports of rapid local and provincial expansion indicate a mobilization just as enthusiastic as that of 1914–15, although considerably better organized. Ontario Division headquarters had to quickly open a second Toronto location to accommodate its expanded activities, a move reminiscent of National Headquarters' August 1914 physical expansion. Editorials, columns, and articles described gifts of labour and money to the Red Cross as patriotic acts, and offered Nazi bombing of Red Cross trains in Europe as familiar proof of the enemy's depravity. One columnist reminded readers of the Red Cross's First World War and interwar "crusade" imagery, finding it especially suited to the new wartime context.[6] Such echoes of the previous conflict were repeated across the country. Within the first two weeks of war the CRCS had once again been positioned by both the grassroots and its own officials as a patriotic, hands-on way for ordinary citizens (especially women) to contribute to the war effort, a position heavily laden with symbolic weight in the landscape of wartime Canada. The First World War had established these links; the Second World War only strengthened them further.

Having survived the Great Depression by the skin of its teeth, financially speaking, the society needed a major injection of new income if it was to provide wartime humanitarian aid on the scale it desired. National Red Cross leaders immediately envisioned major, coordinated national appeals and in early September 1939 established a framework to support them. New national subcommittees for finance, transportation, purchasing and supplies, women's work, campaigns, and publicity were modelled after their First World War predecessors; they were joined by new press, radio, motion picture, and editorial committees, reflecting leaders' recognition of the need to use modern advertising techniques. Publicity and fundraising could no longer be left primarily to locals or amateurs. Adelaide Plumptre left her First World War role of coordinating women's work to the younger Mrs Wallace R. Campbell and assumed the new position of vice-chairman in charge of war activities, but also edited *Despatch* (a modernized version of her First World War *Bulletin*). The main purpose of *Despatch* was to prime the pump for financial appeals by spreading accurate information about CRCS work year-round. A new wartime cooperation agreement with St John Ambulance and the creation of a CRCS War Council that drew together representatives of other leading voluntary organizations completed National Headquarters' mobilization.[7] In contrast to the decentralized, provincially focused society of the interwar years, the CRCS of the Second World War was once again centrally driven and nationally directed.

On 13 November 1939, with slogans including "The Need Is Urgent – Dig in and Give," the society launched its first national fundraising campaign of the war: an appeal for $3,000,000. Images of lovely Red Cross nurses and the Red Cross "flag of mercy" joined text highlighting the need to provide home comforts and the best of health care to Canada's "own courageous sons" who would soon "face danger in defence of our liberty." Canadians responded generously, providing the CRCS with an initial war chest of $5,118,086.31.[8]

The success of the "Dig in and Give" campaign suggested smooth sailing of the kind experienced in First World War CRCS campaigns, but the Canadian charitable landscape had changed dramatically. Seeking to avoid the necessity of any initial bank loans, the CRCS had intended to conduct its campaign shortly after the September declaration of war. These plans had to be altered when representatives of more than forty charities (primarily the municipally based Community Chests which had revolutionized charitable campaigning in the interwar period) insisted that the CRCS wait until the respective conclusions of their October campaigns, and the Poppy Fund's early November campaign, before launching its own appeal. Since the Community Chests had only reluctantly agreed to hold their campaigns in October, leaving November clear for the Red Cross, CRCS leaders felt they must comply.[9] This initial hitch in CRCS plans inaugurated six years of fundraising-related friction between the society, other charities, and the federal government.

Many experienced officers and volunteers helped the CRCS mobilize rapidly. At the national level this included the indefatigable Mrs Plumptre and energetic National Commissioner Dr Frederick Routley. Experience was not always an asset, however. Like Dr Ryerson before him, long-serving Central Council and Executive Committee chairman Norman

Sommerville was ousted in a polite *coup-d'état* at the end of 1940. Certain central councillors felt that the universally respected and naturally diplomatic Justice P.H. Gordon (a long-time Saskatchewan Red Cross supporter and Supreme Court judge since 1935) would be a more effective chair of the wartime Executive Committee than the ailing and sometimes belligerent Sommerville.[10]

Gordon's potential as a positive ambassador for the society bore early fruit: those outside the Red Cross welcomed his election, with one contemporary affiliated with the Canadian Welfare Council deeming him a "level-headed" and "exceptionally fine chap," who would "at all times listen to reason."[11] Of the many organizations with which the CRCS had to work, none was more significant than the new Department of National War Services (NWS), and in this realm the new chairman held a trump card: Gordon had a longstanding personal friendship with former Saskatchewan attorney general and long-time Red Cross supporter T.C. Davis, now serving as deputy minister of NWS. For two years, "Percy" and "Tommy" (as they addressed one another) worked out many kinks in the uneasy triangular relationship between the government, other organizations, and the Red Cross, which might otherwise have proved intractable.

The series of upsets and arguments that Gordon and Davis's friendship helped to smooth over reveals the underlying tension in this period between the traditional moral authority of the Canadian Red Cross and the growing power of the federal government.[12] The First World War had developed a strong, meaningful relationship between the CRCS and ordinary Canadians, and in the absence of a Canadian Patriotic Fund in the new conflict, the Red Cross was *the* pre-eminent Canadian war charity during the Second World War – no small feat in the face of its 3,475 registered competitors for Canadians' time and money. The CPF had fallen victim to its own volunteers' diligent prying into their First World War recipients' financial and domestic arrangements: Mackenzie King's government believed in 1939 that a new CPF "was more likely to deter voluntary enlistment than to encourage it," and shifted the responsibility for meeting emergencies in soldiers' families to the CRCS.[13] As Jeffrey Keshen and Serge Durflinger each demonstrate, Red Cross work was an integral part of the war on the home front, at both the national and community levels. This popular support, plus its traditional dominance in the area of wartime aid to the sick and wounded, led the CRCS to presume that it was therefore entitled to a more or less free hand in fundraising and aid activities. The federal Liberal government of Prime Minister William Lyon Mackenzie King, however, disagreed. Charity, no less than war production, manpower, media, or wages and prices, must submit to the guiding hand of the wartime state.[14]

As Mariana Valverde notes, regulation is one of the government's most effective means of controlling activities it has delegated to the voluntary sector, and this trend was everywhere evident in the mixed social economy of wartime.[15] The government signalled its intent to regulate wartime voluntary work by enacting a new War Charities Act on 13 September 1939, only three days after Canada officially declared war. During the First World War, the federal government had not regulated the unruly realm of Canadian war charities until 1917. In contrast, the 1939 War Charities Act immediately asserted government control over these supposedly non-governmental endeavours by stating that anyone who wished to raise money for a war charitable purpose had to have a licence; no one could appeal for funds without the permission of the secretary of state; and the secretary of state could shut down any fund if he was not satisfied with its procedures. The 1939 act should not have come as a surprise, given its 1917 predecessor, but it nonetheless raised hackles within the CRCS. Whereas the CRCS and the CPF had been exempt from certain key provisions of the 1917 act, no such exemption was offered in 1939. CRCS leaders' protests fell on deaf ears in Ottawa.[16]

In following years the government extended its regulatory regime. The Department of National War Services was created in June 1940 to deal with the country's thousands of war charities and peacetime organizations doing war work, as the government's "limited liability" approach began to shift to "total war" after the fall of France.[17] In late 1941 NWS created a War Charities Funds (WCF) Advisory Board, which oversaw fundraising activities among the largest war charities. The WCF Advisory Board emerged as part of a broader move by NWS to streamline and reduce the fundraising activities of the major national war charities (the Knights of Columbus, YMCA and YWCA, Canadian Legion, Salvation Army, and Canadian Red Cross) between late 1941 and early 1942. Not only would streamlining reduce competition with the government's own Victory Bond campaigns, but it also echoed the shift of peacetime charitable fundraising toward a united appeal or Community Chest model, which used modern business practices to limit administrative inefficiency and reduce the number of appeals to the public.[18] NWS began by suspending all fundraising by national war charities and requiring them to exhaust the remainder of the funds they had raised in 1940–41. The government financed any further budgeted operating costs.[19] Having decided to fund the so-called "auxiliary war services" itself, the government next sought stricter supervision of the money allotted and how it was spent. This was where the WCF Advisory Board's budgetary approval process came in.

The CRCS welcomed the creation of NWS, since it provided a single government department with which to deal, but heartily despised the WCF Advisory Board. One of the board's duties was to review and approve the budgets of the major war charities, a role and process national CRCS leaders found particularly galling. Not only did they resent the government supervision, but they also believed it undermined the society's neutral and independent status – key principles of the international Red Cross movement.[20] However, no amount of protest by national and local Red Cross leaders could convince the government to exempt the CRCS from budget scrutiny.

When the government then proposed a united appeal for all the major war charities in 1942, Red Cross supporters across Canada reacted with outrage. Many believed the society already did what the united appeal would achieve: namely, maximize fundraising efficiency by coordinating one large national appeal instead of many small ones. Moreover, it was already also raising funds for St John Ambulance needs. But more broadly, CRCS supporters flatly refused to be lumped in with everyone else, believing the society's humanitarian goals and international dimension made it unique.[21] Some supporters also believed that by emphasizing its traditional imagery of service and sacrifice in a solo campaign the Red Cross could earn more money than it would as part of a united appeal. Nearly all were afraid of losing the distinct Red Cross identity and thereby also the source of the society's ability to mobilize Canadians' resources and voluntary labour. In an impassioned letter to the minister of NWS, J.T. Thorson, George B. Webster of Toronto wrote, "[The CRCS] has been in a class by itself and commands Universal respect amongst all classes of the Public. It has an appeal which is unique and which is not given to the rags and tags of other Societies, with which the Government is forcing them to merge. All over the Country Women are working very hard for the Red Cross and if this merger goes into effect the spirit which inspiers these women to work to the Red Cross would I am sure be lost [sic]."[22] Red Cross supporters were deadly serious on this issue. Saskatchewan Division reported receiving "a flood of letters from [its] branches stating that they [were] going to disband" rather than be forced into union with other war charities. Luckily for them, in April 1942 Thorson announced that the "international character" and "Geneva Convention obligations" of the CRCS dictated that it be kept separate from the other national auxiliary war services. The Canadian Red Cross would not be financed by government and would be the only major war charity to have its own national appeal for funds in 1942.[23]

Throughout the remainder of the war, the Red Cross continued to fret about losing its identity, its independence, and its authority. It chafed under the restrictions and supervision imposed on it and continually challenged the government's authority by exerting its own. It was by no means a futile effort. Purvis Wood, a civil servant with NWS, recognized the limits of the state's power when he noted that the society had not accepted the government's ruling against a national Red Cross fundraising campaign in 1946. "They haven't agreed to abide by the ruling," he wrote confidentially, "and frankly nobody can stop them if they decide they won't – and they know that." This confidence was bolstered by the individuals who composed the CRCS Executive Committee and larger Central Council: many were well respected in their own fields, such as Canadian nursing leader Jean I. Gunn, and former University of Toronto president Sir Robert Falconer; others were wealthy, connected, and powerful, such as Montreal philanthropist Lady Julia Drummond, and Bank of Montreal manager Jackson Dodds. The current governor general still automatically served as president, while the prime minister and the leader of the opposition lent their names in wartime as honorary vice-presidents. Altogether, twenty-four men and five women sat on the Executive Committee, augmented on Central Council by eighteen provincial representatives (six of them women) and a further nine members at large, including Alice (Mrs C.D.) Howe, wife of the powerful federal minister of munitions and supply.[24]

P.H. Gordon and T.C. Davis exerted a moderating influence within this context of friction and protest. Although the two men did not always see eye to eye, their personal friendship and Davis's support for the Red Cross helped them to smooth over many tensions through to the end of 1942. For instance, in February 1942 Davis urged Gordon to accept the existence of the WCF Advisory Board on the grounds that having the board scrutinize CRCS budgets would offer added legitimacy in fundraising campaigns *and* provide a convenient scapegoat in relations between local branches and National Headquarters. "Any time you want to tell them that something must be done," Davis suggested chummily, "you can blame it on the Board." Gordon wrote of their working relationship, "I do not know what I would do without Tommy Davis," but he eventually had to find out. Davis's departure at the end of 1942 for the position of Canadian high commissioner to Australia may well have contributed to the fact that it took an official order-in-council rather than behind-the-scenes intervention to settle ongoing friction between the CRCS and SJAA over the society's civil defence-inspired move into teaching first aid – traditional SJAA territory. It may also help explain the society's appointment of Major-General B.W. Browne to the new post of assistant national commissioner in Ottawa, charged with liaising between the CRCS and the government. By December 1942 Dr Routley and Justice Gordon were chief among those who recognized that the national wartime CRCS headquarters should be in Ottawa, but by then housing and office space shortages made a move unfeasible. An assistant national commissioner on the spot would have to suffice.[25]

By regulating but maintaining a place for voluntary charitable agencies in the war effort, the government paid lip service to the ideal of citizens' democratic right to support the causes of their choice.[26] It also reaped the benefits of increased morale that came from Canadians working to support their citizen-soldiers, and ensured that the agencies' work fulfilled the state's broader wartime aims. For instance, in the summer 1941 salvage campaign, household aluminum collected by volunteers (often children) was sold to factories for recycling into military aircraft and other war materiel, with the proceeds supporting CRCS work for prisoners of war. In other words, the very same aluminum donation could help save Canadian troops *and* kill the enemy. This troubling example of what John F. Hutchinson calls "militarized charity" seems to have raised no eyebrows among Canadians once again in the warm embrace of Red Cross patriotism.[27]

The society's fundraising for international civilian relief offered further proof of the altered context of the Second World War. The Battle of Britain's indiscriminate bombings of British civilians prompted renewed pangs of imperial sentiment in many Canadians, who then created a host of new funds such as the Queen's Canadian Fund (Halifax) and the British War Victims' Fund (Toronto) that competed for donations with established agencies like the CRCS. P.H. Gordon confided to T.C. Davis that all the competing British bomb victim funds meant a "serious fall-off in revenue for the Society." For example, Nova Scotians made only a single $7.00 contribution to the Red Cross British Bomb Victims' Fund as of late August 1941. By diverting stockpiled comforts and medical supplies not yet needed by military sick and wounded, the society was able to provide assistance to British civilians. Yet the larger problem remained: without money to purchase materials, the female volunteers the CRCS relied on would have nothing to work with – a development Gordon believed would leave the society "shattered," and one that women themselves actively protested.[28]

The rival bomb victim funds represented precisely the sort of overlapping that NWS wished to avoid. So, when Germany attacked its erstwhile ally the Soviet Union in 1941, NWS acted swiftly to prevent a similar mushrooming of funds in aid of the USSR. Ottawa also had explicitly political concerns: among those seeking NWS permission to raise money for Russia were many groups with leftist, socialist, or explicitly communist affiliations – groups either actively suppressed or declared illegal early in the war, in a context of growing public suspicion of "foreign" elements in Canada. The government feared such organizations might use relief money for their own "subversive organizational work," and opted instead to authorize one national campaign, led by a government-approved (read: non-communist) agency. When NWS proposed the CRCS as that agency, the politics of humanitarian aid came to the fore: the Knights of Columbus protested providing any aid because the Soviets were not Christian, while the Salvation Army protested because they were communists. Major Beaton of the YMCA pragmatically argued that aid would boost Russian morale and ultimately "save the lives of British subjects in coming years," an opinion the government seems to have shared. A CRCS-led national appeal for Russian relief was eventually approved, and federal officials encouraged the society to specifically target "the foreign elements" in the Western provinces, where some Anglo-Canadians felt that Eastern European immigrants "were not supporting the War effort, either in men or in a material way." The bureaucrats hoped involvement in the relief campaign might "impose upon [these groups] a sense of responsibility as Canadian citizens."[29] With support from the federal government and Canadian newspapers, the CRCS raised $800,000 by mid-June 1942, which it spent on medical supplies for the USSR. Russian relief was then turned over to a new relief agency supported by Toronto newspaper publishers, the Canadian Aid to Russia Fund. Thanks to countless column inches in the *Toronto Star* and the *Globe and Mail*, the new fund collected double its $1,000,000 objective by February 1943 and began to impinge on the campaigns of other war charities. NWS officials urged the fund's powerful backers to close their campaign but could not convince them to stop printing appeals in their own newspapers.[30] Eliminating charitable competition often proved easier in theory than in fact.

The difficulties surrounding British and Russian relief prompted the federal government in 1943 to create a single umbrella organization to raise money for relief purposes in all Allied nations. The CRCS staked out its territory from the start: the society would not take part unless it was in control of purchasing and allotting relief supplies. Around the same time, Minister of NWS L.R. LaFlèche was told confidentially that there was "strong objection to the Canadian Red Cross Society" among some of the other agencies.[31] Faced with this impasse, NWS allowed the CRCS to continue providing medical, surgical, and hospital supplies to Allied Red Cross societies, while other Allied relief was united under the new Canadian United Allied Relief Fund (CUARF). This arrangement baffled some members of the public, who recognized "assistance to Allies" in the 1944 CRCS campaign material and interpreted it to mean duplication of the CUARF's purpose. The 1944 confusion led NWS to revisit the issue for 1945. As the spectre of a united appeal reared its head again, the CRCS protested that its national charter and international obligations precluded participation in joint fundraising. Inquiries by NWS, however, revealed that "'relief' [was] very definitely not an exclusive field of the Canadian Red Cross,"[32] and NWS initiated serious negotiations in November 1944. CUARF secretary-treasurer Dr Lawrence J. Burpee, reflecting on the frustrating process which ensued, wrote that the CRCS seemed to believe "that they were dealing with a self-constituted body set up in rivalry with the Red Cross and ambitious to do something that the Red Cross believed was their particular prerogative and felt that they were in every way better fitted to do than the CUARF."[33] His assessment was apt. From 1944 to 1946 the society provided ever-increasing amounts of civilian and refugee aid in liberated Europe, so it made sense (as NWS recognized) for the CRCS and the CUARF to join forces. Yet the CRCS was determined throughout to retain the upper hand.

The CUARF member agencies reluctantly accepted the society's terms in December 1944. In March 1945 the CRCS therefore conducted a national appeal "in conjunction with" the CUARF, in which it sought $10,000,000 to fund CRCS, St John Ambulance, and CUARF activities. The terms of agreement gave the CUARF very little active role in fundraising, purchasing, shipping, or distributing relief supplies, but as one CUARF member put it, "half a loaf was better than none." Its member agencies' ultimate purpose – relief of the various Allied countries they represented – was accomplished, and after the Allied victory the CUARF and the CRCS joined the new United Nations Relief and Rehabilitation Administration (UNRRA) in providing desperately needed humanitarian aid to millions of Europeans.[34] However, the CRCS flatly refused to participate in a 1946 CUARF-CRCS appeal. NWS punished the society by refusing permission for a separate national CRCS campaign, but the society successfully fell back on small-scale local fundraising. The CUARF, on the other hand, floundered without funds and swiftly disintegrated.[35] As this example suggests, the constant external pressure on the CRCS to participate in wartime federated fundraising too often showed a less than laudable side of the society. The ease with which the CRCS mobilized Canadians in 1939 encouraged it to imagine it could act as independently as ever, but civilian relief fund competition and increased regulation made that impossible. Fighting the previous war simply would not do.

Supporters, Detractors, and the Objects of Aid

The humanitarian mission and patriotic appeal of the CRCS drew support from as diverse an array of Canadians during the Second World War as they had in the previous war; new segments of the population were successfully mobilized as well. Yet not everyone was a fan of the Red Cross. The society's wartime ubiquity and drift from its core mandate drew criticism from certain quarters, and one critic even dared to question the usefulness of women's traditional war work.

On the positive side, the Second World War brought large numbers of French-speaking Quebecers to the CRCS fold. The Quebec Division of the society had remained largely anglophone during the interwar years, but winning francophone support finally became a conscious objective after September 1939. To further this goal the Quebec publicity and women's work committees appointed joint chairs and sub-convenors of both languages by 1940, and the division's annual reports were printed bilingually for the first time in 1941. The deliberate appeal to both linguistic communities paid off: Geneviève Auger and Raymonde Lamothe estimate that 80 percent of the 35,000 women working for the CRCS in Quebec in 1942 were francophones, and Serge Durflinger notes that in bicultural Verdun, Quebec, francophones participated in Red Cross work "roughly in proportion to the linguistic balance in the community." Quebec Division rapidly expanded, taking up new quarters in Red Cross House on Montreal's St Antoine Street and more than doubling its 1938 budget to a little over $1,100,000 by 1941.[36]

Quebec's religious divides were similarly overcome. The division appointed both the Anglican bishop of Quebec and the Catholic archbishop of Quebec as honorary presidents in 1939. At a crucial moment in the autumn of 1941, the Catholic archbishop, Cardinal Villeneuve, released a public letter in French declaring his support for the CRCS and its work. Dismissing rumours of inefficiency and paid staff, he described the humanitarian work of the Red Cross as Christian in spirit, if not in name, and therefore worthy of Catholics' support. Quebec CRCS leader and Bank of Montreal executive Jackson Dodds believed that Villeneuve's intervention played a vital role in the society's mobilization of French Catholic Quebecers, especially in rural areas. Québécoise volunteer

Madeleine Auger remembered local support for Red Cross work, too: Catholic clergy in her community permitted women to knit on Sundays, without fear of censure, for the duration of the war.[37]

Cardinal Villeneuve was not alone in viewing religion and the Red Cross as highly compatible. Frank Inrig, president of the Baptist Convention of Ontario and Quebec, called the society's work "a God-like service," and other religious leaders agreed. The society asked churches across the country to observe "Red Cross Sunday" with a word of support from the pulpit on 12 November 1939, and again in ensuing years. The accompanying pamphlet for 1940 suggested that the Second World War was "at base a religious war, a war of high ideals against low ideals."[38]

When he accepted the invitation to become an honorary president of the Quebec Division, Cardinal Villeneuve wrote, "Whatever one's sentiment may be towards participation in the war, there is nobody in Canada who does not wish to give Canadian soldiers the fullest possible service both morally and materially." In his opinion, this made the Red Cross "an organization whose purpose is above all discussion."[39] His subtle reference to anti-war sentiment applied not only to francophone Quebecers resistant to overseas service but also to Canada's pacifist Mennonites. The CRCS provided Canadian Mennonites with a means of demonstrating their citizenship in a socially approved manner by providing relief to the suffering, while still upholding their pacifist convictions. Leaders of the Canadian Mennonite Brethren insisted that all Mennonite conscientious objectors who were performing alternative service (instead of enlisting in the military) must assign all wages they received above fifty cents a day to the CRCS. By the end of the war some 7,500 Mennonite conscientious objectors had contributed more than $2,200,000 to the society's relief work for non-combatants. Marlene Epp shows that Mennonite women were equally active in relief-oriented forms of Red Cross work, such as sewing and quilting circles.[40]

While the society's compatibility with Christian virtue was important to many Canadians, its official religious neutrality made it attractive to others. In mid-September 1939 Montreal's various Jewish women's organizations came together to form the "Montreal Jewish Branch" of the CRCS. In her October 1939 appeal for Jewish women to volunteer, President Saidye Bronfman emphasized that the Red Cross's humanitarian work was undertaken "regardless of race or creed," and presented it as an opportunity for Jewish women to "join with all other Canadians to work and serve our Country and Empire." The new branch made relief for European refugees one of its areas of focus. As Robert Rutherdale notes with respect to the First World War, such separate branches reveal that barriers to these groups' full and unquestioned participation still existed.[41] Yet the fact that minority groups participated at all shows that the wartime Red Cross held a broad appeal. This is most concisely demonstrated in the list of groups who contributed funds to the Saskatchewan Division in 1943: among those represented were Irish, French, Finnish, Russian, Czechoslovak, Icelandic, Ukrainian, Greek, Hungarian, Aboriginal, Doukhobour, Mennonite, Jewish, Baptist, Anglican, Lutheran, Nazarene, and United Church organizations, donating amounts that ranged from $1.25 to $1,190.[42]

The CRCS attracted this high level of support because the meanings attached to it remained powerful motivators: Red Cross work was maternal, caring, and patriotic, a "shining beacon in a world of war, disease, darkness and death."[43] Campaign material echoed First World War fight-or-pay rhetoric by emphasizing Canadians' moral obligation to the troops and duty to live up to their example in a reciprocal relationship of sacrifice. "The most we can give will never equal their gift to us," Canadians were reminded in 1940 – but supporting the Red Cross was a good way to try. Announcing a national CRCS appeal, Minister of NWS L.R. LaFlèche argued that since Canadians had been spared from fighting on their own soil, the least they could do was "to see that we in this favoured land contribute to the utmost, in helping those who have suffered the horrors of war in lands beyond this Dominion."[44] The Second World War's devastating impact on civilians and wide geographical scope helped make the work of the CRCS both literally and discursively more international and less narrowly focused on Canadian or British combatants than during the First World War.

Images of red crosses, wounded soldiers, and POWs were common in Red Cross publicity, but perhaps the most frequently used image was the iconic "Red Cross nurse." Dressed to evoke the uniform of a First World War Canadian Nursing Sister, she was always beautiful, frequently reaching out to the viewer in silent appeal for help or pointing at a red cross flag, and gave an impression of maternal-yet-virginal saintliness.[45]

This appealing icon was completely unrepresentative of real CRCS volunteers and their labour, yet conveniently encapsulated the lofty ideals and gendered notions about the society that Canadians had acquired, and the society had encouraged, over the past five-and-a-half decades of Red Cross work in Canada.

Other meanings resurfaced, too, like the First World War-era concept of the Red Cross as an extension of family, doing for those overseas what Canadians on the home front would do if they could. "It is the privilege of the Canadian Red Cross to be there when YOUR soldier needs YOU ... when he's wounded, when he is lonesome – and even when he's a prisoner of war," stated one March 1945 campaign pamphlet.[46] For recent Canadian immigrants with extended family in Europe, this same Red Cross-as-fictive-kin idea no doubt added to the appeal of supporting the society's work for refugees and other civilians in liberated countries. The importance of love and caring as aspects of Red Cross work appeared regularly, for instance when asking a prospective donor to "open [their] heart and purse strings" or praising "unselfish, warm-hearted" volunteers (especially women).[47] In terms of the international Red Cross family, the CRCS worked closely with the BRCS throughout the war and provided substantial grants and concrete supplies to the BRCS, British hospitals, and British POWs, demonstrating the continued strength of Canada's ties to the United Kingdom. However, the CRCS now referred to the BRCS as a "sister" society rather than as the "parent" society and did not fundraise on its behalf.[48] Clearly, a fuller sense of Canadian – and Canadian Red Cross – autonomy had developed since the 1931 Statute of Westminster officially cut Canada's British apron strings.

If these positive reasons did not motivate Canadians to help the CRCS, there was always social pressure to fall back on. One example is preserved in poet Elizabeth Smart's literary account of her 1940s love affair. Unrepentantly unwed and pregnant in wartime Ottawa, her poetic alter ego finds passive-aggressive shaming instead of sympathy in the city: "I am saving my money for the Red Cross. What war-work are you doing, my dear?" she is asked.[49] This kind of pressure helped ensure that Canadian women still dominated the ranks of CRCS volunteers. Meanwhile, some ethnic communities used the CRCS as a vehicle to demonstrate their citizenship in wartime, through well-publicized donations of cash, ambulances, or other items. However, not all such gifts were purely voluntary. Social and economic pressures prompted the generosity of the Italian-Canadian employees of Consolidated Smelter in Traill, British Columbia: a pledge of loyalty to Canada and a monthly payroll deduction for the CRCS were the price of their employer's promise not to lay them off.[50]

Different but no less powerful social pressures brought 874,205 Canadian and Newfoundland children and youth into the Junior Red Cross's wartime labour pool by 1944. After twenty years of promoting the school-based program as a tool for instilling good health and internationalism, the CRCS shifted its emphasis to its third pillar – service – in September 1939. The Junior Red Cross seemed a good fit for many schools already trying to cultivate patriotism and good citizenship in their young charges, and thanks to a combination of adult coercion and children's enthusiasm for actively participating in the new national preoccupation, Junior Red Cross membership across Canada grew dramatically. By 1941, roughly one-quarter of all Canadian youth between five and nineteen years old were enrolled in the Junior Red Cross, almost all of them doing some kind of war work.[51]

While many Canadian girls and boys likely participated because their teachers introduced the Junior Red Cross program into their classrooms, some youth clearly articulated the reasons they found such work meaningful. One Ottawa student wrote in the Glebe Collegiate yearbook that Junior Red Cross work helped students who could not yet enlist deal with the anxiety, frustration, tension, and grief of wartime – making Second World War Junior Red Cross activities precisely the kind of emotional labour Bruce Scates identified in women's First World War voluntary work. When former Juniors from Manitoba were interviewed by Mary Elizabeth Nowlan in the mid-1990s, they explained that they knitted for the CRCS during the war "because it needed to be done."[52] Young people were no less motivated by a sense of duty than the adults around them.

Despite this widespread support, the CRCS had its critics. Surfacing principally between 1939 and 1941, criticisms of the society's attitude and sphere of work, accusations of financial mismanagement, and rumours about sock-selling and high administrative salaries swirled within certain circles – particularly those frequented by Canadian Welfare

Council (CWC) executive director (and future mayor of Ottawa) Charlotte Whitton.

The CWC had an uneasy relationship with the CRCS during the interwar years, and the wartime expansion of the CRCS hardly improved it. Charlotte Whitton respected the society's Geneva Convention obligations and admired the Junior Red Cross, but was suspicious of the CRCS as a whole and resented its infringement on the social welfare field. She studied the relevant Canadian and international legislation in an attempt to pin down the society's legally mandated role, rather than the role it claimed for itself, and concluded that although the CRCS was allowed to cooperate with military medical services in war, and to work for public health in peacetime, nowhere was it set apart as a special auxiliary of the Department of National Defence, nor was it given an exclusive role in wartime or peacetime Canada. She believed its new work for healthy combatants broke international law and argued that the CRCS must cease all "community social work" in order to enjoy the protection of the red cross emblem in wartime.[53]

Whitton raised important questions. The society had evolved substantially since its founding and taken on work its creators did not envision. In light of those changes, what *was* the proper role of a national Red Cross society in wartime? Should it cease its peacetime work entirely? Would there be negative repercussions for national societies who assisted combatants as well as the sick, wounded, and captured? What exactly *was* the society's legal relationship to the government in wartime?

Answers to Whitton's queries arrived from two different sources, and together they help explain why her criticisms never went beyond her own private research and correspondence to provoke a larger reassessment of the CRCS's proper role. Her CWC associate Philip Fisher argued that there was no point in making a fuss. It was up to the federal government or the Germans to respond if they were upset by CRCS aid to combatants, he wrote, and the society's national charter allowed it a social welfare role in peacetime.[54] In turn, National Junior Red Cross director Jean Browne pointed out that public statements about the society's auxiliary role by the governor general and the prime minister, plus Department of National Defence requests for particular services from the CRCS, were "surely as practical a recognition of [the society's] position as an auxiliary as could possibly be made." "I think you will find the Prime Minister's interpretation is quite generally accepted by the people of Canada," she added. Whitton let the matter drop, but actively followed the CRCS's battles with NWS through 1941 and used her position and contacts to try to limit the society's ability to steam-roll other organizations in the name of its auxiliary role.[55]

Whitton was not alone in objecting to CRCS mission drift since 1918. Some within the society also felt the wartime CRCS should strictly adhere to its Geneva Convention role of aiding the sick, wounded, and captured, while others believed the 1919 mandate to relieve suffering and promote health justified CRCS involvement in a much wider range of wartime activities, such as following American Red Cross precedent to provide comforts to combatant troops as a health-promotion measure.[56] This basic dispute was complicated by the further improvement of Canada's military medical service since the First World War, and the King government's regulation of Canada's war effort, both of which greatly limited the society's opportunities to provide direct medical services to the sick and wounded and left it looking for things to do. In January 1940 Victor Sifton, president of the Manitoba Division, wrote to National Headquarters to register Manitoba Division's protest against the use of CRCS funds for recreational services and grants to other agencies in Britain and Finland. The Manitobans urged National Headquarters to firmly adhere to the Geneva Convention mandate and hold onto its money until Canadian troops were actively engaged in combat. Norman Sommerville's seven-page reply on behalf of National Headquarters rationalized the grants on two grounds, one humanitarian, the other financial. First, people were suffering and needed the help. How could the society say no? Second, providing grants to other organizations was the best way to prevent them from competing with the CRCS in Canada.[57] The threat of charitable competition remained ever-present.

By this point the society had achieved – at least in wartime – what John F. Hutchinson later called "sacred cow" status.[58] While some Canadians obviously took issue with aspects of the wartime CRCS, very few publicly voiced their objections. Among the exceptions were Canadian tabloids *Hush* and the *North Toronto Herald*. The *Hush* story was of particular concern: the paper had been popular across Canada since it first appeared in 1927, and specialized in exposing what it considered the hypocrisy of Canada's upper crust.[59] Under the screaming headline

"Red Cross Big Shots Should Disclose Salaries," in March 1941 *Hush* accused the CRCS of "crookedness, graft [and] chiselling," and claimed it kept down hard-working, honest volunteers for the glory and financial gain of its top executives. Calling for full disclosure of supposedly exorbitant staff salaries, the article singled out Fred Routley, Norman Sommerville, and Adelaide Plumptre as particularly suspect.[60] After *Hush* and the *North Toronto Herald* repeated these allegations in October 1941, the Royal Canadian Mounted Police (RCMP) launched an investigation: not of the CRCS, but of the tabloids. The country's wartime censors relied heavily on self-censorship by patriotically minded media outlets in order to keep damaging information out of the public sphere. Although the censors focused primarily on military and economic secrets, the CRCS story had sufficient morale-damaging potential to warrant investigation; furthermore, as RCMP Inspector F.W. Shutz put it, "to besmirch the reputation of the Red Cross" in this manner was "most contemptible" if the claims were untrue.[61]

The investigation revealed that the allegations were "based on anything but fact," with the principal informant a disbarred lawyer with a grievance against a prominent Sarnia, Ontario Red Cross leader. With the weight of the RCMP behind him, P.H. Gordon extracted apologies and printed retractions in February 1942.[62] The society also released a list of salaries paid to CRCS officials to quiet the rumours. Dr Routley, as a full-time employee of the society, earned $9,000 a year (largely to cover his travelling expenses), and Assistant Commissioner Cairns received $2,400 a year. Neither would receive a CRCS pension upon retirement. With the exception of a few clerical staff, all other National Headquarters staff and leaders were unpaid. Nonetheless, this rumour continued to dog the society.[63]

The October 1941 *Hush* article also featured a new version of the old First World War-era sock-selling rumour, once again in circulation. *Hush* had fabricated the specific incident it reported, but the idea that profits might be made from donated labour and skill remained upsetting to ordinary Canadians and CRCS leaders alike. A Montreal-based newspaper, the *Canadian Veteran,* offered a $100 reward to anyone who could provide credible evidence of the CRCS selling goods given to it for the free use of the armed forces, and (like Mrs Plumptre in the First World War) found the few submissions it received to be false.[64] The letters of two veterans who wrote to the Alberta Division Commissioner in 1961 suggest reasons for the rumour's persistence. E.P. Foster swore that he personally bought Red Cross socks during the war, while H.J. McDonald reminded the commissioner that the Red Cross had run canteens where servicemen paid for their food and drink.[65] As in the First World War, the plethora of organizations at home and overseas (including various national Red Cross societies) that provided some sort of service, recreation, or comfort to Allied troops – some for free, some for a small fee – made for all sorts of confusion. The prevalence of wartime black markets also meant that inevitably some supplies *were* sold – but selling comforts was not CRCS policy, was not widespread, and was never condoned. The single documented instance of Red Cross supplies being openly sold took place in the last year of the war, on the Channel Island of Jersey (occupied by Germany through much of the conflict). Canadian and American Red Cross food parcels and clothing for Jersey civilians arrived without clear instructions on distribution, so local residents decided to sell the supplies at low prices. When word trickled back of CRCS supplies being sold in the Channel Islands, the error was rectified – a simple case of miscommunication.[66]

Some Canadians raised concerns about who received CRCS supplies. In response, the society issued a public statement that any money the CRCS forwarded to the ICRC would not be spent in enemy countries, but designated for Allied-friendly causes such as Greek relief. Expressing similar concerns about the uses of CRCS funds, the father of Canadian POW John Denver wrote to Adelaide Plumptre to protest the treatment of German POWs in Canada, whom he heard were "wined and dined and taken on sight-seeing tours" while his son was "handcuffed in Germany." Mrs Plumptre assured him that German POWs were not treated like celebrity tourists and suggested that such stories were German propaganda. In April 1944 the CRCS also clarified, for the benefit of Ontarians who lived near camps housing enemy POWs, that the fruit, skipping ropes, and other "treats" they saw entering the camps came from the German Red Cross, not the CRCS.[67]

Charlotte Whitton contributed one final topic of CRCS controversy. In November 1939 the Maritime Red Cross grapevine reported that Whitton had publicly declared that during the First World War "the battlefields of France were strewn with socks." Norman Sommerville angrily asked Whitton to desist, claiming that her comments would discourage women volunteers and thereby deprive Canada's fighting men of emergency supplies.[68] Whitton felt so strongly that she sent two replies in the same day, attributing the original remark to someone else but agreeing with its basic premise. She questioned whether hand knitting and sewing by inexperienced women was the best option "in a day of mechanized and mass production" and whether it might not throw female employees of textile factories out of work. Whitton wanted Canadian women to stop and think before they used scarce resources and labour, which could perhaps be put to better use.[69]

Even Mrs Plumptre recognized that women's "perfect passion ... to *make* things for the men" could be problematic, since "you cannot build hospitals with socks or feed prisoners on pyjamas." But either Sommerville did not recognize the validity of Whitton's criticism, or he realized he could not properly answer the challenge. He simply defended Red Cross accounting practices and inspection procedures and insisted that "never were there more perfect socks being forwarded than by the Red Cross."[70] His instinctive recoiling was natural, given the society's reliance on its female volunteers, but he failed to see the growing gap between what Canadian women had traditionally done in wartime and the wider possibilities for women's wartime participation recognized by people like Whitton. Traditional Red Cross "women's work" continued to offer an economically valuable and emotionally meaningful outlet for many Canadian women during the Second World War, but others clearly saw opportunities beyond the status quo.

Dig In and Give: Making It Happen on the Home Front

Throughout the war, the generosity of volunteers and donors in Canada enabled the CRCS to provide humanitarian assistance abroad. While Second World War fundraising and women's work closely resembled their First World War counterparts, the second war introduced new avenues of voluntary service through the Blood Donor Service and Canadian Red Cross Corps. Both opportunities sprang from the same changing wartime social context that proved so frustrating to the CRCS in other respects.

Although its voluntary workforce allowed the CRCS to accomplish things on the cheap, in order to successfully fulfill its wartime mandate the society needed money, and lots of it. Within weeks of the outbreak of war, Canadians from coast to coast showed signs of the same ingenuity in raising funds that they had demonstrated during the First World War, with men once again taking a central, although not exclusive, role in this aspect of the society's work. The major nationwide campaigns emphasized workplace collections, door-to-door canvasses, and corporate donations, but at the local level, teas, picnics, card parties, lectures, bake sales, auctions, bazaars, concerts, tag days, and salvage collections featured heavily. Gifts in-kind were popular with cash-poor segments of the population.[71] Many of these small efforts gave ordinary Canadians an opportunity to indulge in guilt-free socializing and entertainment while raising money for a good cause. Prince Edward Island Red Cross volunteers made this clear by describing their goal for a dance in Brackley Beach as "to make a little money for the soldiers and have a good time."[72]

The endless fundraising got on some people's nerves. When Calgary City Council considered a request to copy a successful Banff initiative and use dogs as canvassers at the city's railway and bus stations, one councillor asked, "Isn't the Red Cross getting enough money?" It must have seemed that way to Canadians faced with constant wartime financial appeals. But the need was vast and ongoing, and not all supplies made it to their intended recipients: hundreds of thousands of dollars' worth of Red Cross supplies were sunk by German U-boats in the Atlantic, and at least one of the society's large warehouses in Britain was destroyed in a German bombing raid.[73]

As Eric Keith Walker has demonstrated, the society's major national appeals during the Second World War were elaborate affairs involving tens of thousands of volunteer canvassers, the publicity expertise and resources of patriotically minded businesses, and the support of prominent politicians, religious leaders, and celebrities; they also evolved considerably, becoming more efficient and effective year by year.[74] Following First World War patterns of gendered Red Cross labour, women tended to be responsible for door-to-door canvassing while men solicited donations from business and industry. Billboard space and posters, radio air time and scripts, and film production and screening were provided for free by the relevant firms, while newspaper ad space was paid at a minimum rate and essentially reimbursed by large donations from the newspapers.[75] Also following First World War patterns, campaign publicity highlighted examples of citizens contributing according to their means, whether large donations from the wealthy, a few cents from small children, or in-kind donations from Aboriginal communities. These anecdotes promoted the idea of national unity in sacrifice while presenting the Red Cross as a cause that every Canadian could and should support, regardless of their circumstances. This was a particularly relevant message during the November 1939 campaign, when Canadians were still wearily mired in the Great Depression. The country truly did "dig in and give," as one campaign slogan urged them, in order to oversubscribe the $3,000,000 campaign goal by $2,000,000.[76]

Beginning with the September 1940 campaign in which Hollywood stars joined Prime Minister Mackenzie King in requesting donations to the CRCS, the society made the most of film, radio, and celebrities. A particularly high profile film called "There Too Go I," shown in major theatres across Canada during the 1942 campaign, featured British film star Anna Neagle in the role of a Red Cross nurse and footage of the real Queen Elizabeth visiting the CRCS warehouses in London and admiring the comforts made by Canadian women.[77] Such films, plus still photographs in *Despatch*, encouraged Canadians to continue their efforts by showing them what became of the money and items they donated.

Many factors contributed to the society's fundraising success. Through membership drives and small-scale local events, volunteers raised $4,694,000 over the course of 1941 despite the absence of a professionally coordinated national appeal. The nationwide whirlwind campaigns held each year from 1942 to 1945 raised successively larger sums, culminating in $15,000,000 in 1945 (the equivalent of over $200,000,000 today). Monthly payroll deductions from factory workers helped fuel the increase, as did substantial donations from particular ethnic communities seeking to help their kin in newly liberated regions of Europe after D-Day.[78] A further coup for the CRCS was American president Franklin Roosevelt's 1943 declaration of March as "Red Cross Month." Capitalizing on the ARC's unmatched talent for wartime hoopla and Canadians' consumption of American media, the CRCS secured permission to hold its own 1943 (and subsequent) national appeals in March as well, making March "Red Cross Month" across both nations. Harsh Canadian spring weather made campaigning in March a real challenge, but volunteers persevered.[79] While much of the society's financial success may be attributed to the power of its humanitarian and patriotic appeal in wartime, in 1942 T.C. Davis identified a further reason to expect success each year: by that point the federal government regulated Canadians' opportunities for wartime giving to the point where the Red Cross was one of the only organizations to which Canadians could make large donations deductible for income tax purposes.[80]

Members of the Junior Red Cross were no less generous with their money and labour than adults. Juniors contributed to adult Red Cross funds and non-Red Cross war charities, but also to a special Junior Red Cross War Fund, largely used for child-centred projects like nurseries for injured British war orphans under the age of five, and relief for starving children in Allied countries. Their hands-on work included major salvage drives, knitting and sewing quilts and garments, and making medical supplies, including hundreds of thousands of wooden arm splints. By 1945 Juniors had donated an estimated $3,000,000 in cash in addition to their in-kind donations of goods and labour. They maintained their pre-war health work at the same time.[81]

Women remained the heart and hands of the society in communities of all sizes. Although the Second World War is notable for the mobilization of Canadian women – especially married and middle-class white women – into non-traditional roles, many women stuck with traditional female war work, or combined it with forays into non-traditional territory. Since the late 1930s, popular Canadian women's magazine *Chatelaine* had been emphasizing the importance of women's volunteer work; the emphasis only increased after September 1939, now conveyed by many forms of media. Such encouragement must have primed some women for their quick voluntary response at the outbreak of war.[82] Hundreds of Montreal women and girls queued outside the Quebec Division headquarters to offer their volunteer services on 3 September 1939, and as of 25 September 1939 more than half of the women of tiny Jasper, Alberta were enrolled in the Jasper Park Red Cross League. By 1944 the massive Toronto branch was coordinating the work of 35,000 women in 700 individual groups. The CRCS National Workroom was up and running five days a week by 1 October 1939, providing samples, charts, and patterns to help standardize the production of provincial and local Red Cross sewing groups – an important addition to the small booklets of knitting instructions which once again flooded the country, now in both French and English. Large urban branches made arrangements that suited their local volunteer workforces, for example, opening in the evenings for "business girls" whose days were occupied with paid employment. University-based groups mobilized the labour of faculty wives and female students, while the skilled labour of Nursing Sister veterans of the First World War was directed to the sterilization and packing of surgical dressings. Church groups, bank- and business-based groups, service clubs, and social clubs provided further pools of voluntary labour. Throughout the war both advertisers and the government churned out propaganda highlighting the social necessity of women's domestic work in wartime, and Ottawa created a Women's Voluntary Services division within NWS to help coordinate and control women's voluntary work through thousands of organizations; both developments created a supportive social and political context for women's CRCS work.[83]

Although this mobilization was to a great extent a grassroots phenomenon, the work itself was guided by top-down direction and supervision. Even before the Canadian government officially declared war, CRCS National Headquarters established its National Women's Work Committee to organize the anticipated efforts of Canadian women. Similar committees were established in each provincial division. A national subcommittee of physicians, surgeons, and nurses coordinated surgical dressings and hospital supplies. Collectively, this approach helped standardize the articles women across Canada produced, but did not entirely eliminate acts of resistance. Two women from a small Ontario branch reportedly complained about the rejection of pyjamas they had made which closed from right to left. When they were told that men's clothing always closed from left to right, they argued that "there should be some closing from right to left for the left-handed men!"[84]

As Jeffrey Keshen points out, women's wartime volunteer work "was rarely perceived as a challenge to male authority" and earned lavish praise in the public sphere.[85] The majority of women's Second World War CRCS work should therefore be understood as a counterpoint to the many ways in which Canadian women challenged the gender-based

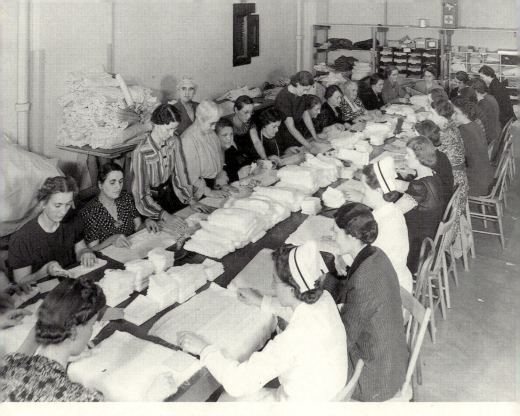

Figure 5.1
A group of largely middle-aged and older women, including two trained graduate
nurses (white caps with black stripe, right) prepare supplementary hospital supplies. The
supervisor (standing, left) and neat piles in the centre of the table illustrate the society's
efforts to maintain consistent standards, while the group setting and monotonous task
speak to the importance of sociability in retaining volunteers over the long term.

status quo in this period. However, this fact should not be allowed to ob-
scure the labour, skill, economic value, or cultural and emotional meaning involved in the work. The records of the well-heeled College Heights
and Rosedale Association (CH&RA), one of the 700 auxiliary groups
working for the Toronto branch, offer a rare glimpse into the grassroots
side of women's CRCS work. The CH&RA was a First World War sewing
group reactivated by surviving members three days after the declaration
of war in 1939. As an independently registered war charity it was self-
directed, but it worked almost exclusively as an auxiliary of the Toronto
branch of the CRCS. In 1943 the CH&RA had 320 active women members, 80 percent of them married. Up to six small auxiliaries supported
the main group's work at any given time – a pattern of large branches
and small affiliates that held true elsewhere as well.[86]

The principal work of the CH&RA took place in the two basement recreation rooms of Mrs Anne Clara Clarke's home in Toronto's wealthy Rosedale neighbourhood – converted for the duration of the war into workrooms open Tuesdays and Wednesdays from 10:00 a.m. to 4:00 p.m. Mrs Clarke was the wife of businessman Lionel H. Clarke, who had been lieutenant-governor of Ontario from 1919 to 1921. Cloth bought in bulk by the CRCS was cut by staff at two local tailoring firms, and between fifty and sixty women gathered at the Clarke home each work day to sew specific pieces (for example, sleeves only), or assemble the finished parts. This adaptation of scientific management to a domestic space worked so well that it made the CH&RA one of Toronto branch's "go-to" groups for rush orders.

The CH&RA's membership of predominantly older, white, married, upper-middle-class women was unrepresentative of the diversity among Red Cross volunteers across Canada, but it demonstrates that such women still found wartime Red Cross work to be a good fit for their abilities and inclinations. CH&RA meetings opened with a Red Cross Prayer which linked the work to love, caring, and patriotism; it also sought wisdom and tolerance, which members required in heated disputes such as whether to allow smoking in the workrooms.[87] As First World War Red Cross volunteers had found, personality conflicts were inevitable as women worked with one another for years at a time in a wider context of strain and stress. When war weariness and charitable fatigue chipped away at workers' dedication, CH&RA leaders used both patriotic and humanitarian appeals to combat them. In their 1941 report, the workroom conveners urged members to work "harder, longer and more often" by invoking the suffering of British civilians during the Battle of Britain. "The Invasion is on! Our boys need our help," proclaimed another notice circulated shortly after D-Day, 6 June 1944. The roughly 30,000 sewn and knitted items recorded in the CH&RA's annual workroom reports – from children's underwear to minesweepers' vests[88] – indicate that whether from love, compassion, or duty, many women still responded to such appeals.

Across Canada, women's efforts earned praise in CRCS materials as well as in the wider public sphere. Reviving First World War language, observers called women Red Cross volunteers the embodiment of "sacrifice and service ... without self-gratification," and described them as vital complements to the fighting men. The economic value of their work earned praise too: as one writer put it, each day they performed "the miracle of converting every dollar they collect into two dollars worth of material mercy."[89] This sleight of hand was prominently displayed in the patchwork quilts CRCS women produced and sent overseas by the thousands to warm bombed British civilians and displaced Europeans. Brackley Beach Red Cross members on Prince Edward Island wrote that "knitted and quilted into every item in hand were prayers, love and concern" for their eventual recipients. Made of leftover scraps of material, CRCS quilts thereby combined clever thrift with comfort and care.[90]

The emotional significance of CRCS comforts and care work is apparent in the wartime work of Nina Cohen. Cohen was in her early thirties, a Mount Allison University graduate married with one son and living near Sydney, Nova Scotia, when the war broke out. She quickly found a wartime outlet for her lifelong community-mindedness through the Sydney Red Cross, and as the branch's publicity and hospitality coordinator, she became a well-known and beloved figure among servicemen in Cape Breton. As a visitor at the local military hospital she dispensed the traditional comforts: cigarettes, toiletries, conversation, and female company. As hospitality coordinator she arranged meals and weekends with local families (including her own) for recuperating servicemen.[91]

Since Sydney was a major assembly point for transatlantic convoys of men, munitions, and supplies, Nina Cohen's "mothering" work had a significant impact. Her warmth, lightheartedness, and intelligence seem to have exemplified hospitality for the young Allied troops who encountered her, and she received a steady stream of letters from grateful (and sometimes smitten) servicemen, unit commanders, and hospital staff throughout the war. British sailor Ernest Bartlett was moved to flowery prose in his letter thanking Mrs Cohen for assisting him and a fellow seaman as they recuperated in Sydney from a torpedoing: "the ditty bags and kind words of your lady helpers were a source of great comfort to us in our distress," he wrote, and "the Cross the symbol of Divine suffering and love was never more nobly borne than on the uniform of the Red Cross Society, we shall always remember you with gratitude."[92] Such testimonials from servicemen indicate the value that simple kindness and caring could hold for soldiers sick, wounded, or simply far from home.

Other women provided similar care as visitors at military hospitals in Canada and overseas, and through the Red Cross lodges. The First World War-era lodge program expanded considerably during the Second World War, with nine new lodges constructed adjacent to the principal veterans' hospitals across Canada. Volunteers worked to make the lodges a home away from home for the walking sick and wounded by providing food, comforts, and entertainment, while volunteer hostesses provided the kind of sisterly companionship and maternal care implied by the "Red Cross nurse" image. The CRCS at its best brought comfort to the vulnerable, and through these programs offered its volunteers coveted hands-on opportunities to provide that service.[93]

Of all the tasks CRCS volunteers tackled during the Second World War, only one could compete with needlework for total volume produced: POW food parcel packing. This most efficiently industrialized activity of all the society's wartime work took place at plants in Winnipeg, Montreal, Toronto, Hamilton, London, and Windsor, Ontario, where blue-smocked female volunteers young and old engaged in a respectable and voluntary form of factory labour. While men too old to fight crated up the finished parcels and prepared them for shipment, the parcel assembly lines were staffed by women volunteers – likely middle-class women who did not need the wages offered by war industry. Women working in the wartime munitions industry and semi-skilled trades represented a more obvious departure from middle-class women's usual tasks; parcel-packing, in contrast, had a tenuous but reassuring connection to traditional female domestic service through its focus on food. As Ian Mosby has shown, food preparation and service were central to the ways Canadian women used voluntary work to demonstrate their wartime patriotism: parcel-packing could be seen as a form of long-distance meal provision.[94] The absence of dangerous equipment or materials also meant that women could wear their usual skirts, hairstyles, and make-up, thus avoiding the overalls, trousers, and bandanas that made women's munitions and trades work threatening to gendered social expectations of women's femininity in other wartime industrial settings.[95] Parcel packing called for precision and speed since the items completely filled the parcels and each woman's item needed to be placed in a very specific spot. At the peak of production a single parcel could be packed in approximately seventeen seconds.[96] Mosby argues that the

CRCS POW parcel program "perhaps more than any other, lived up to the promise made by wartime propaganda that women's individual efforts on the home front would save the lives of soldiers overseas," and points out that "food was the quintessential comfort ... loaded with emotional and symbolic significance in terms of its connection with the home, family, and community." Parcel packing was solidly linked to both traditional women's Red Cross work and women's domestic work, in spite of the factory setting, standardization, and need for speed.[97]

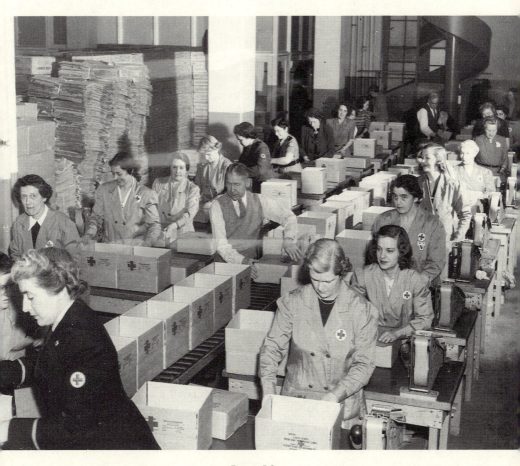

Figure 5.2
Industrialized caring work: women (many wearing the society's sky blue volunteer smocks) and two men seal up filled POW food parcels at one of the CRCS parcel packing plants. The large pile of flattened boxes at left hints at the millions of parcels produced.

The parcel-packing workforce seemed threatened when in 1942 the government strengthened the National Selective Service (NSS) operations meant to regulate Canada's wartime human resources mobilization. A series of regulations compelled the registration of unemployed men (May 1942), instituted an NSS permission requirement for men and women entering any form of employment (June 1942), expanded the permit system to seeking, taking, or leaving employment (August 1942), and created a national system of priority classification for different work (August 1942). The question of whether people who worked six to eight hours a day in a voluntary capacity would be considered unemployed in the eyes of NSS (and therefore compelled to take a job in industry or enlist in the military) concerned not only the coordinators of parcel packing plants, blood clinics, and women's workrooms, but volunteers themselves: P.H. Gordon reported that some volunteers had begun leaving these time-consuming venues "because they say it would be far better for them to select their own job than have one selected for them." Both T.C. Davis and NSS officials offered Gordon the partial reassurance that the government would not immediately compel women to do anything, but even if it came to that, women working full time in important Red Cross work would be "considered to be in an essential industry already and not disturbed." Michael D. Stevenson's examination of the NSS demonstrates that the government's commitment to gradualism and voluntarism made its human resource mobilization for industry, agriculture, and the military inefficient and sometimes ineffective, but this same commitment was a boon to wartime voluntary organizations like the CRCS which relied on Canadians' freedom to direct their own time and labour.[98]

The NSS was not the only threat to the society's voluntary workforce. Other organizations, paid employment, and the armed forces beckoned, each using clever propaganda to attract new recruits. Even within the CRCS itself, different types of work vied for volunteers. By 1944 the Women's Work Committee instituted a badge of recognition for its volunteers in hopes of stemming the tide of desertions to the blood and POW departments, whose work was more directly life-saving.[99] And although wartime propaganda paid lip service to the importance of women's domestic and voluntary work, the work was sometimes undervalued in ways reminiscent of the First World War. For instance, in her 1942 book-

let *Canadian Women in the War Effort*, Charlotte Whitton acknowledged
– despite her reservations on the subject – that women's "rapid and rea-
sonably effective" mobilization into traditional volunteer channels
"contributed very definitely to the nation's war service."[100] The statistics
she provided showed hundreds of thousands more women providing
voluntary service than any other form of war work: in 1942, the largest
single mobilizer of women's labour was the CRCS, with an estimated
750,000 women working directly for it, plus the indirect labour of
many other women's organizations like the Women's Institutes and
IODE. Yet Whitton's booklet foregrounded women's wartime work in
manufacturing, on farms, as military nurses, and in the new women's
armed forces – work that took women into a variety of historically
"male" spaces. Many scholars have shown that this movement of women
into non-traditional roles was undermined by pervasive discourses of
women's beauty, charm, and softness, and the temporary nature of their
efforts, but it remained groundbreaking.[101] Conversely, as Jeffrey Keshen
notes, the ways in which women's wartime voluntary and domestic
work for organizations like the CRCS "meshed naturally with patriarchal
constructions" meant they did not prompt "major and lasting changes
to the traditional gendered order."[102] Whereas women's First World
War-era voluntary work helped some women attain more powerful and
public roles, by the 1940s the frontier of social change for women in
Canada had moved well beyond volunteering.

As the war progressed, the declining supply of male labour increased
the necessity of, and competition for, female labour: by the end of 1944,
full-time paid non-agricultural work employed over a million women,
while nearly 50,000 enlisted in the armed services, and hundreds of
thousands took on part- or full-time agricultural labour.[103] Canadian
women produced 415,000 fewer sewn and knitted items in 1943 than
in 1942, and CRCS leaders recognized that women's increased participation in paid employment meant less time for Red Cross work. Nevertheless, they did not accept this as an excuse for decreased production.
In an early 1944 radio broadcast, Quebec Division's Ruth (Mrs Andrew)
Fleming told listeners that with an Allied invasion of Europe anticipated
that year, it was "the *duty* of every Red Cross worker to keep our fighting men supplied with the comforts they need" [italics added].[104] Such
emotionally and patriotically coercive calls for renewed effort were

heeded, and in spite of war weariness and the lure of paid employment and military service, Canadian women and children produced more than 53,000,000 CRCS comfort and relief items during the six years of war.[105]

Although older women seemed content to do traditional Red Cross war work, many younger women gravitated toward the other opportunities Charlotte Whitton championed – women like the unnamed Winnipeg resident who recalled decades later, "I wasn't going to sit and knit!"[106] The society's answer to this challenge was the Canadian Red Cross Corps, a uniformed, highly disciplined corps of women volunteers trained for emergency service.

Inspired by uniformed British Red Cross volunteers, the CRCS took preliminary steps early in 1940 to train and mobilize a women's transport service of uniformed volunteer drivers.[107] The motor service subsequently expanded to become a Canadian Red Cross Corps of four distinct sections, each of which likely attracted women already experienced or interested in that area: transport, nursing auxiliary, office administration, and food administration. Dressed in smart, military-style uniforms, members were subject to a hierarchical chain of command, practised military drill, and acquired specialized mechanical, VAD, clerical, and mass feeding skills relevant to their particular section. The corps was created to augment the society's own work with a versatile and dedicated pool of specialist-trained female labour that knew how to take orders, but CRCS leaders anticipated that these attributes might also lead corps members into service for the government or military[108] – a patriotic and practical expectation, but not a particularly neutral, humanitarian one. Prior to the creation of the women's branches of the armed forces (beginning August 1941), many women from female paramilitaries like the British Columbia Women's Service Corps transferred to the Canadian Red Cross Corps. They were joined throughout the war by others who wished to take a trained, active role in the war effort, although given the society-wide unease surrounding women in the armed forces, perhaps not a military one. By 1942 the CRCS reported forty-five corps detachments in existence.[109]

The corps seems to have filled a socially acceptable space between traditional Red Cross volunteer work and the more controversial field of actual military service; at any rate, it successfully appealed to a portion of the eighteen- to forty-five-year-old demographic at which it was targeted. Corps members' work largely upheld gendered expectations of the period: they cooked and served in canteens for servicemen and munitions factory workers, filled clerical positions within CRCS departments, provided VAD service in understaffed civilian hospitals, helped with blood clinics, and drove trucks and bloodmobiles.[110] The corps therefore offered women an important space for active service and camaraderie as well as a uniform that publicly signalled the wearer's involvement in vital war work, but did not fundamentally challenge prevailing notions of women as supportive nurturers and preservers of life even in a context of war. In her discussion of the numerous paramilitary organizations created by Canadian women after September 1939 – organizations that, like the corps, wore uniforms, used military rank, practised military drill, and trained for wartime emergencies – Ruth Pierson attributes some of the members' enthusiasm to "a fascination with all things military" and "the mystique of the uniform."[111] The appeal was apparent even at the time. Lest prospective recruits be wooed solely by the romance of uniformed service in wartime, Ontario Commandant Isobel Pepall stressed, "the Red Cross Corps does not want 'deadwood' and it is not an organization in which members merely wear a uniform and look snappy on the street."[112] In fact, the cost of the self-purchased uniform may have deterred some potential recruits. Members came and went, but 15,000 women reportedly enrolled in the corps at some point over the course of the war, with some 6,000 enrolled during the corps' peak year of 1944.[113]

Women and men alike were central to the success of a momentous new chapter of the society's history, which opened in 1940 with the inauguration of the CRCS Blood Donor Service (BDS). The society served as a conduit for home-front blood donations needed by Canadian troops overseas, and in the process became a voluntary, charitable component in the much broader Second World War militarization of science and medicine.[114] Direct arm-to-arm blood transfusions had proven their value in the First World War, and transfusion therapy slowly came into general practice during the 1930s. As the clouds of war gathered during the late 1930s, research scientists in many countries focused on solving the anticipated challenges of more effectively getting bottled blood (which had a short shelf-life) from civilian donors to military recipients on battlefields that might be half a world away. Canadian surgeon Norman

Bethune was among those experimenting with blood transfusion, famously using media attention in Canada to raise funds for his mobile blood transfusion unit in the Spanish Civil War in 1936–37. By 1939 University of Toronto professor and insulin co-discoverer Charles H. Best and his colleagues at the Connaught Laboratories had developed a homegrown Canadian solution to the challenge of long distance blood provision: dried blood serum. This processed derivative of the clear plasma found in whole blood could be efficiently transported overseas and easily reconstituted for use with patients of all blood types, and lasted much longer than whole blood. Among Canada's major wartime allies – each independently experimenting with blood transfusion technologies – Britain and the United States preferred plasma as a blood substitute, while Australia, like Canada, favoured serum (a more processed version of plasma). The two were equally effective in treatment, and successful voluntary blood collection systems for military purposes were established in all four countries during the war.[115]

Next came the question of supply. Canada's existing hospital-based blood collection was both limited and completely uncoordinated, and the provincial jurisdiction over health made it difficult for the federal government to establish a national civilian blood collection system itself. Drawing on Canada's tradition of a mixed social economy, Ottawa turned to the voluntary sector and asked the CRCS to take up the challenge. A few Ontario branches had experimented with blood banking in the late 1930s, and the BRCS had been involved in British blood donation since 1910, so the CRCS had precedents when it agreed to take on this new role.[116]

Canada's first national blood donation service brought together specialists and amateurs, professionals and volunteers. The Connaught group processed most of the serum, while the CRCS handled donor recruitment, blood collection, and eventually some partial processing.[117] The first BDS blood clinic opened on 29 January 1940 in Toronto; by September 1943 the BDS was collecting in every province, with forty permanent clinics in major urban centres from Vancouver to Charlottetown. Soon mobile clinics took the BDS to Canadians outside the biggest cities and the whole service grew to 662 clinics by the end of the war. Blood donors came from all walks of life, and ranged in age from eighteen to sixty-five. Initially only men could donate, but by 1942 demand

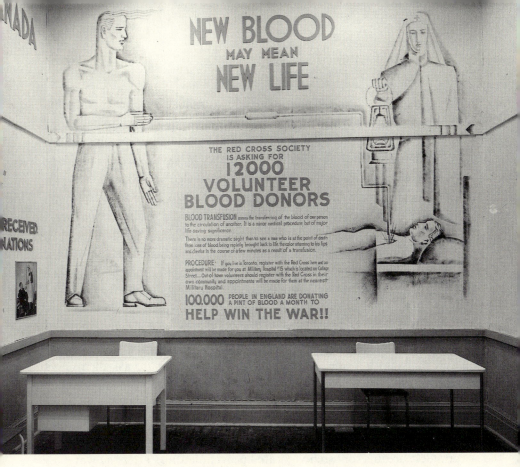

Figure 5.3

This Toronto display seeks 12,000 wartime blood donors. The stylized image shows
a healthy man physically connected by a tube to a man in bed watched over by a
Nightingale-esque "Red Cross nurse," while the slogan equates blood donation with
direct life-saving. England's 100,000 donors are held up as an example to be emulated,
and fearful donors are reassured that donating is a minor procedure with major impact,
a point reinforced by photos of actual donations on the left-hand wall.

outstripped any lingering concerns about women's delicate health, so
women were permitted to donate also. The CRCS collected 2,338,533 units
of blood between January 1940 and August 1945, more than 1,000,000
of them in 1944 alone, the year the Allies invaded Europe.[118]

This generosity was prompted at least in part by emotional appeals
emphasizing the life-saving power of blood transfusions and Canadians'
duty to provide them. A blunt advertisement in Dauphin, Manitoba informed readers that if they did not donate sufficient blood, wounded
Canadians on active service would "die because the people at home have

failed them." As the CRCS information pamphlet for potential donors proclaimed on its cover, blood donation allowed civilians to engage in a meaningful, reciprocal relationship of protection with citizen-soldiers, performing "Front Line Service in Canada" by saving their protectors' lives. Since donating blood for wounded servicemen was framed as a patriotic and charitable act, no one was paid for their blood.[119] Even the nurses and supervising physician at each clinic provided their services for free.

Countless servicemen's lives were saved by civilians' blood. Moreover, the low cost of the entirely voluntary BDS (approximately $2.20 per transfusion) helped outweigh what Richard Kapp describes as "the many drawbacks involved in making an army of part-time volunteers responsible for the technically complicated procedure of blood donation." The wartime BDS was such a success that by 1944 a growing number of Canadians both inside and outside the society began to ask themselves why such a system did not exist for the benefit of Canadians at home.[120] Like the Canadian Red Cross Corps, the BDS had been created in response to specific wartime needs, but of all the society's home-front work during the Second World War, these two activities inspired the grandest dreams for a reinvigorated peacetime CRCS after the war.

Eleven Pounds of Heaven: Humanitarian Aid Overseas

From 1939 to 1945 the Canadian Red Cross Society quietly carried on its public health work at home, but what really mattered was humanitarian aid overseas. Like all such humanitarian efforts, the society's work was imperfect and limited: at times a drop in the sea of need; at others a best possible response under difficult circumstances. Nevertheless, it provided real aid that made a difference for many.

The nerve centre of the society's overseas work was its central office on Berkeley Square in London, England. Like its First World War predecessor, this new overseas headquarters grew to encompass departments for POWs; hospital visits; excursions; newspapers and other Canadian reading material; the receipt, storage, and distribution of comforts and medical supplies; and information on the sick, wounded, and missing. The office also coordinated new CRCS handicraft training – a form of occupational therapy – in military hospitals, and established a branch office at Aldershot offering similar comforts and services to the thousands of Canadian troops stationed there.[121] The assistant commissioner for France was withdrawn after the May 1940 Dunkirk evacuation, and Britain remained the centre of CRCS overseas activity until Allied advances in 1944–45 made regional CRCS work possible and necessary in Rome, Brussels, and Paris. The overseas headquarters worked through British voluntary agencies, the three Canadian armed services, and Canadian military hospitals to channel its supplies and comforts to British civilians, Canadian combatants, and the sick and wounded, respectively.[122] In Europe, the ICRC facilitated the collection of POW information and the distribution of CRCS parcels to Canadian and Allied prisoners.[123]

The society's overseas operations during the Second World War were built on a bedrock of First World War experience, and CRCS leaders strove to avoid the difficulties that had cropped up in the first war. To this end, National Headquarters immediately organized an Overseas Advisory Committee chaired by former prime minister R.B. Bennett, now retired to Britain and elevated to the peerage as Viscount Bennett of Mickleham and Hopewell. Bennett was joined on the committee by other expatriate Canadian men resident in Britain, including managers of Canadian banks and representatives of Canadian industry; the purpose of the committee was to open doors for the society overseas and supervise the operations of the London headquarters in conjunction with an overseas commissioner.

Although R.B. Bennett's energy and social status were assets to the CRCS, neither he nor the full committee proved easy to get along with.[124] The first overseas commissioner appointed, Colonel George Nasmith of Toronto, engaged in unproductive power struggles with the advisory committee, and when CRCS National Headquarters insisted that the committee continue to limit his power of independent action, Nasmith resigned in November 1940.[125] His replacement, Major Scott, also had some difficulty working with Bennett and the committee. Scott was succeeded, to everyone's relief, by the level-headed, capable Major-General C.B. Price of Montreal, who managed to maintain good relations with the committee while coordinating the daily operations of the overseas headquarters.[126] Price soon assumed the role of chief CRCS spokesman in Britain, replacing an ailing Bennett. The change eased tensions between the CRCS and Canada House in London, which had resulted from (Conservative) Bennett's animosity toward (Liberal) Canadian high commissioner Vincent Massey. Fortunately, these personality conflicts overseas took place largely out of the public eye.

Meanwhile, Canadian military hospitals overseas spent the first few years of the war dealing primarily with victims of road accidents (as Canadians tried to negotiate unmarked English country lanes in the blackout), routine sickness and accidents among the Canadian troops restlessly accumulating in Britain, and civilian bombing casualties of the Battle of Britain.[127] With no great demand for medical supplies for troops, CRCS supplementary hospital supplies initially sat unused in London warehouses. The society therefore decided early on, seemingly for both humanitarian and pragmatic reasons, to follow the example of the military hospitals and turn its attention to the civilian victims of the Battle of Britain. This decision marked a departure from past practice, but pro-British popular sentiment in Canada and the increasingly blurred line between home front and battle front probably encouraged the change.[128] Conveniently, the shift also provided a focus for Canadians' home-front Red Cross work until offensives in France and Italy produced large numbers of sick, wounded, or captured Canadian servicemen.

In the field of military medical care provision, the Second World War muddied further the ever-unclear waters of the society's relationship to wartime nursing. Like their First World War predecessors, Second World War Canadian military nurses were enlisted in the Royal Canadian Army Medical Corps (RCAMC), and later in the separate naval and air force nursing services, at the rank of officer, where they performed skilled nursing work for sick and wounded troops in surgical, convalescent, and palliative contexts. In response to a request from the Scottish Ministry of Health in 1941, the CRCS recruited and transported a unit of roughly twenty Canadian nurses who served for the duration in the orthopaedic unit at Hairmyers Hospital in East Kilbride, Scotland. As of 1944 it also provided Canadian Red Cross Corps uniforms for them. However, they were paid by the Scottish government and not officially part of the CRCS.[129] VADs once more provided supplementary volunteer nursing assistance in both civilian and military hospitals in Canada in order to free trained nurses for more skilled work. As in the previous war, VADs tackled the dirtiest, least skilled, and most unglamorous aspects of nursing work, from emptying bedpans and cleaning equipment to changing bandages and delivering meals. But in this war, women seeking to serve as VADs had two options: they could enlist with either the St John Ambulance Brigade (as in the First World War), or with the new Nursing Auxiliary section of the Canadian Red Cross Corps.[130]

The addition of the corps' Nursing Auxiliary members to the ranks of VADs meant there *were* Canadian Red Cross nurses of a sort from 1939 to 1945, but the popular image of the "Red Cross nurse" remained more fiction than fact. The persistence of the "Red Cross nurse" image echoes the experience of Canadian Nursing Sisters in this period. Although military nurses traded their starched white aprons and veils for khaki trousers and boots when nursing in active theatres of war, Cynthia Toman's research shows that they remained "women first, and nurses second," portrayed in official discourse as models of respectable femininity who boosted morale while providing nursing care.[131] This connection between wartime nursing and a range of positive and feminine qualities similar to those associated with the CRCS is probably what led the society's publicity department to use "Red Cross nurse" images in its campaign materials as frequently as it did.

The Canadian government prohibited the creation of private hospitals and rest homes during the Second World War, so whereas the society had provided and equipped a number of hospitals and rest homes in England and France during the First World War, its hospital provision this time around was concentrated in one institution which it built, equipped, and immediately turned over to the RCAMC to run: a new state-of-the-art, 600-bed general hospital (usually referred to in this war as Taplow Hospital) on the Astor family's Cliveden estate near Taplow, England. All but one of the hastily erected pavilion-style buildings remaining from the First World War CRCS hospital at Cliveden were demolished and replaced by the new hospital, a series of forty-one steel and concrete hut buildings with central heating and sunrooms that cost nearly $1,000,000.[132] The society proudly furnished Taplow with the latest medical technology and a "home-like atmosphere" courtesy of maple furniture and scarlet red blankets. In his speech at the official July 1940 opening of the hospital, R.B. Bennett emphasized that Taplow was "a concrete expression of the loving thought and affectionate regard of Canadians," which would put modern science at the service of the nation's citizen-soldiers. Bennett also ventured into Red Cross patriotism territory. "[Taplow] expresses the hopes, aspirations and determination of the Canadian people," he argued: "their affection and concern for their fellows; their pride and confidence in the [democratic] institutions they have established and their determination to work out their great destiny as part of the British Empire."[133] More than 25,000 patients were treated at Taplow between 1940 and 1945, and after the war it was donated to Britain's new National Health Service.[134]

Much of the society's aid for soldiers and civilians overseas fell squarely into the category of emergency humanitarian relief for populations in distress. By war's end the society had provided forty mobile kitchen units equipped to travel into bombed areas and feed hundreds of workers at a time, forty-one smaller mobile canteens, 355 ambulances, twenty station wagons, and fifty trucks for delivering POW parcels in Europe. It distributed food, children's shoes, and millions of articles of clothing to air raid victims in Britain and (after liberation) European countries. It also provided millions of supplementary medical and surgical supplies, from hospital trousers to operating room linens, requisitioned by Canadian military hospitals. At the same time, the society's First World War–era concern to provide care and comfort of less tangible varieties continued to guide some of its overseas work. The jam, jelly, and honey produced in Canada by CRCS and Women's Institute volunteers made their way to Britain as invalid foods for the sick and wounded, and as a treat for combatant troops.[135] The CRCS operated several recreational centres in London for service personnel on leave – the popular Maple Leaf Clubs – and once again ran an Enquiry Bureau, which tried to comfort families in Canada by seeking out and providing information on missing, wounded, and captured servicemen. At the end of the war, several dozen CRC Corps members provided support services as escorts to British and European war brides and their children during the Atlantic crossing.[136] All this work required volunteers, but in 1940 the Canadian government prohibited Canadian women from travelling to the war zone unless they were on official business.[137] Since there was no First World War-style pool of Canadian servicemen's wives in Britain from which to draw volunteers, the society turned to a combination of

British and expatriate Canadian volunteers, some seconded Canadian servicemen, and members of the Canadian Red Cross Corps. Together, they kept CRCS overseas services running.

The fear of a direct attack on Canada may have lurked behind the organization of the CRC Corps in 1940, but no such emergency materialized. Instead, some corps members moved on to the women's armed forces and others were dispatched overseas by the society itself. By the end of the war, 641 women had gained a coveted spot in the corps' Overseas Detachment. Most served in Britain, but some followed the Allied advance into continental Europe. The CRCS also posted a handful of corps members and Assistant Commissioner Mona Wilson to the neighbouring Dominion of Newfoundland, which was transformed after autumn 1940 into a North Atlantic military outpost. With its major Canadian and American military installations, Newfoundland was a prime site from which the CRCS could assist members of the Canadian and Allied navies, merchant seamen, and survivors of U-boat attacks who landed in St John's.[138]

Much like their sisters in the armed forces, corps members' hands-on work overseas for the CRCS, military and civilian hospitals, and servicemen's clubs did not break much new ground for women. The corps' hierarchy of local, sectional, and national commandants did offer a new outlet for strong female leadership, but its welfare work for the troops upheld gendered notions of appropriate "women's work" and drew on members' existing domestic and professional experience. Even driving ambulances and trucks had First World War precedents. As Ruth Pierson notes of the Canadian Women's Army Corps in the same period, "the military regimen, parades, barracks, and mess halls constituted the main change from their civilian work experience" for Overseas Detachment members.[139] Still, the women of the CRC Corps were a new kind of Red Cross volunteer: they worked extremely hard through bombing raids, food shortages, and the personal loss of loved ones, and they were fiercely proud of the overseas service that allowed them to get closer than most Canadian women to the battlefields. During the latter years of the war, the society's visibility in the eyes of both Canadian servicemen and British civilians was increased by the uniformed presence of corps members in London and elsewhere, and their efficient service in a variety of contexts. Throughout their work, members had to negotiate

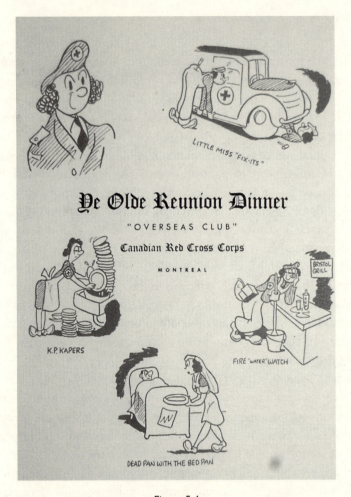

Figure 5.4

Members of the Overseas Detachment held annual gatherings
for sixty years after the war's end. The cover of their 1993 reunion
program – recycled from the third reunion, in 1948 – plays up their
distinctive uniform and the varieties of work they did, but also their
strong sense of camaraderie.

the challenges of remaining "feminine" in appearance and behaviour
despite the military trappings of the corps, while also holding an in-
between status, which was neither military nor strictly civilian. In the
process, they managed to impress observers with their ingenuity, professionalism, and work ethic. Corps members' overseas memoirs reveal
that they found their work demanding but very rewarding, and its overseas context both exciting and meaningful.[140]

Occupational therapy proved its worth in military hospitals during the First World War and made great strides toward professionalization during the interwar years, but it seems to have been the arts and crafts work of CRC Corps members that reminded the RCAMC of the field's value in the Second World War. Arts and crafts work was a form of occupational therapy that used activities like leather work and toy-making to provide a diversion for convalescing soldiers while also contributing to their overall physical and psychological rehabilitation. Corps members first introduced it at Taplow Hospital in 1940, and its success helped pave the way for trained occupational therapists with a wider array of therapies to be posted overseas by the RCAMC beginning in February 1944. Nearly two dozen corps members were recruited to assist the newly arrived professionals, and the two groups worked together to provide occupational therapy to nearly 4,000 patients each month by 1945.[141]

The society's largest single category of wartime expense was its work for POWs. Only blood collection matched the life-saving potential of POW work, and its morale-boosting and alliance-reinforcing abilities were unsurpassed. As Daniel Pomerleau argues, media coverage of the conditions POWs faced and the publication of POW lists and letters from prisoners created widespread empathy for POWs. This in turn fuelled broad-based support for CRCS work to help them.[142] Unfortunately, the arrangements made by government and the voluntary sector as early as November 1939 proved unwieldy and inefficient after the 1942 Dieppe raid produced substantial numbers of Canadian POWs. In the wake of Dieppe, the society created its Enquiry Bureau in Ottawa and London, England, hoping to provide comfort and assurance to prisoners' families as it had done during the First World War. Instead, families faced a confusing choice between the CRCS Enquiry Bureau, the Department of National War Services' POW Next-of-Kin Division, and the Department of National Defence's Office of the Special Assistant to the Adjutant-General, all of which performed similar functions with a great deal of overlap. Combined with inter-agency distrust, this overlap sometimes led to unnecessary delays in acquiring information for anxious next-of-kin.[143]

The work of aiding the prisoners themselves was also hindered by organizational competition. The CRCS, with its First World War experience and ICRC access to POW camps, initially dominated the field, but was challenged as the war progressed by the War Prisoners' Aid of the World's Committee of YMCAs, which provided educational, recreational, cultural, and spiritual relief to POWs, and the Canadian POW Relatives' Association, which kept next-of-kin updated on regulations and assisted them with the provision of next-of-kin parcels. All three relief agencies were well-intentioned but frequently obstructionist. Around 1943 Ottawa realized a central government-led umbrella committee to coordinate the POW system would help, but by then it was too late: the existing parties were entrenched and unwilling to budge. It was a bureaucratic mess that reflected poorly on everyone, and as Jonathan Vance notes, "in some ways it is a wonder that anything was achieved at all."[144]

The CRCS did shine in its provision of POW food parcels. The society strove throughout the war to provide one parcel per Canadian prisoner per week, and since Canada had extensive resources and relatively few of its own prisoners – approximately 10,000 by war's end – it could afford to help feed other Allied POWs, too. By 1942 the CRCS regularly produced extra parcels for the British, Australian, and New Zealand Red Cross societies, and considered this its contribution to the BRCS goal of caring for prisoners from every part of the British Commonwealth.[145] The massive ARC was able to supply American POWs on its own, but in time the CRCS also supplied parcels to French, Belgian, Polish, and Yugoslav POWs (with CUARF, Canadian, and Allied government support) and was packing 149,600 parcels per week in 1945. As overseas commissioner, General Price pushed heavily for this expansion. By 1944 the Cabinet War Committee agreed: parcels offered proof of Canada's assistance to her allies, and would pave the way for further Allied relief after the war. Prime Minister Mackenzie King came to believe that "every dollar spent on this form of assistance" to ordinary Allied POWs "may be far more effective ... than a hundred or perhaps a thousand given to a government," and he was keen to ensure that the parcels were clearly labelled as gifts of Canada.[146] In this way the Canadian Red Cross once more served as a channel for demonstrations of Allied solidarity in wartime.

The Allies proposed further Red Cross cooperation – now in the Pacific theatre of war – beginning in 1942. Unfortunately, their schemes

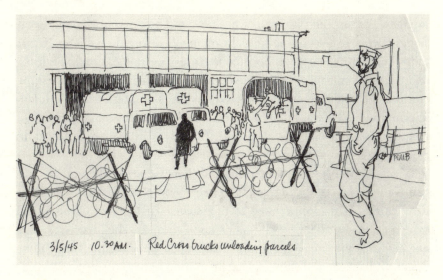

Figure 5.5

Canadian POW Robert Marshall Buckham's pen and ink sketch of ICRC trucks delivering food parcels to his camp, 3 May 1945, testifies to the parcels' value as a boost to prisoners' diet and morale. Their arrival was also a notable incident in the monotonous camp life.

for joint CRCS, BRCS, and ARC provision of food parcels and clothing for Allied prisoners and civilian internees in East Asia ultimately had little impact: Japan had not signed the 1929 Geneva Convention governing the treatment of POWs, and Japanese military culture (which viewed capture as shameful) did not encourage favourable treatment of enemy prisoners.[147] Although the Japanese government agreed in principle to respect the Geneva Conventions and accept shipments via the ICRC in September 1942, it stonewalled most of the Allied proposals for actual relief shipments and frequently did not distribute the supplies it allowed in. The appeals of Allied Red Cross societies, the ICRC, and others left the Japanese government and Japanese Red Cross unmoved.[148] Roughly 225,000 Red Cross parcels, plus limited medicine and clothing, landed in East Asia during the war, and Canadian and American civilian internees in Hong Kong were exchanged for Japanese civilian internees held by the US in late 1943, but little aid reached the malnourished and disease-ridden POWs themselves. Many parcels were used or sold by the

Japanese; others simply sat in warehouses. The few parcels and occasional twenty-five-word messages from home conveyed by the Red Cross that did reach the captives boosted their morale immeasurably, but the entire East Asia POW relief effort was a frustrating and often fruitless exercise, which painfully demonstrated the limits of international humanitarian law.[149] If a warring government had no interest in observing the niceties of the Geneva Conventions, there was little anyone could do aside from securing the prisoners' release by winning the war.

Germany and Italy largely respected their Geneva Convention obligations and the ICRC did its best to keep food parcels arriving in their POW camps. This contributed to the success of the Red Cross parcel campaign in Europe, but so too, Vance argues, did the fact that it was not plagued with an overabundance of relief agencies: the CRCS alone designed, packed, and shipped Canadian food parcels for POWs.[150] CRCS parcels made the most of both Canada's vast agricultural resources and the latest nutritional science. Dr Frederick Tisdall and his research team at the University of Toronto's Department of Pediatrics carefully formulated them to supplement German rations, cramming 2,070 calories and as many essential vitamins and minerals as possible into the internationally authorized eleven-pound package.[151] CRCS volunteers packed 16,310,592 of the parcels during the course of the war, and as Vance notes, the scale of the venture and its significance to the men on the receiving end meant that "the Red Cross food parcel has become the symbol of Canada's relief effort in aid of POWs."[152] One prisoner wrote that "without Canadian parcels, life, already grim, would be almost impossible."[153] Unlike some countries' parcels, CRCS food parcels' contents never varied. This bored some prisoners, but 80 percent of Canadian POWs surveyed in 1945 remembered Canadian parcels as their favourites because they contained the most items. With characteristic ingenuity, prisoners found creative uses for every item included: cigarettes, chocolate, and soap became camp currency, and former POW Harry Crease recalled men in his camp using the tin from KLIM powdered milk containers to create everything from cups and dishware to escape tunnel air ducts and homemade furnaces.[154] As in the First World War, CRCS parcels made a real difference to Second World War POWs.

One of the society's greatest assets during the Second World War remained its ability to create a tangible sense of connection between the people at home and those they cared about overseas. CRCS campaign publicity often reminded Canadians that POW parcels could reach someone they knew: "There's a lad from your home town perhaps ... a neighbour, an old school chum who will really mean YOU when he says a prayer for the Red Cross as he opens a box containing eleven pounds of heaven," announced one 1945 radio script. The society's pride in its scientifically researched and nutritionally complete parcels speaks not only to the increased professionalization of Red Cross work and to changes in Canadians' understandings of healthy eating and malnutrition but also to the cultural and emotional significance of food in wartime.[155] Supplementing the meagre diet of Canadian POWs was as much a national outpouring of care for the country's imprisoned warriors as it was a dietary intervention for imprisoned men needing more to eat. This symbolic dimension made the Allies' inability to reach POWs held by the Japanese even more upsetting.

✤

The Second World War constituted both a Golden Age and a time of profound struggle for the Canadian Red Cross Society. It brought the CRCS back into the mainstream of Canadian society and made it matter in a way it rarely had for twenty years. Building on its record of First World War activity and interwar public health work, the society raised more money, enlisted more volunteers, provided more aid, acted more professionally, and held more authority and prestige in Canada and overseas than ever before. But certain factors in its First World War success could not simply be reproduced on a bigger scale. Some women sought new wartime roles, and Japanese non-compliance tested the limits of international humanitarian law. The CRCS lost some of its independence, squared off against rival organizations, and found its wartime moral authority countered by the growing power of an interventionist state. These were years of transition and renegotiation.

By consistently arguing its own exceptionality when faced with greater state regulation, making use of the personal relationship between P.H. Gordon and T.C. Davis, and moving into new avenues of service such as the CRC Corps and blood collection, the CRCS survived – and mostly overcame – the challenges of the war years. But it would soon find that those challenges did not end with Allied victory in 1945, whereas much of the wartime moral authority of the Red Cross did. Key Red Cross leaders and supporters may have thought that their organization was back in its destined role, but this reversion to a previous incarnation of the society was short-lived. Another transformation would be needed if the CRCS intended to survive in a rapidly changing, post-1945 world of Cold War and the welfare state.

6

MID-CENTURY MODERN RED CROSS, 1946–1970

For three weeks during the summer of 1952, the world came to Toronto for the Eighteenth International Red Cross Conference. The Canadian Red Cross Society, primed for success with elaborately staged water safety demonstrations, day-trips to the majestic horseshoe falls at Niagara, and nine smartly dressed detachments of the CRC Corps, welcomed some 3,000 international delegates, clerical and technical staff, volunteer aides, and members of the press. The IRC offered the CRCS this opportunity to host in recognition of the society's growing international profile. No longer a British Red Cross tag-along, the post-Second World War CRCS felt mature, independent, and ready to participate fully in the world of international humanitarian aid. But when the delegates arrived in Toronto, they brought with them not only the warmth of humanitarian idealism but also the chill of the Cold War. General sessions exploded into shouting matches over the same issues rocking the new United Nations – China, Korea, Germany – and the credibility of the global Red Cross movement, predicated on rising above politics in the pursuit of humanitarian ends, seemed to hang in the balance.[1] The Cold War era (1947–91) presented serious challenges for the venerable Red Cross movement, as it did for the international community as a whole, but the international tensions on display in the summer of 1952 proved to be only a slight annoyance to the CRCS compared to the major domestic challenges it faced after 1945.

On the surface, the two-and-a-half decades of Canadian economic prosperity that immediately followed the Second World War brought about an interlude of serene domestic equilibrium for the society. CRCS annual reports, campaign literature, and budgets took on a sameness during these years, with core areas of peacetime programming like water safety, blood transfusion, Junior Red Cross, and disaster services giving an initial impression of steady expansion and achievement. But not far below the surface the CRCS – like Canadian society – was changing. The CRCS began to rely more and more on paid professionals, faced financial strains that required new relationships with government, and struggled to ensure its own long-term survival. Between 1946 and 1970 the society transformed, often painfully, into the modern voluntary-humanitarian organization it would be through the remainder of the twentieth century. It was a transformation deeply marked by both the optimism and the angst of Canada's 1950s and 1960s.

Postwar Prosperity?

The reluctance to demobilize and sense of possibility that led the CRCS of 1918 to enter peacetime public health work once again animated the society in 1945–46. In an address to the annual meeting of the Alberta Division in March 1946, CRCS national commissioner Dr Frederick Routley urged the society's "great army" of nearly 3 million junior and senior wartime members to continue working together for a common goal. Canadians' health needs had been starkly highlighted in a national report submitted to the Rowell-Sirois Commission of 1939, and now that the war was over, it was time to address those needs. Routley believed the new era of peace offered "a far better work of reconstruction, of improvement of health, of working for the betterment of [Canadians] and their greater happiness" if everyone did their part.[2] The challenge of the immediate postwar decades would be to translate such idealism into action. Would Canadians dig in or drift away?

The society's dramatic decline in membership and financial support after the First World War shaped its approach to its 1945–46 peacetime transition. In hopes that Canadians' interest in the Red Cross would not be "allowed to lapse in the way it did after the last war," former Central Council chairman Jackson Dodds urged the Quebec Division to make a concerted effort "to enlist the services of men and women in the younger age bracket, particularly those who have demonstrated administrative ability, possibly in the services during the war." This concern with recruiting and retaining a younger age group would resurface more dramatically during the 1960s. Dodds also hoped that Quebec Division's wartime success in crossing the province's linguistic and religious divides could be sustained.[3] Others had their own ideas on how to retain volunteers. The chair of the national Women's Work Committee, Mrs Clara McEachren, believed that "any voluntary organization for the most part must depend for its support on the women" and stressed the urgency of finding new outlets for women's needlework. Some leaders advocated expanding programs already successful in one region – for example, the Sick Room Supplies Loan Service, which loaned items like crutches for short-term home use. Others looked to fill gaps in existing services, through a breast milk bank, for instance.[4] Collectively, CRCS leaders seem to have been seeking a "magic bullet": one single program that would keep small branches active, attract donors and volunteers, and make a valuable contribution to Canadians' health and welfare.

The postwar scramble to find this magic bullet belied the fact that the society (like the federal government) had begun preparing for peacetime well before the war ended. Spurred into action by a May 1943 invitation to join the British Red Cross in Commonwealth-wide postwar reconstruction discussions, the CRCS began its own planning in September of that year. At its inaugural meeting, the CRCS Postwar Planning Committee established two central principles that underscore the society's ever-increasing sense of independence and desire to pursue its own path: first, "contributions made by the Canadian Red Cross Society must be distinctly designated as such" even if pursued in cooperation with British relief plans; second, the CRCS would take the lead in its own postwar planning.[5] Yet, over the course of 1944, the winds of ambiguity surrounding Canada's shifting relationships with Britain and the United States buffeted this initial determination to pursue a distinctly Canadian path in postwar European relief. First the committee planned to pursue the work "on an Empire basis," then wanted to cooperate with the new United Nations Relief and Rehabilitation Administration (UNRRA), then decided to withdraw from UNRRA in favour of independent relief work through the League of Red Cross Societies. Committee members argued that "a much larger field of work would be open to the Red Cross outside UNRRA, through the League," and leaned heavily on the example of the American Red Cross, which refused to be submerged into the general body of UNRRA workers.[6] As 1944 gave way to 1945, the committee changed focus and directed its full attention to domestic planning. Suggestions received from divisions and local branches ranged from mental health work to the teaching of dressmaking. The committee's final recommendations to Central Council, presented in early May 1945, outlined an ambitious postwar program that drew on the society's prewar and wartime strengths as well as venturing into new fields. In addition to the society's existing public health work the committee envisioned new programs in water safety and nutrition; the continuation of the CRC Corps, the Blood Donor Service, and recreational handicraft work with sick and wounded veterans; transatlantic CRC Corps escort service for war brides and children; and (in a shift away from using community halls, homes, and rental premises), the establishment of permanent bricks-and-mortar Red Cross branches across Canada, to serve as hubs for local activities.[7]

Mindful of the challenges of the 1920s, Jackson Dodds wrote to Philip Fisher of the Canadian Welfare Council in October 1945 to reassure him that the CRCS intended to "continue to be pioneers in some fields and help in others, but not by 'butting in' or trying to 'hog' projects." He offered Quebec Division's new school lunch project in Montreal's Rosemount district as an example of the society demonstrating the worth of specific endeavours prior to handing them over to "some other proper body."[8] Diverse, regionally created postwar initiatives like the Rosemount school lunches reveal that the standards of living and availability of health care in Canada continued to vary widely – not only by province but also along the urban-rural divide. They also highlight the society's postwar return to a more decentralized, provincially autonomous manner of functioning.

The ultimate success or failure of the new peacetime program rested on the shoulders of the society's volunteer workers and donors. Adult CRCS membership numbers reported between 1945 and 1964 suggest fairly steady peacetime growth: after an initial postwar decline from more than two million members in 1945 to one million by 1948, membership increased steadily, hitting a postwar high in 1964 of 1.8 million (13.9 percent of the 1961 adult population). However, this impression does not survive scrutiny. Instead of submitting concrete figures as in former years, more and more provincial divisions began submitting rounded-off (and often unchanging) estimates, so that the 1.8 million of 1964 could represent a certain amount of wishful thinking. No adult membership numbers were reported at all as of 1965.[9] And even if they were accurate, membership numbers usually indicated only the number of people who made a minimum one-dollar contribution to a financial campaign. Saskatchewan Division's 1964 report that it had 5,500 active *volunteers* – as compared to its estimated 115,000 *members* – shows that membership alone was a poor indicator of more active voluntary engagement.[10]

The number of CRCS branches across Canada tells a more revealing story: the 2,499 branches of 1945 declined to 1,307 by 1950, then to 1,152 by 1960, and finally to 935 by 1970. The most precipitous drop occurred at the end of the Second World War, with 539 branches closing in 1946 alone – a sign of many Canadians' eagerness to leave the war behind. The steady decline in branch numbers also shows that the society failed in its search for a magic bullet program: Canadians remained less compelled by peacetime domestic public health than by wartime patriotism and compassion for citizen-soldiers.[11] However, despite losing both branches and supporters in the postwar period, the society demonstrably grew in one respect: it gained a tenth provincial division in 1950, after Newfoundlanders narrowly voted to join Canadian Confederation in 1949. Newfoundlanders had no peacetime Red Cross history before 1947 (when they established a branch of the British Red Cross Society), but members of the Newfoundland Women's Patriotic Association had sewn for the BRCS during the First World War, and both the Canadian and American Red Cross societies were active on the island in support of their countries' servicemen during the Second World War. Red Cross responsiveness to local and regional public health needs promised to make it a useful tool (joining the famous Grenfell Mission and other pre-Confederation voluntary and government initiatives) in addressing some of the many nutritional shortfalls and deficiencies in health care provision facing outport Newfoundlanders.[12]

Although many wartime volunteers carried on into the postwar period, death or retirement produced significant personnel turnover within the ranks of CRCS leadership in the later 1940s. Adelaide Plumptre – referred to by Dr Routley as "one of the greatest of all Canadian Red Cross workers" – was incapacitated by a serious illness in 1944, and did not recover prior to her death in 1948.[13] Fred Routley retired from his position as national commissioner in 1947 and died in 1951. Other longtime leaders at the local, provincial, and national levels similarly left the society through death or retirement in this period. The postwar decades would be shaped by a new cohort for whom either the heady days of the Second World War or the postwar period itself constituted their formative Red Cross experience. Dr Routley's post-retirement remarks to Central Council in October 1948 highlight the importance of this generational change. "Red Cross has been a crusade with me," he told the assembled councillors. "Those of us who are not in Red Cross as a crusade ought to step out."[14] Routley had taken to heart the health crusade imagery of the interwar years, and he seems to have sensed a weakening of this understanding of the CRCS by mid-century. The humanitarian idealism and broad, flexible mandate of the CRCS would continue to inspire many future donors, volunteers, and staff, but Dr Routley, like Mrs Plumptre, represented a particular kind of early twentieth-century volunteer who took the Red Cross message to heart and saw it not as a mere charity, but as a calling. The second half of the century would see a long, slow shift away from this model, as the ethos of associational life and community service declined and modern business practices and professionalization reoriented how the organization worked. In the long term, Routley's plea for a renewal of the passion he and others had felt for the Red Cross crusade in the interwar years could not compete with the impact of changing social values and an altered charitable landscape.

Among these changes were new peacetime roles for National Headquarters and a growing reliance on paid professionals – for instance, the proliferation of new national director positions. One by one, the volunteer committees responsible for major nationwide programs lobbied for paid directors who could offer much-needed full-time professional support and interprovincial coordination to their programs. Occasional attempts to save money by cutting such positions failed to check the overall trend. The provinces followed suit: Nova Scotia Division's regular staff members reportedly "increased 20-fold" between 1945 and 1975.[15]

Most crucially, the role of (paid) national commissioner gained new importance and influence after 1945. Leading the CRCS had become a full-time job, and during the interwar years many functions once played by the president shifted to the full-time, paid national commissioner. The national commissioner took direction from the society's volunteer officers and councillors, but held significant authority in supervising the society's daily affairs, advised the provincial commissioners, and after 1945 largely replaced the chairs of the Executive Committee and Central Council as the public face of the society. He also provided crucial continuity and institutional memory. Between 1946 and 1970 the Executive Committee was chaired by thirteen men, and Central Council by sixteen, while only four men worked as national commissioner in the same period: Dr Routley to 1947; Dr W. Stuart Stanbury, 1948–62 (cut off by his untimely death from a heart attack); acting commissioner Dr J.T. Phair, 1962–63; and Major-General A.E. Wrinch, 1963–75. Wrinch's brisk military efficiency made him an excellent national commissioner, but the defining figure of the postwar CRCS was unquestionably his predecessor Dr Stanbury, described in 1963 by Dr Phair as a man "who epitomized Red Cross both nationally and internationally."[16] As chief architect of the society's free blood transfusion service and tireless champion of greater CRCS engagement on the international stage, Dr Stanbury became the third major figure (after Dr Ryerson and Mrs Plumptre) to place his unmistakable stamp on the entire CRCS.

After being lauded in wartime media, ordinary branch-level CRCS volunteers largely disappear from the historical record after 1945, making it difficult to say with any precision who they were. National and provincial CRCS leaders, on the other hand, can at least be sketched in some measure. The CRCS hierarchy did not reflect Canada's growing postwar ethnic diversity: leaders at both the provincial and national levels remained overwhelmingly Anglo-Celtic up to 1970. The society did, however, capitalize on its wartime success in francophone Quebec by including at least one francophone among the national officers from 1945 to 1970.[17]

Earlier debates around truly "nationalizing" the national CRCS resolved themselves by 1945, so that both Central Council and the Executive Committee included representatives of each province at all times. Yet the country's vast geography remained a challenge, and a Toronto-based national Sub-Executive Committee arose during the Second World

War to handle decisions requiring a quick response or regular monitoring. At the same time, the national commissioner and increasing numbers of national program directors took more and more of the day-to-day responsibilities upon themselves. The increased regional representation in the society's governing bodies, therefore, had less impact than its advocates had hoped.[18]

The CRCS drew many of its mid-twentieth-century leaders from the same professions it had at the end of the nineteenth century, suggesting a continuing affinity among these groups for the society's work, and perhaps also the influence of professional networks in attracting new leaders. Among those leaders whose professions can be traced, military men, physicians, surgeons, nurses, lawyers, judges, businessmen, and accountants feature prominently. After 1945 medical professionals tended to fill medically or scientifically related advisory roles, while the top executive positions went to businessmen, lawyers, and accountants. Even among volunteer leaders, professionalization was at work.[19]

From 1945 to 1970 the highest ranks of CRCS leadership remained largely a boys' club. The internal gender dynamics are difficult to assess, but a few indicators suggest that women temporarily lost status in the national society after the Second World War. Historians Ruth Pierson, Veronica Strong-Boag, and Jennifer Stephen have convincingly shown that there was intense pressure on women to give up their wartime jobs and other gains in favour of building a domestic paradise in the suburbs after 1945. Within this broader context, the postwar decline in women's Red Cross engagement is unsurprising. Women may also have begun to join other organizations instead of the CRCS, leading to an overall decline in women volunteers eligible for leadership positions.[20] However, the trend began even before the war. Women's vital contributions during the South African War and the First World War helped them break into the closed club of national CRCS leadership, but their progress stalled during the interwar years, despite wider women's rights achievements including (partial) federal voting rights in 1918 and legal "personhood" in 1929.[21] Tracking women's proportional representation on Central Council, the Executive Committee, and among the national officers further reveals that women had a stronger voice at the national level of the CRCS in the early 1930s and again during the Second World War than they did in 1970. They were best represented on Central

Council (elected as provincial representatives), but even there women members constituted on average less than 15 percent of Central Council through the 1960s, a full 10 percent less than in the early 1920s.[22]

The same trend appears among the society's annual honourees. Beginning in 1930, the CRCS awarded honorary counsellorships for outstanding national service, and honorary memberships for outstanding provincial service, awarding 921 provincial awards and sixty-one national awards between 1930 and 1970. Overall, 51.5 percent of provincial awards went to women, but the proportion declined decade by decade: from a high of 75 percent in the 1930s (which included both First World War and interwar service) to only 34 percent during the 1960s. Of the sixty-one national honourees, only sixteen were women (26 percent); thirteen were honoured in the 1930s and 1940s, and only three in the 1950s and 1960s.[23] Two explanations seem equally plausible: the Baby Boom and slow but steady increase of women working in paid employment may have decreased the number of women able to give "outstanding" amounts of voluntary service; or perhaps as the society became more heavily influenced by modern business practices, women's contributions through domestic work and hands-on service lost status compared to the white collar exertions of finance committees.

Although the provincial divisions offered women greater access to leadership positions, there too they faced glass ceilings. Between 1945 and 1970 women generally filled from one-eighth to one-quarter of the officer positions in provincial divisions, being consistently best represented in Nova Scotia and worst represented in Quebec, but were overwhelmingly relegated to vice president or honorary secretary. Only Manitoba, Saskatchewan, and Nova Scotia ever (briefly) had a woman as president, and the sole female provincial commissioner was Prince Edward Island's formidable Miss Iphegenie Arsenault, a Summerside native who held the position for thirty-four years and worked for the CRCS in either a voluntary or paid capacity for seventy years. The provincial committees usually chaired by women constituted a "pink collar ghetto" embracing the CRC Corps, nursing, women's work, homemakers, veterans and hospital visiting, voluntary services, or some aspect of awards and uniforms.[24]

At the local level, the exact proportion of female to male volunteers in mixed-gender CRCS programs like water safety, disaster services, or the blood transfusion service is impossible to pin down in the absence of records, but the continuous activity from 1945 to 1970 of local women's work committees, hospital visitors (traditionally gendered female), and CRC Corps detachments shows that women remained crucial contributors to the society's programs and services. Collectively, these indicators suggest that in the postwar period the CRCS, while still owing a massive debt to female voluntary labour, publicly honoured their labour less often and offered them access to positions of authority in ways every bit as constrained by prevailing gender roles as in previous generations.

Money stood alongside volunteers as the other key to success for the postwar Canadian Red Cross. The society's interwar experience had demonstrated the folly of handing over to others money it might find difficult to replace, so it did not replicate its early 1920s grants to other Canadian public health organizations. But neither could the CRCS use its leftover wartime funds on peacetime public health activities: unlike its First World War predecessor, the War Charities Act of 1939 included a stipulation that funds raised through wartime appeals must be used for war-related purposes. The society therefore spent its remaining war chest on overseas relief and Canadian veterans through 1949,[25] and had to rely on new fundraising to launch its ambitious new peacetime program.

The success of the society's wartime campaigns fundamentally altered its approach to raising money. Every year from 1947 to 1970 the society held a major national whirlwind campaign, still piggybacking on ARC efforts south of the border by designating March as "Red Cross Month." But unlike the consistently oversubscribed wartime campaigns, postwar campaigns fell short of their objectives in twenty of twenty-three years. Since the under-subscribed campaigns still reached, on average, 95 percent of their goal, the society managed to cover the rest of its expenses through interest from small endowments, modest fees for a few services (such as those at outpost hospitals), government grants, and regular budget trimming. The society's consistent failure to meet its campaign objectives (which from 1952 onward were carefully calculated to cover its projected expenses), and the constantly rising costs of providing CRCS services caused serious and ongoing concern. Although the society raised more money over the years in simple terms ($7.15 million in 1969 versus $5.7 million in 1959 or $4.65 million in 1949), by 1969 it also relied far more heavily on off-setting revenue (grants, fees, and re-imbursements) and its own reserve funds. Of the $20.4 million spent by the society in 1970, for example, only $7.1 million came from that year's campaign receipts. When compared to the same figures for 1949, the difference is striking: 60 percent donation-funded in 1949, versus 35 percent in 1970. The largest portion of off-setting revenue in 1970 came from the federal and provincial governments: roughly $6 million for the technical costs of the CRCS Blood Transfusion Service (BTS). Governments began contributing to various CRCS efforts during the South African War, and more consistently during the interwar years, but did not contribute any funding toward BTS technical costs until the end of the 1950s.[26]

Shifts in how the society marketed itself to raise money each year reveal changes in both CRCS perceptions of Canadians' motivations for giving, and the tactics it used to mobilize them. The society's peacetime record after 1918 saved it from having to justify its existence after 1945, so it initially traded on its war work and simply reminded Canadians of what else it did. From 1946 to 1949 the society's March campaign ads featured the familiar "Red Cross nurse" with outstretched hand appealing to Canadians, usually reminding them that "The Work of Mercy Never Ends." Publicity materials listed the society's wide range of public health services at home and postwar relief work in Europe. The proposed nationwide blood system appeared often, its promise to "serve Canadians coast-to-coast" as a "national life-saving system" likely finding traction among Canadians for whom a decade and a half of Depression and war had created an openness to greater collective action in pursuit of a "more stable and equitable society."[27]

In 1950 the CRCS jettisoned all images and slogans evocative of wartime, but the new approach did not initially take hold in the public mind. In 1953 an Ontario Division leader observed that "despite some very clever and constant publicity, the public still associates Red Cross with war time activity." By the middle of the decade, however, the society had firmly committed to new ways of thinking about and promoting the Canadian Red Cross.[28] Phrases like "people helping people" and "whenever and wherever help is needed" expressed a new set of universalist values in the society. CRCS work had traditionally been grounded in so-called "care values," which assumed that some citizens were more vulnerable than others – sick and wounded soldiers, for instance – and made them the objects of its work. But by the 1950s, as Shirley Tillotson points out, "universalist values were in the ascendant." The CRCS now presented itself as offering a full range of programs that served Canadians "of all ages and in all walks of life" across the country[29] – not unlike the new family allowance and old age pension programs of the postwar Canadian welfare state. The society's 1950s "Across the Street, Across the Nation, Across the World" slogan also signalled its move onto the international Red Cross stage, extending its universalism beyond Canada. Significantly, the word "humanitarian" (previously implied but rarely stated) first began appearing in CRCS publicity on a regular basis during the late 1950s, often in the context of "humanitarian obligation."[30]

A second group of CRCS slogans attempted to address fundraising shortfalls and declining numbers of volunteers by expanding on the nature of voluntary work and charitable giving. "Everyone helps and everyone benefits" suggested that because the CRCS served all Canadians, all Canadians should be contributing to the CRCS – a kind of universalism of contribution. Meanwhile, "You Serve by Giving," and "Red Cross Serves for You" simultaneously suggested that money was an acceptable substitute for labour and harkened back to the Red Cross's wartime function of extending a citizen's reach beyond his or her community. In the words of a December 1953 report, the society "quietly and competently did what you would have done yourself, had you been there."[31]

These basic concepts remained staples of national CRCS publicity and campaign appeals through the 1960s, perhaps best summarized by the CRCS's 1967 French-language slogan, "C'est vous, c'est moi, c'est nous tous" – It's you, it's me, it's all of us. Donor self-interest joined this universalism after 1960, in slogans like "You help yourself and you help others when you help the Red Cross." Two major milestones also produced a tendency to look backward and forward at the same time: the society's fiftieth anniversary of incorporation (1959), and Canada's centennial year (1967). CRCS leaders spoke of the society having kept pace with a growing, changing Canada, while other supporters wrote of the Red Cross as "a vital part of our way of life" or praised the efforts of volunteers who pursued "the traditional work of the Red Cross in a modern setting."[32]

The society's new articulation of itself as an explicitly humanitarian organization received a boost during the mid-1960s when the International Red Cross formally adopted its Seven Fundamental Principles: humanity, impartiality, neutrality, independence, voluntary service, unity, and universality.[33] As the ideological linchpin of CRCS work, the 1919 mandate to improve health, prevent disease, and mitigate suffering gave way after 1965 to the Seven Fundamental Principles. Although the fundamental principles represented *ways* of working, rather than specific *fields* of work, they nonetheless retained the earlier three-point mandate's broadly empowering nature. With the cause of humanity as its purpose, the CRCS could justify future involvement in diverse fields at home and abroad.

Still, no campaign slogan, no matter how clever, could make post-1945 fundraising easy. The CRCS had always existed within a context of competing voluntary organizations and charities, but the postwar period saw the emergence of formidable new competition. International humanitarian aid organizations like CARE, World Vision, and Oxfam Canada emerged to claim a share of overseas relief and rehabilitation work.[34] At home, "dread disease" charities tapped into Canadians' fears for their own and their loved ones' health, and during the 1950s the annual fundraising calendar filled up with campaigns for the Canadian Cancer Society, the Canadian Arthritis and Rheumatism Society, the Heart and Stroke Foundation of Canada, the Canadian Diabetes Association, and more.[35] North Americans enthusiastically joined associations in the 1950s and 1960s,[36] but with so many new competitors for labour and funds, older voluntary organizations like the Red Cross felt the pinch.

The pressure of fundraising competition forced the society to finally come to terms with federated fundraising. Although charity survived the Second World War to become, in Shirley Tillotson's words, "part of the welfare state rather than its alternative," the pressure to streamline charitable fundraising only grew after 1945. In 1939 eleven Canadian cities undertook federated fundraising; by 1948 that number had grown to forty-seven.[37] The society began the postwar years committed to resisting the trend, offering the same arguments it had raised in wartime about international obligations, a loss of identity, and lower campaign returns, plus a new argument borrowed from the dread disease charities: an independent campaign raised not only money but also public awareness and volunteer support. "We have a good story, and we must be able to tell it," argued CRCS National Campaign Committee Chair Bruce Shaw in 1955.[38] But federated fundraising had momentum in the postwar years, and for every small Red Cross branch that agreed to follow national policy and drop out of a joint appeal, another joined. These exceptions to the rule gave the Community Chest movement a stick with which to beat other Red Cross branches when they refused to join their local federated appeal. In May 1956, after a year in which united appeal organizers in Vancouver and Toronto specifically targeted the CRCS with pressure tactics, the ramparts crumbled at last. The society's enviable solo fundraising record could not overcome the weight of its declining number of branches, its growing campaign shortfalls, an increasingly crowded charitable field, and a public perception that the new, tax-funded social services of the postwar welfare state offered a fair and efficient alternative.[39] After a period of institutional soul-searching, the society came to the belated realization that "consolidation was a trend of the times" and it was better to join from a position of relative strength than be forced in later, when it might be impossible to negotiate any privileges. Branches were now *allowed* to join united appeals, but not *encouraged* to do so. And the terms on which they were to join included the same demands for organizational autonomy, decision-making authority, and freedom to spend as had been forced on the CUARF at the end of the Second World War. Luckily, many federated appeals had begun offering an "open door" policy in 1948 that allowed precisely these sorts of flexible terms.[40]

The CRCS entered the postwar period riding a wave of public support and, in historian John F. Hutchinson's view, "an implicit belief that the Red Cross was beyond criticism." Hutchinson's postwar Toronto boyhood included singing at the Sunnybrook Red Cross lodge, playing the Junior Red Cross health game, and taking Red Cross swimming lessons in the summer – common childhood experiences, he argued, which led his generation to give the society little conscious or critical thought: "One knew that the Red Cross existed and that its existence was a good thing, but one took it and its goodness entirely for granted." (It was precisely this kind of unthinking support for the CRCS that irked social worker Charlotte Whitton during the late 1930s.) However, Hutchinson noted that like most of his generation, his adult Red Cross involvement was limited to occasional blood donations.[41] The very success of the blood transfusion service became a problem for the society in the postwar period: not only did it gobble up CRCS funds but it also seemed to detract from some Canadians' financial support for the Red Cross. In a 1965 submission to the federal Advisory Committee on Hospital Insurance and Diagnostic Services, the society explained, "A substantial number of people say, 'I give my blood to the Red Cross and my money to … '" Federated appeals could not completely overcome this problem. Thus, after 1945 the society faced declining adult membership, financial strains, and a blood service that seemed to compete with the larger society itself. The CRCS may have been a "sacred cow" in postwar Canadian society, as Hutchinson argues, but that status by no means assured it untroubled prosperity.[42]

Something Old, Something New: The CRCS at Home

The postwar public health program of the Canadian Red Cross Society played out across Canada against this backdrop of institutional struggle. Many of the society's interwar-era programs had quietly carried on during the Second World War, but regained prominence in the postwar period. Other postwar programs grew out of Second World War initiatives, and only one was a completely new creation. Collectively, they contributed to the health and welfare of Canadians in diverse contexts, while asserting that volunteers and charity still had a place (albeit a changing one) in a postwar landscape of professionals and the welfare state.

Some postwar programs offered humble forms of service in quiet ways, drawing little attention. The CRC Corps, for instance, remained visually distinctive in uniform, but now channelled its members' service into regular Red Cross programs. Local Women's Work committees produced supplies for international relief. The interwar home nursing classes carried on, now linked to the society's wartime first aid instruction program as two components of Cold War civil defence preparation. The Visiting

Homemaker Service flourished in British Columbia, Nova Scotia, and Ontario divisions, where government funding propelled it forward.[43] The Canadian government's determination to do better by its veterans than after the First World War led to the creation of a generous package of training, education, health, and home-buying entitlements,[44] but the CRCS retained a role in veteran care through hospital visiting, Red Cross lodges, therapeutic arts and crafts work, and a film service.

The society continued to provide outpost hospitals and nursing stations in rural and remote areas, but steadily relinquished them – and its remaining Crippled Children's Hospitals – during this period. The phase-out took place gradually and without significant resistance in the CRCS because outposts had always been designed as temporary measures. The introduction of publicly funded hospital insurance (first in Saskatchewan in 1948, then federally in 1957) seems to have sped up the transfer of most outposts to either community or provincial hands, or their replacement by new provincial facilities. In some places the CRCS continued to operate outposts even after it ceased to pay for them: the society had twenty-seven outposts in five provinces still under its care at the end of 1970. Despite the replacement of dogsleds with helicopters, outpost nurses still braved long treks to remote homes in order to care for their patients.[45]

The Junior Red Cross boomed during the 1950s and early 1960s. After a brief postwar dip, Junior membership (which, unlike adult membership, was closely tracked) exceeded its wartime heights in 1949 – just as the first Baby Boomers entered elementary school. The Baby Boom fuelled growth until 1964, but membership slowly declined thereafter, as Boomers reached school-leaving age. Postwar childhood remained a prime site for adult nation-building efforts, and the program's democratic format, emphasis on good health and service to the community, and association with wartime patriotism likely made it attractive to adults concerned with ensuring that young Canadians avoided the era's perceived dangers of communism and juvenile delinquency.[46]

CRCS disaster relief – previously an uncoordinated, locally driven activity – became a growth area during the Second World War, with emergency response plans and interagency cooperation fuelled by fears of enemy sabotage, bombing, and invasion. Happily, no major disasters or invasions occurred, and the CRCS dissolved its national advisory com-

mittee on disaster relief in 1945. Two years later, the national committee was revived – possibly as a response to the emerging Cold War threat
of the Soviet Union, or perhaps inspired by the way disaster relief helped
the American Red Cross retain public support in peacetime. A series of
major floods and fires in 1948 proved the need for national advice, coordination, and large-scale planning,[47] and over the course of the 1950s
disaster services became a significant component of CRCS postwar work.
Local CRCS branches responded to hundreds of single house fires, while
river flooding, tidal waves, tornados, and forest fires occupied volunteers across regions. Manitoba's massive Red River Flood of spring 1950
provoked the society's largest peacetime disaster response effort up to
1970, and the society's responses to Hurricane Hazel (which devastated
Toronto on 15 October 1954) and the rescue efforts following Nova
Scotia's Springhill Mine Disasters of 1956 and 1958 similarly garnered
national attention, support, and enthusiastic volunteers for CRCS Disaster Services, making it one of the society's higher-profile activities.
Working in conjunction with the Canadian army and other relief agencies, the CRCS established an accepted role for itself in registering, feeding, clothing, sheltering, and providing medical care for both evacuees
and rescue workers.[48]

After this enthusiastic beginning, the society's attitude toward its disaster services took a sharp turn in the 1960s. Where 1950s reports
proudly trumpeted the thousands of individuals helped by the CRCS,
1960s reports celebrated the *decreased* numbers who received aid. The
culprit: the society's financial problems. CRCS leaders used the familiar
rhetoric of trying to avoid duplication and overlapping, bolstered by a
new theme of state responsibility to support "persons in need, whatever
the cause," but the real bottom line was financial. The society remained
committed to offering its expertise and voluntary service in disasters,
but seized on the expanding range of municipal and provincial government social welfare provisions as a means of reducing the money it spent
on emergency relief. Since state agencies had money to spend on disaster assistance, there was no good reason to use scarce CRCS resources
that could be used by other programs.[49]

The society's continuation or expansion of these older programs after
1945 arose out of a conviction that they met important needs and filled
gaps in existing public health provisions. At the same time, the society's

search for a magic bullet program to keep the CRCS vital and its volunteers engaged joined its organizational ethos of promoting health and
saving lives to produce two new initiatives. These two programs, more
than any others, would imprint the CRCS in the minds of postwar Canadians: Swimming and Water Safety, and the nationwide free Blood
Transfusion Service (BTS).

The Swimming and Water Safety program responded to the steady
growth in popularity of water-based recreation over the first half of the
twentieth century. Around the turn of the century, transportation developments within and from urban areas helped city dwellers get to wa-
terfronts and new indoor YMCA pools more easily, while small craft
sailing became popular with segments of the growing middle class. But,
as the work of historians Nancy Bouchier and Ken Cruikshank shows,
late nineteenth- and early twentieth-century public debates about swimming places primarily revolved around finding unpolluted places where
citizens – especially children – could enjoy water and fresh air in a respectable context. The possibility of drowning rarely surfaced.[50] Post-
Second World War prosperity then increased many Canadians' leisure
time and disposable income, prompting a 1950s surge of pool construction and a spike in small craft sales and waterway use. At the same
time, the Baby Boom increased the number of children and teenagers
looking to cool off in the summer heat. With earlier moral concerns
now settled and water-based recreation more popular than ever, the
issue of drowning finally came to the fore after 1945. During the late
1940s, an average of 1,000 Canadians drowned each year (compared
to 1,600 deaths by automobile accident), and only an estimated one in
ten Canadians knew how to swim. Even fewer knew rudimentary life-
saving techniques.[51]

The obvious choice to address this deficiency was the Royal Life
Saving Society (RLSS), which awarded its first Bronze Medallion in
1896, the year the CRCS was created. But while the Red Cross grew and
evolved after 1896, the RLSS remained a small organization dedicated
solely to teaching lifesaving.[52] In 1945, Ontario RLSS representatives approached CRCS leaders with the idea of a Red Cross water safety program: the CRCS network of branches in small communities gave it access
to citizens neither the RLSS nor the urban YMCA/YWCA could reach.
Seeing a way to keep small CRCS branches alive, and encouraged by the

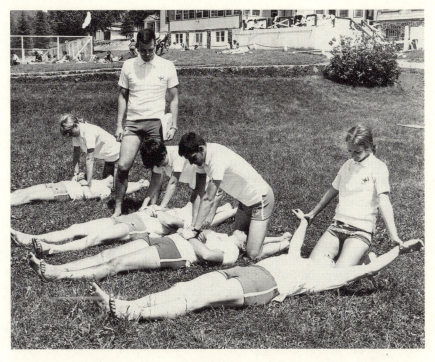

Figure 6.1

Eight teenagers practise rescue and resuscitation techniques under the watchful eye
of a Red Cross swimming instructor, on the lawn beside a public pool. The teens'
matching Red Cross outfits suggest they may be instructors-in-training.

successful American Red Cross water safety program, the CRCS agreed
to focus on swimming instruction and instructor training, while the RLSS
would continue to teach lifesaving. The CRCS planned to train instructors at its own expense, then send them back to their communities to
offer free swimming lessons that emphasized safe recreation.[53]

The new program dramatically increased the availability of swimming
instruction across the country and led to the first efforts to standardize
all instruction and examinations across Canada.[54] The program initially
functioned as designed, and within two years of the national launch the
society had trained 2,158 instructors who had gone on to provide free
lessons for nearly 43,000 children and youth. Small communities were
particularly receptive, but universities, schools, service clubs, church
groups, summer camps, and other community organizations also offered

various forms of endorsement and support. Red Cross-trained instructors gave lessons in pools, rivers, millponds, on the radio, and even in a grain wagon lined with canvas. Publicity images showed male and female instructors and pupils in roughly equal proportion, making it clear that this program was aimed at a population defined by age group (children and youth), rather than gender.[55]

Complications clouded this sunny picture by the early 1950s. Not all Red Cross-trained instructors were willing to offer lessons for free, or at all, and the society could not compel them to do so. Some enthusiastic local branches began paying to rent pools for lessons. Provincial divisions appointed directors to promote and coordinate the program in their regions, and between paid staff, instructor training, badges for successful pupils, and publicity for Water Safety Week, costs quickly mounted. Meanwhile, in larger urban areas where the YMCA and RLSS offered their own swimming or lifesaving programs, charges of duplication and overlapping sometimes led to friction with the other agencies, or with potential donors at campaign time.[56] Tensions especially grew between the CRCS and a reorganized, expanded RLSS after 1960: the RLSS claimed a much longer history of lifesaving work, but the CRCS had become the country's leader in swimming education since 1945. In 1963 the two agencies began negotiating an agreement delineating their specific spheres of work, but it took five years to overcome the distrust and organizational pride on both sides. The eventual 1968 agreement determined that the CRCS would teach swimming in a series of graded levels from basic safety to more advanced skills; the RLSS would then teach experienced swimmers more advanced lifesaving skills; and, finally, the CRCS would teach swimmers with lifesaving certification how to be instructors. The names of both organizations would appear on all certifications. With some minor tweaking, this arrangement remained intact for the rest of the twentieth century, in time giving birth to the National Lifeguard Service and bringing the CRCS into the lives of tens of thousands of children and youth each year.[57]

Swimming and Water Safety made a valuable and well-received contribution to postwar Canada, but ultimately took a backseat to the society's other major new initiative after 1945: the nationwide Blood Transfusion Service. No program demonstrates the society's early postwar ambition or subsequent reliance on the welfare state better than this

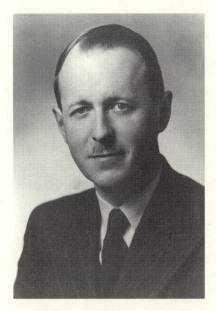

Figure 6.2
Dr W. Stuart Stanbury, architect of
Canada's first peacetime, nationwide free blood transfusion service.
As national commissioner, he
brought the society into sustained
international aid after 1945.

flagship postwar endeavour. The BTS grew directly out of the wartime
Blood Donor Service: Dr J.T. Phair's final task as chairman of the BDS
in October 1945 was the presentation of a report on the status of civilian blood transfusion services in Canada, based on a survey of Canadian
hospitals undertaken in 1944 by Dr W. Stuart Stanbury.

Stanbury was a thirty-nine-year-old Canadian haematologist and former University of Leeds lecturer who had served as the British Ministry
of Health's transfusion officer for northeast England since 1940, supplying much of the whole blood required by the Royal Navy, the Canadian and British armies in Europe, and air raid victims in that part of
Britain. By September 1944 the CRCS National Blood Donor Committee had ascertained (via informal questionnaire) that a clear majority of
Canadian hospitals would welcome a national peacetime blood bank
run by an agency like the Red Cross. Having secured tentative support
from the wider CRCS, a joint committee of the CRCS, the Canadian Hospital Council, and the National Research Council then sought "the best
possible" medical man to spearhead an investigation into the feasibility
of this idea. They unanimously chose Stuart Stanbury.[58]

Stanbury's survey covered more than 80 percent of the general hospital beds in Canada, and although undertaken for a specific purpose, it

was nonetheless a full and honest account of what he found. His exacting standards of personal integrity would allow nothing less. After commending the "outstanding success" of the wartime BDS, Stanbury noted the lifesaving potential and ever-widening applications of transfusion therapy in civilian medicine. In this era before publicly funded health care, Stanbury's survey revealed that blood transfusions were inaccessible to huge numbers of Canadians by virtue of either economic status or geography. Large hospitals often lacked the equipment, the trained personnel, or the blood required. Even the largest urban hospitals sometimes struggled to secure sufficient blood donors to meet their needs, while vast areas of the country had no transfusion facilities whatsoever. Meanwhile, most small hospitals and their patients simply could not afford the therapy: it cost the patient an average of $25 (equivalent to more than $300 today) for one bottle of blood, with an additional $5 to $10 service charge if the patient could not supply friends or relatives to make a replacement donation. Even having a prepaid hospital care plan did not help: none included significant coverage for blood transfusion.[59] Where individual hospitals and patients fell short, the CRCS might step in. Stanbury proposed that the CRCS create a nationwide peacetime blood transfusion service to provide blood and blood products to all Canadians – for free.

There *were* other options, and both Britain and the United States were constructing their own peacetime civilian blood systems concurrently with Canada. The United States established a mixed system of blood collection, which included voluntary donors to the American Red Cross and community blood banks, paid donors to commercial firms, and a cost to most patients who received transfusions. The League of Red Cross Societies likewise initially took it for granted that a Red Cross-run blood transfusion service would involve the exchange of money in order to make the system self-supporting. Stanbury clearly wanted to avoid this model. Conversely, Britain established a purely voluntary collection network and provided blood free of charge to patients. After significant wartime involvement by the BRCS, British blood collection was taken over by the state in 1948 with the establishment of the National Health Service.[60] While no evidence has been uncovered to suggest that the CRCS took its cues from the emerging British model, Stanbury's wartime work in British blood collection likely meant he had personal and professional ties with British colleagues as the two systems were independently being constructed. These contacts may have reinforced his own convictions on the subject of blood collection.

Canada's wartime BDS set a precedent for a blood system that relied on unpaid donors, did not charge fees to patients or hospitals, and was permanently run by a non-governmental voluntary organization. But commercially based blood collection was an equally viable option, and the fact that the CRCS did not pursue this path largely reflects the steely determination of Dr Stanbury. The CRCS commissioner's Red Cross involvement dominates the few existing biographical portraits of him to such an extent that little is known about his earlier life and formative influences. This makes it difficult to determine the origins of his beliefs about blood (or his interest in Eastern Europe, discussed in a subsequent section of this chapter). However, reading between the lines of some of his official reports, the outline of an idea emerges. To use Immanuel Kant's distinction, Dr Stanbury seems to have viewed blood as something with "dignity" rather than "value." Kant wrote that "whatever has value can be replaced by something else which is equivalent; whatever on the other hand is above value and therefore admits no equivalent has a dignity."[61] By this definition, human blood had a dignity: there was neither an adequate substitute for it, nor a non-human source from which to procure it. Since the fluid itself had dignity and the therapy possessed extraordinary healing power, Stanbury understood the act of blood donation as a fundamentally moral act. Blood "cannot, or should not, be bought and sold as a commercial commodity," he wrote in 1945, "for it represents the free gift of one man to another in order that life may be saved."[62] Accordingly, Stanbury designed a system that would support his vision of blood freely given and equally freely received.

The plan was ambitious, born of a heady mixture of wartime accomplishment and postwar optimism about a bright national future – and perhaps a measure of ignorance. Dr Stanbury confided to a group of colleagues in 1948 that he felt the provincial divisions "[did] not fully appreciate the magnitude of the job that [had] been undertaken."[63] The CRCS BTS proposed to supply every hospital in Canada with fresh whole blood (and dried plasma as a backup) along with sterile administration sets. Once in place, the nationwide BTS would offer every Canadian free and equal access to blood transfusion therapy – the only universal feature in an otherwise highly inequitable patchwork of health care provision across the country. Since the provinces held (and jealously guarded) constitutional jurisdiction over health matters, the federal government could not establish such a system in 1945. A national voluntary organization coming off of six years of widely supported war work, however, just might manage it.

The plan required cooperation from provincial departments of health, hospitals, the CRCS, and ordinary citizens. The provinces were asked to supply and maintain central blood depot laboratories for processing and centralized distribution; each hospital had to agree not to charge patients for the blood supplied; the CRCS would operate the whole service, providing equipment, transport, and medical, nursing, and technical personnel; Canadians, it was hoped, would voluntarily give their blood on a regular basis. Donated blood would move around the country in two directions. First, CRCS teams would collect it through mobile or permanent clinics in communities across the country, and send it to the provincial depots to be grouped and tested for communicable disease (primarily syphilis). Second, it would be sent out from the depots to the larger hospitals for use, or for further transfer to smaller hospitals. Blood would be parachuted into extremely remote locations. The BDS's wartime partner, the Connaught laboratories at the University of Toronto, would process unused whole blood into blood products – initially dried plasma, and later blood protein fractions like plasma albumin, fibrinogen, and gamma globulin. In October 1945 the CRCS Central Council adopted Stanbury's plan. Armed with public endorsements from the Canadian Medical Association and Minister of National Health and Welfare Paul Martin, the CRCS officially embarked on a significant new phase of its institutional life.[64]

The BTS would involve CRCS volunteers, staff, and branches in every province, but it would be primarily a National Headquarters responsibility. Dr Stanbury was named first national director of the BTS and although he then replaced Dr Routley as national commissioner in 1949, he remained personally active in expanding and fostering the success of the BTS. The ink was scarcely dry on the last wartime BDS reports when the first provincial unit of the new, peacetime BTS set up shop in Vancouver on 3 February 1947. The service expanded throughout Alberta later that year, and to Nova Scotia and Prince Edward Island in 1948.

The following year Ontario and Quebec got their first blood depots, and in 1950 the Manitoba and New Brunswick depots opened their doors.[65]

The steady march of BTS expansion came to a halt after the opening of the Saint John depot in January 1950, when two thorny issues became impossible to ignore. The first was active resistance by some hospitals, including those in parts of Ontario and Quebec whose large populations could not be served solely by the existing depots. Other areas that *did* want to join the BTS came up against the second problem: insufficient funds. The very success of the already established portions of the BTS hindered the completion of the national network, since they devoured CRCS funds: the BTS reportedly consumed "40 cents of every campaign dollar" by the mid-1950s.[66] Saskatchewan received its two regional depots in 1952 but a Central Council moratorium on further expansion meant that Newfoundland had to wait until 1958 and the eastern and western portions of southern Ontario until 1959. Not until the establishment of the Quebec City depot in 1961 did the CRCS consider itself to have finally achieved national coverage. Dr Stanbury's pride – and relief – in this milestone are palpable in his description of the "sixteen long and hard years, not infrequently touched with frustration and adversity" that led up to the accomplishment of the task he and the society had set themselves, a task that "sometimes seemed impossible."[67]

During those sixteen years, the landscape of health care provision in Canada changed dramatically. The first provinces to be organized for the BTS pre-dated any provincial hospital insurance or health care system beyond basic public health departments, but by the mid-1950s there were government agencies to liaise with. The records of the Ontario Hospital Services Commission provide a useful glimpse into the issues that hindered BTS expansion in Central Canada by the 1950s, and the crucial role that the state played in helping to complete Canada's purportedly non-governmental national blood system.

Even after the 1949 establishment of a Toronto depot, the BTS served only a small portion of Ontario. Population-dense southern Ontario seemed better able to supply its own blood needs without the BTS than more thinly populated areas of the country, and in Sarnia, Sudbury, Sault Ste Marie, and Toronto, powerful hospital-based blood banks refused to join the new service. They resented the loss of income that would attend a BTS monopoly.[68] On the other side of the coin, the cost of further expansion frightened the already struggling CRCS. Each new depot meant new staff salaries and transportation costs, while greater supply seemed to fuel greater demand: the new availability of blood fed surgical advances and research into new therapies. By 1950, the CRCS Budget Committee recognized that the society's "future solvency depended to a large extent on what decision was made with regard to the Blood Transfusion Service."[69] At this point BTS expansion ground to a halt.

Meanwhile, the success of Saskatchewan's experiment in provincially funded universal hospital insurance led to a federal scheme to cost-share a similar program with any interested provinces. The Ontario Hospital Services Commission (OHSC) began meeting in July 1956, just prior to the new national Hospital Insurance Act taking effect in 1957. Any arrangements to extend BTS service in Ontario now came under its jurisdiction. The first tentative CRCS-OHSC discussions in July 1957 explicitly included the possibility of federal-provincial cost sharing with the Red Cross,[70] and this new willingness on the part of the two levels of government to pay for health-related services emerged at a crucial moment for the CRCS. The BTS was simply too expensive for the CRCS to support on its own indefinitely, so by 1956 the society had three main options: abandon the whole BTS project, accept a mixed system that allowed hospital fees and payment for donations, or acquire government grants to maintain and complete the system.[71] No one voiced a fourth possibility – shutter every other CRCS program and become solely a blood transfusion agency – since that would have run counter to the international mandate of the Red Cross. Dr Stanbury went cap in hand to the federal and provincial governments that year to appeal for funding – the first such request since the creation of the BTS – and made his case, emphasizing how efficient and cost-effective the BTS was compared to hospital blood banks. Luckily, federal-provincial discussions in Ottawa in 1957–58 approved considering blood as a "biological" suitable for financial support, opening the door for a favourable response to Stanbury's appeal. Any amount of government funding for the BTS would ease the society's financial burden and facilitate the completion of the nationwide blood system.[72]

Each hold-out hospital capitulated for its own reasons, in its own time, but the advent of publicly funded health care in Canada helped break the impasse between the CRCS and the Toronto hospitals. "It is not our concern, nor is it the concern of the public," Dr Stanbury assured the CRCS Executive Committee in January 1949, "whether or not the hospitals are making money. The public is concerned, and we are concerned, that every person who requires a transfusion should receive it."[73] This principled stand kept the Toronto hospitals from joining the service until 1958 when, as part of a deal brokered by the provincial government to extend the BTS in Ontario, the CRCS finally agreed to allow the Toronto hospitals to levy up to a $5 service charge for administering blood. This concession must have been a bitter pill for Dr Stanbury since it thwarted the basic principle of a free BTS, but the timing of the concession was likely significant: government-funded Medicare was already being discussed as a likely development in the next few years, and would probably erase this type of hospital service charge. Similarly, if some of the hospitals had been concerned (like one Toronto pathologist) that the BTS was "an opening wedge for State medicine," then the introduction of hospital insurance, and then Medicare, rendered the point moot.[74]

By April 1959 the federal and provincial governments agreed, for the first time, to help pay for the BTS. This initial arrangement saw public funds cover 30 percent of the technical costs associated with the BTS (as opposed to the donor procurement costs) – a godsend at the time, but one that quickly fell short. In 1961 the society was back, requesting a dramatic increase – ideally to cover the entire technical cost of the BTS. As national commissioner, Dr Stanbury had to make the society's case before the federal-provincial Advisory Committee on Hospital Insurance and Diagnostic Services. In his brief he compared the Canadian BTS with the Australian, British, Netherlands, and American blood systems. Each was arranged differently, but all of the non-Canadian systems received more outside funding (largely from government) to cover the combined technical and donor procurement costs than did the CRCS. Stanbury's carefully compiled statistics and behind-the-scenes diplomacy won a government funding increase to 60 percent of BTS technical costs in 1962.[75] However, government officials did not passively acquiesce to the society's requests for funding, nor unquestioningly accept its claims of financial need. Over more than a decade, OHSC commissioner of finance E.P. McGavin crunched the numbers and asked probing questions about BTS efficiency, rates of hospital blood use, and the workings of the wider CRCS.[76] Some of his lines of inquiry highlight a fundamental difference in how the CRCS and the OHSC (and likely other government bodies) viewed the BTS. In the society's view, the BTS drained resources from other CRCS work; for the OHSC, the society's other work and its national administration drained resources from the BTS. The difference highlights their divergent views of what this particular element of the mixed social economy was supposed to accomplish.

The society's 1965 request for another funding increase takes on heightened significance in hindsight: for the first time, rising costs seemed to be affecting the safety and standards of the BTS. Citing a need to invest in more modern equipment, hire specialists, undertake certain research, and replace its reusable glass bottles with safer disposable plastic packs, the CRCS asked for 75 percent technical funding. It had already hired the firm of Woods, Gordon and Co. to study the BTS and recommend ways to make it better and more efficient. Rising BTS costs largely came from annual wage and salary increases across Canada, so the Woods, Gordon report's recommendations could not offer much help on that score. They did, however, help win the OHSC's support in 1967 when the society returned to ask for a further funding increase to 82.5 percent of technical costs. "It seems to me," E.P. McGavin wrote to OHSC chairman S.W. Martin, "that the Blood Transfusion Service is a service which should keep improving and there are sound reasons for leaving it in the hands of the Red Cross."[77] By 1974 the federal and provincial governments covered the entire technical costs of the BTS, but the intertwined problems of how to pay for Canadians' access to free blood and how to maintain the highest standards of safety and service were far from solved.

Paying for the BTS was only one of the challenges the new program brought with it. Some critics at large urban hospitals complained of intermittent blood shortages after joining the BTS, while others asked why the BTS had to be national. Shortages could be avoided with the benefit of greater experience; the national question Dr Stanbury met with the same logic that has motivated many Canadian projects, from prairie wheat pools to federal transfer payments: centralized collection and redistribution meant everyone had greater access to the resources they needed regardless of location, ability to pay, or rarity of blood type. Nationally standardized equipment and procedures (useful from a civil defence perspective) were a bonus.[78]

One Vancouver physician believed that without tapping into the pool of emotionally overwrought friends and family on the spot (as hospital blood banks did), the BTS would never satisfy peacetime blood requirements.[79] Determined to prove such detractors wrong, the CRCS made procuring blood donors and treating them well a primary concern after 1945. Volunteers (usually women) played a crucial role at blood donor clinics, providing refreshments, good cheer, and gratitude in hopes of making a donor's experience pleasant enough to "cope with the fear complex" and make the donor feel she or he had done "something really wonderful." The technical demands of blood donation and loss of the wartime emergency, however, meant that the BTS also required "a highly trained, disciplined and paid staff" of medical and technical personnel, and could not rely exclusively on volunteers in the same way it had during the Second World War.[80]

Simply getting donors *to* the clinic was hard work, and a combination of local and national publicity campaigns worked to transform the society's stirring wartime BDS appeals into an equally motivating peacetime equivalent. The earliest nationally supplied materials framed blood donation as a "privilege," an "opportunity," and a "personal responsibility" of only slight inconvenience to the donor, and made direct, emotional appeals on behalf of the lives that would be saved, often putting faces on the recipients through illustrations of bedridden men, women, and children receiving transfusions. J.N. Kelly, the society's public relations supervisor, concluded by 1949 that appealing to the public to give blood in order to save a life was insufficient – something further was needed. BTS publicity would evolve in many directions over the ensuing decades in search of that elusive element. Meanwhile, the basic humanitarian appeal to "give blood that others may live" remained the beating heart of BTS donor recruitment advertising.[81]

The CRCS did not struggle alone in its quest to convince Canadians to roll up their sleeves on one another's behalf: blood donor recruitment and retention challenged the ingenuity and perseverance of blood system staff and volunteers worldwide.[82] It is difficult to say why individual donors donated, but the fact that the whole system got up and running indicates that significant numbers of Canadians were in fact willing to give their blood for free even without a wartime emergency to motivate them. And as the BTS expanded its geographical reach, its hardworking volunteers

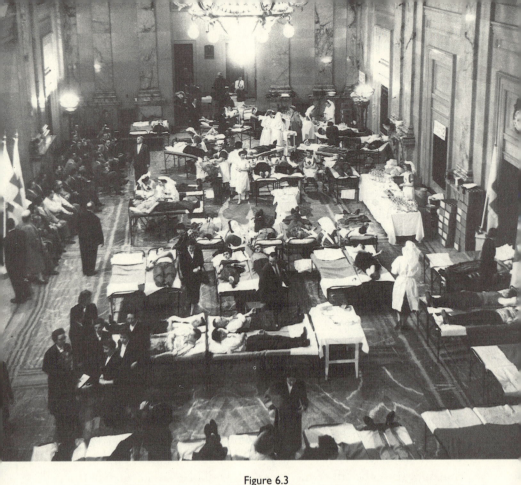

Figure 6.3
A busy New Year's Day mobile blood donor clinic in Montreal during the 1960s.
Trained nurses, Corps members, and volunteers in "Red Cross nurse" costume
(all female) attend to the largely male donors present at this moment in the multi-hour
clinic. Wooing donors like the sixty plus shown here required constant and persuasive
advertising campaigns.

also expanded its donor pool. The 261 clinics held in 1947 garnered an average 122 bottles per clinic; by 1960, 3,761 clinics averaged 170 bottles each.[83] The realization of Dr Stanbury's vision of a nationwide free blood transfusion service stands as an impressive achievement not just for the CRCS but for all Canadians. The free gift of blood from one stranger to another remains an audacious vision worth upholding, even in light of the Tainted Blood tragedy, which brought this chapter of the society's history to a close at the end of the century.

Although volunteers who worked in the BTS and other CRCS programs often became strongly attached to their specific area of Red Cross work, Dr Stanbury emphasized in 1962 that the CRCS must be a pioneer organization, identifying needs and responding to them, then turning over the work to public health authorities at appropriate times.[84] In that year Stanbury and his National Headquarters colleagues Margaret Wilson (national executive secretary) and Anna Horvath (national librarian) researched and wrote an exhaustive brief for the Royal Commission on Health Services which was then assessing the state of health care in Canada and what future role the federal government should play. The recommendations presented in the brief demonstrate that although the idea of Medicare produced uncertainty within the CRCS, the society's national leaders did not perceive it as a threat. Stanbury, Wilson, and Horvath argued that the state would "never be able to cover the whole field of public health" and claimed that this was a good thing, since voluntary organizations usefully channelled citizens' desires to help one another and in the process strengthened the entire nation. The CRCS had worked within a framework of local and provincial public health legislation, funding, and provision since the turn of the twentieth century; further expansion of that state framework would not undermine the role of the CRCS, simply redirect it. Stanbury, Wilson, and Horvath suggested that CRCS dental clinics, outpost nursing stations, and Sickroom Supply Loan Service should be entirely taken over by the state, but wished to continue its veterans' programs "as long as the Society has the means to support them" since the use of volunteers not only kept costs down but also provided a "friendly atmosphere and extra services" crucial to veteran work. Similarly, the CRCS felt "uniquely equipped to operate and administer" the BTS "based on the voluntary principle" and recommended that the present partnership continue: a CRCS-run BTS supported by "adequate financial assistance from the federal and provincial governments."[85] Perhaps encouraged by the survival of charitable social welfare agencies after the advent of family allowances, old age pensions, and other aspects of the welfare state, early 1960s Red Cross leaders had confidence in the continued relevance of voluntary health work even in the face of Medicare.

Help in a Hurry: CRCS Humanitarian Aid Goes Global

As the CRCS juggled its varied domestic work, its attitude toward the rest of the world underwent a sea change. The society had occasionally contributed to international relief work before 1945 – most notably in the wake of the First World War – but was primarily a Canadian-focused humanitarian and public health organization which took little part in the wider work of the IRC. The First World War had recreated the society as a genuinely national organization; now the post-Second World War period transformed it into a truly internationally engaged one. By 1950 new Newfoundland commissioner L.J. Harnum explained that Red Cross volunteers and donors needed "to think in terms of charity at home *and abroad*" [italics added]. The postwar years awakened in the entire CRCS what Harnum called the "Red Cross conscience" – a peacetime humanitarianism no longer limited by Canada's geographical boundaries.[86]

Historians and other scholars have yet to examine in any detail the multitude of individual postwar CRCS international relief efforts (each with a complex history), making this a field ripe for study. Unfortunately, without knowing the detailed reasons for intervention, kinds of relief provided, and challenges or successes in the field, what follows here is, of necessity, an incomplete account of CRCS international relief after 1945. Using national CRCS records and the wider context of Canada's growing postwar engagement on the world stage, this section sketches out the institutional framework within which the society's international work unfolded, in hopes that it will be useful for (and perhaps inspire) future research, and to suggest the impact of this international work on the CRCS itself.

The society's overseas humanitarian awakening took place in several phases between 1945 and 1970, jointly influenced by CRCS commissioners' interests, global developments, and the state of the society's finances. The first stage involved postwar reconstruction in the late 1940s. The society's humanitarian desire to do civilian relief work in Britain and Europe benefited from the fact that this was one of few acceptable outlets for its substantial remaining war funds (which, under the terms of the War Charities Act, had to be spent on war-related purposes). The CRCS contribution was only one component of a massive, multi-organization, and multi-government relief and rehabilitation effort, but every gift mattered to the recipients.[87] For instance, the thank-you letters and "Arbre de Noël" booklet written and illustrated by French schoolchildren from a small village in Normandy, France express both adult-prompted gratitude and childish glee in new clothes from the Red Cross. Nine-year-old Monique Nicol's effusions over a pretty pink dress and sweater are characteristic: "vive le Canada j'aime le canada et ma jolie robe rose, et mon pullover. J'envoie de gros besers et je dis merci [sic]," she wrote.[88]

By October 1946, the CRCS had purchased and sent close to $5 million worth of supplies for European relief in conjunction with the CUARF, in addition to clothing and supplies from its wartime stocks. Canadian Red Cross leaders considered this earliest foray into postwar international relief work merely another component of the society's war effort. In the same way, the wartime Red Cross Enquiry Bureau continued to accept and trace inquiries about family members. In both cases, however, temporary war work grew into an ongoing peacetime engagement. The renamed National Inquiry Bureau expanded its mandate to include disaster as well as war, and handled hundreds of cases each year after 1945.[89] At the same time, the Canadian government gave the CRCS a stiff nudge in the direction of new forms of international work. The minister of national war services asked the society to spend a further million dollars on European relief before the end of 1947, and in the autumn of the same year the Department of External Affairs encouraged the society to respond to anticipated epidemics and food shortages in newly independent and partitioned India and Pakistan.[90] The society's response (penicillin supplies) was tiny in comparison to the relief it provided to Europe in the same year, but it nonetheless represented the society's first significant postwar response to a crisis outside of Europe or North America. In doing so, it inaugurated a tradition that has come to be central to the work of the twenty-first century CRCS. It also represents an early example of what would become a growing trend in postwar Canadian foreign relations: government use of humanitarian aid as a tool for diplomacy.[91] In 1948–49 the CRCS expanded its relief work to include aid to refugees or natural disaster victims in Palestine, Lebanon, Ecuador, and the Philippines.

The transition of international work from an outgrowth of war work into an accepted, important, and permanent feature of CRCS peacetime work during the 1950s can largely be attributed to the vision and energy of new national commissioner Stuart Stanbury. In this second stage, Dr Stanbury consistently emphasized Canadians' moral obligation to care beyond their own borders, and made international work a significant part of both the commissioner's and National Headquarters' roles in the society. He also pioneered an approach he called "help in a hurry." "Unmindful of the time of day or night," recalled one colleague, "he cut red tape, shattered traditions and worked with initiative and speed to get the job done." In its memorial tribute to Dr Stanbury, the society's magazine *Despatch* asserted that the CRCS stood in the ranks of global Red Cross leaders by 1962 "because of [Stanbury's] belief that it should be in that position."[92] Two important resources facilitated this expansion into the international field: the re-purposed Junior Red Cross War Fund and local Women's Work committees. The Junior Red Cross money largely funded child-focused relief and health promotion, while Women's Work supplies translated a wartime tradition of mothering the nation's fighting men into a form of global mothering to all in need.[93] The hand of the CRCS extended ever further around the globe, embracing the wider Middle East, parts of South and Central America, the Caribbean, Japan, Southeast Asia, and North Africa by the end of the 1950s. Europe remained a focus, but increasingly only in response to natural disasters, as formerly war-devastated countries recovered thanks to Marshall Plan aid.

The third stage of the society's international engagement unfolded during the 1960s. Peacetime international work had become normalized by this time, with the vast majority of aid sent to non-European countries, but Dr Stanbury sounded a note of warning in 1960. The designated funds had been all but drained, and future international work would have to be paid for in a different way.[94] Given his personal role in advocating for greater involvement, Stanbury's unexpected death in 1962 could also have jeopardized international work, but by then the CRCS had become proud of its role on the international stage. New CRCS commissioner Major-General A.E. Wrinch took up Stanbury's mantle and made it his own. Wrinch took a personal interest in the welfare of newly decolonizing Africa, and under his guidance the CRCS divided its resources between disaster relief and longer-term infrastructure projects increasingly known as "development" work. Wrinch believed that only

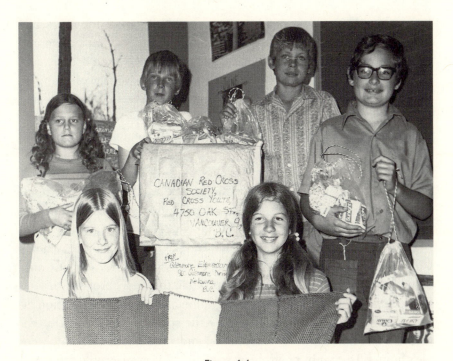

Figure 6.4

These students from Glenmore Elementary School in Kelowna, British Columbia are sending kit bags of toiletries, and a knitted quilt (like those of Second World War Juniors) to Vancouver, to be forwarded overseas for CRCS international aid work.

swift and adequate development work could stave off "an explosion, or a series of explosions, that will cause present-day difficulties [in under-developed countries] to pale into insignificance," and personally visited East and West African countries to observe the challenges involved and initiatives underway.[95] As the 1960s wore on, more and more African countries joined the list of CRCS aid recipients, and the CRCS began allocating a portion of its campaign income to the work. But it also found that high-profile humanitarian crises like the intensifying war in Vietnam or the Nigerian/Biafran conflict attracted designated donations from individuals, corporations, specially created relief funds, and other aid organizations. The Canadian government also began contributing substantially to CRCS international work: first through general donations to disaster relief campaigns; then, beginning in 1968, by providing funds for disaster relief and development through the new Canadian

International Development Agency (CIDA).[96] By 1970 the CRCS had matured into a truly international humanitarian aid organization and assumed the funding model that would prevail thereafter: a basic core of funds from the annual budget, supplemented by an ever-changing array of partnerships with other agencies, plus individual donations designated for international work.

The growth in postwar CRCS international humanitarian aid work was very much in line with the tenor of the times. Scholar John W. Holmes writes that in the postwar world, "isolation from the world's problems ... was no longer a possibility."[97] Canada's horizons broadened after the Second World War, its participation in multilateral organizations and programs, including the North Atlantic Treaty Organization (NATO), the United Nations (UN), and the British Commonwealth's Colombo Plan, bringing international events to the forefront of Canadian life. Canadians' global awareness began to quietly broaden beyond Europe in the face of increased immigration and growing population diversity in large urban areas, aided by the spread of modern telecommunications that brought war, famine, and suffering directly into people's homes. Dr Stanbury wrote in 1952 that "with telegraph, radio and now television, no one can profess ignorance of world conditions." This meant that "surely not the hardest heart can disclaim some measure of obligation." The CRCS was only one of many humanitarian organizations in the postwar period to "discover" the non-Western world. As political scientist Michael Barnett writes, once Europe was back on its feet, "agencies that once practised a politics of identity and profiling, helping those like them and not many others, now practised a politics of impartiality."[98] The outlines of a "global village" were emerging.

In the Cold War which quickly followed the Second World War, Canada allied itself with the American-led democratic-capitalist West and, like other Western countries, came to recognize relief and development work in so-called "Third World" countries as a weapon in the battle to contain the spread of communism. Early on, Prime Minister Louis St Laurent explicitly included international aid as one of the strategies by which Canada should fight the Cold War, alongside military defence and anti-communist measures at home.[99] Ottawa's creation of CIDA in 1968 merely entrenched an already existing priority. Western governments' post-1945 adoption of humanitarian aid as a Cold War weapon raises the question of how well the CRCS upheld its neutral, impartial ideals in this period. Since he was the driving force behind the society's move into international work, Dr Stanbury's attitude toward the Cold War inevitably influenced CRCS decisions about where and who and how to help. Although no fan of communism, Stanbury was first and foremost a humanitarian and a moderate. Communism grew out of "fear, want and suspicion," he wrote, and until the hungry and hopeless millions were given the means to live and flourish as they deserved, it was "useless" to preach democracy. He believed the polarized postwar world needed "mutual understanding" more than ever, and worked to maintain the IRC as a network of active cooperation above politicking. He took special pride in visits between Canadian and communist leaders, and in Red Cross cooperation across the Iron Curtain for purposes of disaster relief and reuniting families separated by war.[100] Stanbury's natural tact and ability to disarm potentially hostile counterparts played a large part in building these small bridges between the CRCS and national Red Cross societies in communist countries. Following Stanbury's lead, the CRCS paid only minimal attention to Cold War politics when pursuing its national and international activities.

Like all humanitarian organizations, the CRCS became vulnerable to being used as a tool of political influence when it served as a channel for government relief funds. Still, it worked to maintain its neutrality in the ways it could.[101] When the CRCS substantially increased its aid to war-torn Vietnam via the LRCS in 1966, it split its $20,000 gift equally between the Communist north and Western-backed south. It continued to split equally all donations from its own international budget through 1970. However, ordinary Canadian donors and government officials still found ways to use the CRCS (as they had in previous wars) as a channel for the aid they wished to provide to specific groups. Through the CRCS, the Canadian government sent $78,000 worth of cash and medical personnel to South Vietnam in 1968, while in 1969 private donations added $22,000 to South Vietnamese relief and only $100 to North Vietnamese aid.[102] As this example suggests, the CRCS of the early Cold War decades attempted to direct its sails by the winds of neutral humanitarianism, East-West cooperation, and mutual understanding, but the state and ordinary Canadians nudged the rudder enough to produce a discernible drift toward the West.

Not only CRCS money and supplies but also CRCS people made a splash in the postwar world, as the society, like Canada, actively engaged in global councils and sought to play an influential role as a Middle Power. After 1945 the society consistently sent a modest delegation to IRC conferences and, in recognition of the society's massive Second World War effort, Dr Routley was appointed to the League of Red Cross Societies' Board of Governors in 1946. This honour was followed by a steady increase in Canadian Red Cross participation in the LRCS, culminating in Manitoban John A. MacAulay's chairmanship of the LRCS Board of Governors from 1959 to 1965, on whose behalf he accepted the 1963 Nobel Peace Prize.[103]

Dr Stanbury believed that Canada served as "a model of what can be accomplished through tolerance and mutual respect" and that Canadian men and women were "ideally fitted as ambassadors of good-will," not only through leadership in the IRC but also by providing "trained personnel for foreign service" as a supplement to material aid.[104] Beginning in the 1950s, CRCS personnel served overseas as on-site directors of relief for the LRCS, and the CRCS began to send trained personnel to do on-the-ground disaster response work. The first group was a medical-social team of three men that provided civilian aid in Korea in 1951; the CRCS subsequently recruited teams of Canadian medical and social work professionals to respond to the refugee crisis associated with the 1956 Hungarian Uprising, the Moroccan paralysis disaster of 1959 (10,000 people left paralyzed by adulterated cooking oil), and the medical emergency in war-torn, newly decolonized Congo in 1960. The society's reputation as a leader in the postwar International Red Cross grew with each overseas mission.[105]

Not all Red Cross work abroad strengthened the society's already positive reputation in this period. Although the CRCS itself did not send personnel to deal with the suffering and starvation that resulted from the Nigerian Civil War in 1968–69, it did send substantial aid – much of it thanks to Canadians' donations. The ICRC was given responsibility for the aid effort in this complex conflict, but its relative inexperience in major on-the-ground relief and cumbersome management structure back in Switzerland soon caused problems. Meanwhile, the military and political strategies of both the Nigerian state and Biafran rebels hindered the provision of aid, as each sought to control these crucial aid resources. The complexity of the situation, when combined with the ICRC's internal weaknesses, undermined the relief effort, and the entire Red Cross movement suffered a temporary decline in public approval.[106] Saturated by images of tiny Nigerian children with swollen bellies and stick-figure arms and legs, Canadians were as vocal as any in the Western world about brooking no excuse for the ICRC's failure to help more effectively. As a direct result of ICRC missteps in Nigeria, General Wrinch received reports of a small number of Canadians ceasing to work for, donate money to, or even give blood to the CRCS.[107] But overall, in spite of this negative publicity, the society's postwar embrace of international involvement marked, in Dr Stanbury's words, a "coming of age" for the Canadian Red Cross.

Few developments demonstrated the society's transformation after 1945 quite as plainly as its role during the Korean War (1950–53). The CRCS provided supplementary aid and comfort to Canadian military personnel overseas during the conflict, but the scale, scope, content, and context differed dramatically from that of only five years earlier. Few Canadians felt a personal connection to the Korean conflict and their financial contributions to CRCS war work were accordingly much smaller. The Department of National Defence asked the CRCS to fill specific requirements for the Canadian contingent: a variety of hospital supplies to be made up by the existing Women's Work committees, and 10,000 bottles of dried blood plasma with apparatus to reconstitute it on site. On its own initiative, the CRCS also met returning veterans in Vancouver and sent shipments of basic comforts (Canadian cigarettes, Canadian newspapers, "ditty bags" of personal hygiene and comfort items) to British Commonwealth hospitals in Japan.[108]

Several dozen Canadian women – known as the Far East Welfare Team (FEWT) – carried the CRCS banner into the war zone. Although inspired by the Second World War CRC Corps Overseas Detachment, the FEWT exhibited telling differences from its predecessor. Early in 1952, Defence Minister Brooke Claxton officially requested that the CRCS provide a team of female Red Cross workers for service in East Asia. The Department of National Defence broke with tradition and designated the CRCS as the only voluntary organization to provide welfare services to Canadian troops overseas, but the role came with restrictions: FEWT members were to be trained social workers, occupational therapists, nurses, personnel managers in industry, or former members of either the armed forces or the CRC Corps Overseas Detachment, and half had to be bilingual (English/French).[109] Overseas, members of the FEWT provided health, welfare, and recreation services to Canadian and other Commonwealth troops at several locations in Japan and South Korea. They viewed their work as an opportunity to serve their country, help care for Canadian soldiers in a tangible way, and travel to an exotic part of the world. Observers praised their professionalism and efficiency, and reported that morale went up and discipline problems decreased once the team arrived.[110] One unnamed team member offered a candid view of her role in a private letter to a friend back in Canada: "The main purpose of your being there is because *you are a white girl* (!), a reminder of Canada, its women and its standards" – in other words, to help combat the high rates of venereal disease among Canadian soldiers on leave in Japan. "Your work," she wrote, "is to try to bring back to them a bit of the stability of home life and good female companionship." The introduction of a FEWT counsellor for Canadian-Japanese couples and "Canadian lessons" for approved Japanese brides attests to the official concern around interracial liaisons and suggests that the letter-writer's assessment was correct: not only FEWT members' professional skills but also the intersection of their gender and race motivated the government's desire to have them serve overseas.[111]

The FEWT and the entire CRCS Korean War effort demonstrated that the Second World War had marked a last hurrah for the old model of wartime CRCS work. In future, citizen engagement with Red Cross war work would be limited, and Canadian military participation would not guarantee a flood of money and volunteers to the CRCS fold. At the same time, the government would prescribe very particular small areas of involvement for voluntary organizations like the CRCS, designed to meet its own needs. The relatively wide field of activity the society had enjoyed during the Second World War ultimately could not be sustained in the face of increased government regulation and without the particular social context of total war.

A Slight Chill: The Cold War and the CRCS

The Cold War was never a primary motivating factor in post-1945 CRCS activity or decision-making, but it was nonetheless a reality the society had to deal with and played a minor role in shaping the society's postwar work. Canada awoke to its Cold War vulnerability in September 1945 when Soviet embassy cipher clerk Igor Gouzenko exposed the presence of an extensive Soviet spy ring in Canada. By June 1946 Canadian and American military officials on the Permanent Joint Board of Defence agreed that, as James Eayrs summarizes it, "geography no longer conferred upon North America the luxury of immunity from major attack by a hostile power." By 1950, the planners estimated, increasingly sophisticated aircraft, submarines, and guided missiles would soon be able to deliver deadly chemical, biological, and nuclear weapons into the heartlands of the continent. Heavily populated cities, centres of government, and areas of industrial production would be the most likely targets.[112] The threat of war suddenly appeared on Canada's very doorstep, and civil defence (plans for protecting civilians and/or coping with a nuclear attack) became a pressing issue. What role would the CRCS play in a frightening new world where the home front *was* the frontline?

A March 1951 public statement issued by Minister of National Health and Welfare Paul Martin clarified the government's expectation that the CRCS would play some part in civil defence planning and implementation, although firmly under "governmental direction, control and financial responsibility." The government anticipated three major areas of CRCS activity: first, providing mass care (food, clothing, temporary shelter), victim registration, and an inquiry service in the aftermath of an attack; second, expanding and operating the BTS; third, teaching first aid and home nursing in conjunction with the St John Ambulance Association. CRCS Executive Committee chairman Leopold Macaulay further encouraged local CRCS leaders to participate in their local civil defence organizations, calling it "quite proper and desirable" that they do so.[113]

Martin's reference to cooperation between the Red Cross and St John Ambulance came as a direct result of federal government intervention in their perennially thorny relationship. After unhappy temporary partnerships during both world wars, the newly re-divorced CRCS and SJAA continued to irk each other: the CRCS resented SJAA work in blood typing, while the SJAA faced direct competition from CRCS first aid courses in some areas.[114] Under the terms of their government-brokered 1951 agreement, the CRCS gained a clear field in blood collection and typing and the SJAA gained sole dominion over government and industrial first aid training, with its certification becoming the Canadian standard. As Deanna Toxopeus shows, the federal government benefited by paving the way for a single-agency national blood system and a single standard of first aid training – both valuable components of civil defence.[115] The CRCS and SJAA repeatedly renewed the agreement until 1973, each surrendering a little in order to gain a lot.

As Andrew Burtch demonstrates, Canadian civil defence planning unfolded through three stages as the destructive capabilities of nuclear weaponry advanced and the reality of what nuclear war would mean became increasingly clear.[116] There was ample opportunity for CRCS involvement in each phase. The initial city-focused self-help strategy (1948–54) mimicked the response to Second World War–era bombing campaigns in Britain and Germany, and could have drawn on many traditional Red Cross wartime services: canteen service, relief supplies, tracing and reunion work, and the trained, efficient service of the CRC Corps.

The subsequent evacuation strategy (1954–59) involved removing civilians from targeted cities on short notice, and government planners valued the society's growing experience in disaster relief. Feedback received from the CRCS and other voluntary groups and organizations associated with civil defence contributed to Howard Graham's 1958–59 critique of the government's mass evacuation policy – a report that eventually led to a third and final strategy.[117] The new national survival strategy (1959–62) acknowledged the impossibility of mass evacuation and instead encouraged families to build their own backyard fallout shelters. In this scenario, CRCS first aid and home nursing courses offered citizens (particularly women) a chance to arm themselves with basic health care training – all the health care that would be available to them in their family shelters, should the worst happen. Tarah Brookfield explains that for many women, civil defence had "enormous appeal … in the early stages of the Cold War." During the late 1940s and 1950s, women "registered in droves to take courses in disaster management," which might help them in case of natural disaster or accident as well as in the terrible event of a nuclear war, when they might have to deal with atomic, biological, and/or chemical weaponry resulting in physical destruction and high casualty rates.[118] After 1963 government emergency planning shifted away from its earlier reliance on auxiliary volunteers, and major budget cuts in 1968 led the federal Emergency Measures Organization (which had coordinated civil defence) to focus on local planning and ordinary disaster relief – often in conjunction with the CRCS. As late-1960s détente thawed Cold War tensions a little, civil defence faded quietly into the background of Canadian public life.[119]

The Cold War came to Canada in a tangible way when the CRCS hosted the Eighteenth International Red Cross conference from 23 July to 9 August 1952. The IRC Conference, held every four years, brought together voting delegates from national Red Cross societies; voting delegates or non-voting observers from governments signatory to the Geneva Conventions (the most recent of which were signed in 1949 and were still being ratified in 1952); observers from international organizations like the UN and its World Health Organization (WHO); representatives of the League of Red Cross Societies; and the entire ICRC. In technical sessions the delegates considered matters of mutual interest such as new developments in vaccination or artificial respiration, while in general sessions the delegates debated broader humanitarian issues and passed non-binding resolutions to express the collective voice of the many actors who made up the Red Cross movement around the world.

In an era in which international Cold War tensions were prone to pop up in ice hockey as frequently as in the UN, no one should have been surprised that the conference very quickly turned political. Since communist countries had not attended the first postwar IRC conference in 1948, 1952 marked the first true Cold War IRC conference. The so-called Iron Curtain was firmly drawn across Europe and communism had recently expanded into mainland China and North Korea; tensions between East and West were playing out in the ongoing Korean War. The American, British, and other British Commonwealth governments staked an early public claim to the moral high ground at the 1952 IRC conference by sending observers instead of voting delegates, but the move – supposedly intended to avoid political battles – accomplished little.[120] The first and largely ceremonial general session of the conference disintegrated into complete uproar over the seating of Communist Chinese and Nationalist

Chinese delegates. Subsequent general sessions saw the Soviet Union accuse the ICRC of being a tool of the West, while the Communist Chinese and North Koreans accused UN forces (by which they meant the United States) of using bacteriological warfare against China and North Korea in the Korean War. Some Western delegates and journalists concluded that the "Red" delegations had attended simply to cause trouble.[121]

After the conference, the CRCS emphasized the technical committees' success and the fact that despite the uproar the communist countries did not entirely withdraw from the Red Cross movement. The fact remained, however, that this was not the kind of publicity the Red Cross movement desired, especially in the wake of the ICRC's recent failure to do anything substantial about Second World War Nazi concentration camps.[122] The society's three weeks at the centre of the international stage demonstrated that self-described neutral international humanitarian organizations would be affected by the Cold War just like everything else in the postwar world. However, this same conference also saw the IRC assert its ideals of apolitical humanitarianism. Although the move went largely unremarked in press coverage at the time, the 1952 conference voted to reaffirm the set of humanitarian values the LRCS had identified in 1946 as grounding the work of the Red Cross movement. These principles, systematically defined and analysed by Jean Pictet in 1955, were re-codified and proclaimed by the IRC in 1965 as the Seven Fundamental Principles of the Red Cross movement.[123] Despite its harrowing moments, the 1952 IRC conference in Toronto ultimately expressed the humanitarian world's persistent idealism in the face of gritty political realities.

Growing Pains: Social Change and Organizational Angst

For the Canadian Red Cross Society, the years 1945 to 1970 were marked by a curious mixture of self-confidence and persistent hand wringing over its present and future well-being. The organization began to engage in institutional self-reflection in new ways, asking the kinds of questions Charlotte Whitton raised during the Second World War: what was the CRCS officially mandated to do? What was it actually doing, and why? *Should* the Red Cross be doing these things? This new self-consciousness inaugurated a parallel process of deliberate institutional assessment and planning that would continue into the twenty-first century.

The society was not alone in its concern with the future. The trend toward infusing domestic charity with modern business practices before 1939 included an emphasis on long-term planning, and as Michael Barnett shows, "planning" became a buzzword among international humanitarian aid agencies during the Second World War. The trend only increased in ensuing decades, as aid organizations centralized, bureaucratized, and professionalized in hopes of saving more lives and provoking lasting change, rather than improvising solutions to emergency situations. In 1946 the CRCS created its first national budget committee, a form of accounting control that was seen as "a necessary part of public spending, whether of charity or of tax dollars" by the 1950s.[124] If approved by Central Council, the Budget Committee's recommendations became the financial basis of the next year's national operations, so the committee members took their task very seriously. But while the committee consistently advocated fiscal restraint, central councillors passionately defended the Red Cross programs and principles they felt were compromised by cutbacks and reallocated resources. The minutes of annual meetings from this period often give the impression of an organization whose head was at war with its heart. For example, when in 1953 the Budget Committee recommended phasing out the Swimming and Water Safety program over five years in order to cut costs, a contingent of central councillors quickly rose to defend the program, citing its popularity and usefulness in keeping small rural branches alive. After pointing out water safety's comparatively low cost, they accused the BTS of eating up the national budget. Their impassioned defence saved the program.[125]

The BTS became a particular sticking point in these discussions. No one disputed its importance or the fact that budget cuts to the BTS could result in reduced service and potentially endanger lives, but it quickly became clear that it was a hugely expensive undertaking with significant unavoidable costs. As early as 1948 the Budget Committee rang the alarm bells, announcing to Central Council in October that the CRCS was "fast getting beyond its depth" and had "gone beyond all reason" in its postwar program. The committee explained that it "could not suggest to Central Council that [the BTS] be curtailed, but something would have to be curtailed if there was to be enough money to carry on," adding with disapproval that the society was "taking on too much work of governments in health work, hospitalization, dentistry, etc." – a suggestion indicative of the degree to which many Canadians had come to accept and expect a state role in health and welfare provision by the late 1940s.[126]

In 1958, Central Council created the Program Evaluation Committee to consider its peacetime work as a whole. Charged with evaluating the national and international importance of all CRCS programs, their relative importance within different provinces, and whether any programs "could be turned over to other agencies," the committee took a full year to complete its task. Its lengthy list of recommendations, however, primarily promised greater effectiveness, efficiency, and national coordination. Only a few small, usually regionally specific, programs were flagged as suitable to be turned over to others.[127] As a consciousness-raising exercise the evaluation succeeded; as a means of significantly reducing expenses it was a bust. Luckily, concurrent discussions with the federal and provincial governments to partially fund BTS technical costs alleviated the sense of immediate financial crisis.

Even with partial government funding for the BTS, a crisis mentality crept back in, this time broadening beyond mere finances. One after another, individual programs and policies began undergoing broad assessments and by the late 1960s another hard look at the big picture seemed to be in order. But this time the study would address not only the society's programs but also its people and the organization's place in the broader landscape of Canadian society. The CRCS national officers who first proposed the study envisioned a grand fact-finding mission that could make recommendations and long-term plans along the lines of the recent seven-year plan drawn up by the BTS as a result of the Woods, Gordon study. The society thus closed out the turbulent 1960s by embarking on its most comprehensive exercise in self-assessment to-date: the CRCS Long Range Planning Committee, whose landmark report would be published in 1973 under the title *And Who Is My Stranger* (discussed in the next chapter). General Wrinch described 1970 as a year of planning and assessing that offered an opportunity to move forward "to a new horizon in Red Cross."[128]

Money was obviously a big part of the problem, but the society's post-war angst also sprang from changes in the voluntary work and activism of Canadian women and youth. Although women remained highly active in organizational life throughout the postwar years, Tarah Brookfield points out that the *kinds* of organizations they chose to be part of changed noticeably over the course of the 1960s. In that decade membership in Canada's largest women's organizations – long-time Red Cross allies like the IODE, Women's Institutes, and National Council of Women of Canada – declined, while women's involvement in electoral politics, unions, and new civil rights and women's liberation organizations increased. Not only did younger women drift away from older voluntary organizations but those who did join often did not possess the domestic skills that had traditionally fuelled Women's Work committees and produced millions of relief supplies on the cheap.[129] The society first created a national Voluntary Services Committee in 1948 as wartime volunteers dropped off in droves, indicative of an early shift in the direction of the "volunteer resource management" model which would prevail by the end of the twentieth century. It studied volunteer services in nationwide programs in 1953, but focused on using volunteers more effectively to reduce staff salaries, rather than the art of wooing and hanging onto volunteers.[130]

Even the Junior Red Cross – the traditional source of hope for the future vibrancy of the CRCS – offered a somewhat gloomy prospect by the mid-1960s. The decade began with promise: French Catholic educational authorities had kept the Junior Red Cross out of francophone schools in Quebec for decades, but beginning in 1962 the doors were opened for individual teachers to adopt the program if they wished, as the Lesage government modernized the province's education system. Since francophones constituted approximately 83 percent of Quebec's student population, this represented a major breakthrough. Quebec Division adapted the program to suit the province's bilingual, bicultural population as well as to respond to educational trends and competition from new youth organizations like the Canadian University Service Overseas (CUSO). This translated into less focus on personal health, a renewed emphasis on service projects, and a reinterpretation of the program's internationalist goals to include fostering cross-cultural youth friendship *within* Quebec.[131] In September 1962 the CRCS proudly promoted a Junior membership figure of nearly 1,500,000 children and youth in 43,000 classrooms across the country: at 27.9 percent of the 1961 population aged five to nineteen, that number represented nearly the same proportion of Canadian youth the Junior Red Cross had boasted during the Second World War. But a troubling decades-old problem marred the triumph: the overwhelming majority of Juniors stopped their Red Cross activities upon leaving school. The crux of the problem lay with high school Juniors and making the transition to senior Red Cross work. In 1963 national Junior Red Cross director Ralph Wendeborn identified "a continuing knotty problem which is the provision of interesting projects and activities" for older youth. The oldest Baby Boomers' enthusiasm for hands-on service can be seen in the fact that even with Montreal's many blood donor clinics, hospitals, and similar institutions, the Montreal Red Cross branch sometimes had great difficulty finding sufficient volunteer placements to satisfy the youthful demand.[132] This problem was hardly unique to the CRCS. Stuart Henderson characterizes the impact of the Baby Boom as a "massive, full-scale societal, cultural, and political shift towards accommodating young people." Their sheer numbers sent "a shockwave ... through Canadian institutions, forcing them to adapt or be crushed."[133]

The society attempted to respond to the rapidly changing social landscape of the 1960s by changing the name of the program in 1966 from Junior Red Cross (with its implications of unequal status) to Red Cross Youth and convening several International Study Centres. Other youth organizations were pursuing similar strategies: the Boy Scouts, for instance, held large Arctic Jamborees in 1968 and 1970 in an effort to bring together scouts from southern and northern regions of Canada. The largest Red Cross Youth gathering of the 1960s, Ottawa-based "Rendezvous '67," brought together some 260 teens from across Canada plus ninety youth from forty-five countries, and served as the society's major project to celebrate Canada's centennial year. Like the wider centennial celebrations, Rendezvous '67 expressed a sense of national pride and hope for the future, as well as a deliberate engagement with the rest of the world.[134] But these measures failed to satisfy the young Baby Boomers. In 1967 National Commissioner General Wrinch warned his provincial counterparts that "more and more youth demand more and more service jobs and the right of doing a lot of their own planning" – something that older CRCS staff found "difficult." Wrinch observed that fundraising opportunities and local charity projects were easy to come by, but "the difficult part of the program is the service to others and broadening the service to include not only people in hospitals at home but abroad." As Ian McKay has pointed out, the young leftists of the late 1960s wanted to root their activism in the global scene rather than the local, and if the CRCS could not accommodate them, newer, more internationally or politically engaged organizations like CUSO and Oxfam Canada would.[135]

In 1969 Ruth Wilson and Gene Miki, two prominent members of Red Cross Youth in the Toronto area, spoke to the CRCS Volunteer Registration and Orientation Services Committee about what youth wanted from the senior CRCS. Wilson said she had no desire to move from Red Cross Youth to the senior society because "there was no opportunity for innovation in the Senior Red Cross," while Miki told the committee his peers wanted "to work out new programs and from here go on and present them to the adult members of the Society." The subsequent discussion highlighted a growing criticism of the CRCS as a whole: that senior members were "emotionally attached" to programs their generation created, whereas young people wanted to serve in ways more meaningful to themselves.[136] The popular Miles for Millions walkathons of the late 1960s and early 1970s offer one example of the meaningful connection young people sought: as Tamara Myers explains, Miles for Millions deliberately pushed youthful walkers to their physical limits as a way to identify with suffering people around the world. Red Cross Youth who tried to innovate in this way often faced opposition from adult CRCS staff. The "go-go clinic" organized by a Red Cross Youth group of law students from McGill University and the Université de Montréal in 1968 met adult resistance, but the members persevered. Volunteer Michael Worsoff proudly claimed that this "combination blood clinic and psychedelic dance" had attracted "representatives of the black and the white, the rich and the poor, the English and the French, the squares and the hippies."[137] This was not your grandmother's Red Cross.

Psychedelic blood clinics did not become the norm – Worsoff had to admit the attendance was lower than expected – but clearly change had come calling. Addressing and trying to overcome the challenges posed by

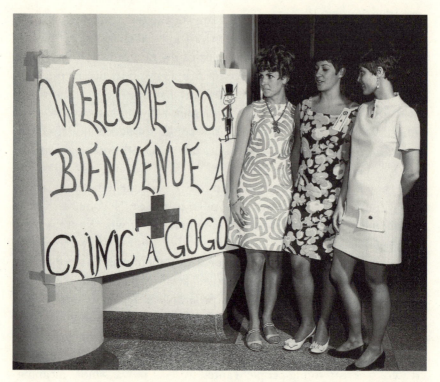

Figure 6.5
The hip, youthful vibe is tangible as volunteers pose at the entrance to the Clinic à
Go-Go organized in 1968 by Red Cross youth groups in the law schools of
McGill University and the Université de Montréal.

a new generation for whom the traditional Red Cross model held limited appeal, and the implications of that for the organization's future,
preoccupied the society as the late 1960s gave way to the early 1970s.
No future war could be expected to bring Canadians back to the organization, as had happened in 1939. The days of the Canadian Red Cross
Society as a significant adjunct to battlefield medicine were now past,
and the language of duty and sacrifice no longer sufficed. The future lay
in some other direction.

+

The years 1945 to 1970 offered stiff challenges and rewarding successes for the CRCS. Organizational postwar prosperity proved more elusive than supporters initially hoped, with the interwar pattern of diminishing volunteers and financial struggles repeating itself. Still, the society retained sufficient public favour to sustain its work. New programs in water safety and civilian blood transfusion saved lives and imprinted the Red Cross onto the consciousness of new generations of Canadians, and the advent of the welfare state altered but did not fundamentally undermine the place of the CRCS in Canadian society. The violence and upheaval of decolonization and a never-ending litany of natural disasters provided opportunities for the CRCS to forge a reputation for Canada as a leader in the field of international humanitarian aid and to finally put into practice around the world the values of humanity and universality the CRCS had long espoused.

The society ended the 1960s engaged in a new kind of formal assessment, but the impulse behind the exercise was nearly as old as the organization: evolve or face obsolescence. In the seventy-four years since Dr Ryerson and his friends founded the society it had lost the flexibility which made possible the spontaneous transformations that characterized its earliest years. The Long Range Planning Committee's study therefore *would* lead to change, but not the radical sort some CRCS leaders may have hoped for or feared. In fact, although the report produced new approaches to staffing and organizational life – partly to deal with new demands from women and youth – by 1970 the basic outlines of the late twentieth-century CRCS were in place: its major programs, its reliance on both private donations and public funding, its understanding of itself as an organization that pioneered programs and filled gaps at home and had a moral obligation to serve as a channel of Canadians' humanitarian impulses overseas, its self-proclaimed "wherever and whenever" mandate to help. The Canadian Red Cross had become its modern self – even to the point of increasingly dropping the old-fashioned "Society" from its name. As it charted a course for the future, the Long Range Planning Committee could look to the society's past and marvel at how far it had come since 1885: from battlefield medicine to civilian blood collection – and well beyond.

CONCLUSION

"Red Cross is a tough old chicken!"[1]

At their meeting of 26 June 1967, the national officers of the Canadian Red Cross Society raised the possibility of creating "something in the nature of a Royal Commission" to map a course for the society's future. The International Red Cross as a whole engaged in a similar exercise in the early 1970s, suggesting a sense throughout the movement that the social, cultural, political, and military changes of the 1960s warranted a re-evaluation of how the Red Cross could best translate its humanitarian ideals into action.[2] The CRCS Long Range Planning Committee (as the proposed "royal commission" was named) pursued a multi-year project of internal reviews and public consultations to assess the society's current state and suggest future directions. This elaborate exercise indicates that by the late 1960s the CRCS was increasingly conscious of its need to adapt. It therefore serves as a useful point in time to step back and assess the history of the Canadian Red Cross Society up to the 1970s, as well as to look ahead at what came next and why.

Time to Transform ... Again

Some Canadians had come to consider the CRCS the "Cadillac of the charitable and social service organizations" by the early 1970s,[3] but the well-appointed Cadillac exterior disguised growing problems under the hood. The Long Range Planning Committee's final report, published in 1973 under the title *And Who Is My Stranger: Exploring Red Cross Policies, Strategies and Priorities for the Seventies,* identified "turbulent

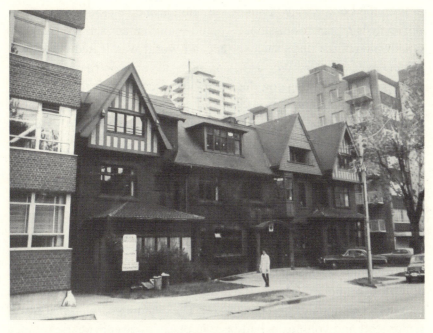

Figure 7.1
The society first rented this handsome Toronto mansion at 95 Wellesley in 1940, needing more space for its wartime national headquarters. Once surrounded by similarly grand homes, by the 1960s it was instead nestled among modern apartment blocks – a visual metaphor for the organization's late-1960s fear that it was falling out of step with Canadian society.

times," "weakened voluntarism," and "financial stringency" as the three factors that made a "radical re-definition" of the society's course not only timely but imperative. Social values had already changed and were continuing to do so; the growth of the welfare state now seemed to threaten "the very viability of voluntarism"; and charitable giving – even through the once-vaunted strategy of federated fundraising – was not keeping up with inflation. Secondarily, "professionalism and bureaucracy" had affected the society over previous decades and needed to be assessed. The committee argued that like people, organizations age: the Canadian Red Cross needed to keep itself oriented toward the future or else it would become inflexible, ineffective, and irrelevant.[4]

Both the Long Range Planning Committee and its report were themselves signs of the professionalism and management science that had quietly altered the CRCS since the Second World War. If Red Cross supporters expected *And Who Is My Stranger* to focus on the financial issues that had been dogging the society for decades, they were in for a surprise. Although the report identified several financial strategies (government grants, bequests, fees) the society might pursue, it focused primarily on ways to make CRCS programs and personnel more effective. This meant more testing of ideas through pilot projects, engaging in more frequent program evaluations, and weeding out programs that were being maintained "just because" (or that had become personal fiefdoms). It also meant revamping the society's complex and somewhat insular organizational structure and creating a more integrated organization through more frequent and meaningful communication, a less rigid hierarchy, and stronger relationships between national, provincial, and local branches. Above all, it meant renewed leadership and increased professionalization at all levels. The committee found that many senior staff and volunteers had been in place for twenty years or more and were not demographically representative of the Canadian population, while the best volunteers were burnt out, a wave of retirements could soon be expected, and the grassroots perceived CRCS policy-making as tightly controlled at the upper levels. If the CRCS was to thrive as an organization and attract capable, enthusiastic people to its ranks – especially younger people – staff and volunteers needed better training, higher rates of turnover, standard criteria for recruitment, and possibilities for advancement within the organization.[5] Observers in the Community Chest movement had already been whispering among themselves that the CRCS needed to move away from the hierarchically oriented "'army' type" and recruit staff with "improved background and sensitivity in the use and understanding of volunteers."[6] The committee's report turned these outside mutterings into a bold internal call to action that required the society to abandon as much as possible the last vestiges of its elite, clubbish, nineteenth-century roots.

Balancing this call for greater efficiency and professionalization, *And Who Is My Stranger* also argued that it was important for the society to value people's desire to give something of themselves (whether time, talents, blood, or labour) beyond money. It reaffirmed a longstanding CRCS belief that the Red Cross mission to help the vulnerable expressed a special, almost sacred, relationship between helpers and those who were helped. But instead of turning (as earlier twentieth-century Red Cross leaders and volunteers had often done) to either religious principles or secular humanitarianism to ground this argument, the CRCS committee drew on the highly influential work of British social scientist Richard Titmuss. In his landmark 1970 study *The Gift Relationship*, Titmuss analysed the very different blood donation systems in Britain (free and state-run) and the United States (a mixture of free and for-profit) to demonstrate that altruism was "both morally sound and economically efficient."[7] His study was launched by two questions: "Why give to strangers?" and "who is my stranger in the relatively affluent, acquisitive and divisive societies of the twentieth century?" The CRCS committee members not only incorporated these questions in their report title but also seem to have taken them to heart. The "gift relationship" of Titmuss's title expressed his view (very similar to Dr Stanbury's) that the free gift of blood from one person to another – even when that recipient was unknown – created a bond of fellowship between them, and a nationwide, free blood donation system magnified that relationship, serving as an integrating force within a society.[8] Applied broadly, Titmuss's study suggested that many forms of voluntary service, not just blood donation, made societies more cohesive – an idea that clearly animated the CRCS committee's recommendations for strengthening the CRCS so that it could continue to play this role for decades to come.

The society gamely took up the report's calls to action throughout the 1970s and 1980s, and by the time I showed up as a summer student in the late 1990s, local branch activity took place under a system of professional fund developers, volunteer resource managers, standardized human resource policies, annual funding grant applications, vulnerability capacity assessments, and a network of "regions" and "zones" that replaced the old provincial divisions. National Headquarters had finally relocated to Ottawa, the word "society" had been dropped from everyday use, and local branches had been consolidated into fewer but more active locations with small numbers of permanent paid staff coordinating the work of volunteers. These changes reflected the growing professionalization and expansion of the charitable sector, increased public expectations of accountability and efficiency, and the decline of voluntarism in Canadian society during the late twentieth century, as well as broader international trends toward centralization and bureaucratization in the field of humanitarian aid.[9]

Although the society's late-twentieth century professionalization marked a distinct and conscious departure from previous practice, the "radical re-definition" urged on the CRCS in the early 1970s was not actually very radical: instead, change and innovation were the defining features of the organization's entire history. Pragmatic assessments of the social context, expansive and flexible definitions of "health," and the willingness and ability to redirect Red Cross resources in creative ways marked the society's most successful initiatives and, ultimately, contributed greatly to its enduring place in Canadian society. The Long Range Planning Committee had to envision a role for the society in the face of a new and troublesome series of challenges, but its ultimate purpose was not so different from that of George Sterling Ryerson, who turned to the Red Cross as a means of addressing a deficiency in Canada's military medical provisions; or Adelaide Plumptre, who drafted the society's first peacetime public health policy in 1919; or Stuart Stanbury, who envisioned a postwar CRCS that could provide a free national blood transfusion service at home *and* humanitarian aid around the world. Many times throughout its history, those in the CRCS saw a need – whether in Canada, the world, or the CRCS itself – and enlarged or altered the society's understanding of its own mission in order to address that need. This kind of mission drift frequently proved unpopular with other voluntary and charitable organizations, social workers, and government departments, but it almost always succeeded in helping the CRCS weather its intermittent crises. The recommendations of the Long-Range Planning Committee, like these earlier reinventions, helped the society cope with its latest challenges and retain its prominent place in Canadian society.

Tainted Blood, Tainted Reputation?

The CRCS was heading toward some very rough waters as it sailed into the 1970s. No amount of long-range planning could counteract the reality that competition for the charitable dollar and volunteer labour increased as the twentieth century entered its final decades. Welfare state provisions led some to predict that charities like the CRCS would soon be unnecessary, and CRCS volunteer numbers were perceived to be in decline. In the absence of statistics it is impossible to determine to what degree this perception was correct, but the perception itself pervaded all levels and all provincial divisions of the society and therefore deserves some credence. The statistics gathered by Theda Skocpol and her colleagues for Harvard University's Civic Engagement Project support this perception: in the American context, three-quarters of the twenty largest American associations (ranging from the Freemasons and American Bowling Congress to the Boy Scouts and United Methodist Women) experienced significant declines in their membership share of the adult population between 1955 and 1995. The decline first became noticeable in the 1960s and 1970s as social movements, advocacy groups, and other non-profits proliferated and began to shift Americans' expectations of what it meant to "support" an organization: many of the new associations required little or no volunteer effort and instead relied on supporters' money to fund a small body of paid staff. Mirroring this American trend, Canadians continued to share their money with the CRCS from the 1960s onward, but ever-more "dread disease" charities, advocacy groups, and non-profits drew support away from older organizations and causes.[10] By the end of the century, government cutbacks in funding to social programs and cultural institutions further increased the competition for charitable and philanthropic donations. At the same time, the rapid pace of medical advances (particularly in the field of surgery) meant an ever-increasing demand for blood and blood products.

As discussed in chapter 6, the BTS became an expensive responsibility for the society almost as soon as it was established. In the face of persistent fundraising difficulties the CRCS struggled to pay for its share of the program, despite funding arrangements with the federal and provincial governments. Brigadier W.E. Huckvale, a leader in the Alberta Division CRCS, claimed in 1958 that in the BTS the society had "a tiger by the tail," and unless something changed dramatically, the BTS would eventually devour all the society's financial resources.[11] Huckvale's concerns were legitimate, but greater threats of a biological nature would prove the undoing of the CRCS BTS: human immunodeficiency virus (HIV) and hepatitis C. During the 1980s infected blood transfusions resulted in roughly 2,000 Canadians contracting HIV and an estimated 20,000 contracting hepatitis C – many of them haemophiliacs.[12] This was arguably Canada's greatest preventable public health disaster to date, and the resulting national scandal provoked much finger pointing, a Royal Commission of Inquiry, and numerous court cases. The federal government and the CRCS eventually provided financial compensation to victims of both diseases, and in 2001 the Supreme Court of Canada upheld an Ontario ruling that the CRCS had been negligent in its donor screening during the early years of HIV/AIDS emergence.[13] Canada was not alone in this: similar tainted blood tragedies unfolded in other industrialized countries including Britain, France, Japan, and the United States, and in those countries, too, citizens infected by tainted blood mobilized to expose official negligence, forced the reform of national blood systems and policies, and won both financial compensation and moral victories.[14] In Canada, long years of courtroom wrangling and sensationalistic media coverage fed some Canadians' appetite for scandal and retribution. But more importantly, behind this public spectacle lay the personal devastation experienced by the recipients of infected blood transfusions, and their loved ones. Their anguish runs through Kat Lanteigne's play *Tainted*, which premiered in Toronto in October 2013 and moved many audience members to tears.[15]

This is not the place to re-examine the specific decisions and complex circumstances that led to the tragic end that came to be known in Canada as the "Tainted Blood Scandal," or to re-hash the voluminous evidence collected by the Royal Commission of Inquiry into Canada's Blood System (popularly known as the Krever Inquiry) between 1993 and 1997. Interested readers may examine the commission's findings, a journalistic history, or a number of scholarly dissertations on the subject.[16] But it seems evident, from a historical perspective, that the seeds of this unhappy chapter in Canadian and CRCS history were sown early in the postwar period. Perhaps, as the federal government believed during the Second World War, creating a nation-wide system for blood collection was not something that could be accomplished by the state, and the CRCS – or an organization like it – was the most practical alternative. But leaving the financial maintenance of the system in the hands of a charitable organization, whether dependent on unpredictable public donations, fluctuating government subsidies, or a combination of both, proved unsustainable and eventually highly dysfunctional.

For most countries, the history of Red Cross blood services, tainted blood scandals, and the resulting changes in blood collection and provision remain to be written. With the passage of time, new studies and new perspectives will provide the material for comparison with the Canadian experience. In the meantime, the Australian case offers another illustration of how national contexts can significantly shape Red Cross history. As Melanie Oppenheimer explains, the Australian Red Cross's voluntary blood donation system was rocked in the early 1980s, like its peers around the world, by the revelation that an unknown number of patients had contracted HIV or hepatitis C through infected blood products. Plummeting public confidence, legal proceedings, and financial settlements ensued. However, the Australian Blood Service was at the global forefront of adopting new screening techniques and ultimately managed to weather both the controversy and litigation. Spurred by pressure from both state and national government levels, the Australian Red Cross underwent a series of major reforms and restructuring, emerging in the twenty-first century with a stronger, centralized blood system to replace the previous state-based version. Blood collection remains a jewel in the crown of Australian Red Cross programs.[17]

In stark contrast, after the Krever Inquiry reported in 1997, the CRCS declined its option to play a role in the overhauled and revamped Canadian blood system and pulled out of blood collection entirely. After roughly a half-century of advertisements and public service announcements urging people to donate blood to the Red Cross, blood had become central to many Canadians' image of the CRCS, and it was hard to imagine the agency carrying on without its flagship program. Was this the end of the Canadian Red Cross? Not so. The CRCS had created the BTS, not the other way around; the Red Cross was always more than its blood program. As an organization the CRCS limped away from the Tainted Blood Scandal deeply wounded, but it retained a core of devoted volunteers, donors, and staff, and as a smaller, somewhat demoralized organization, it began a process of reassessment not unlike that of the Long Range Planning Committee thirty years earlier.[18] The same multiplicity and diversity of activities that had sometimes frustrated government officials and the personnel of other agencies in earlier periods now showed itself to be one of the Canadian Red Cross's enduring strengths. Relinquishing the BTS did not spell the end of the CRCS any more than had the turning over of outpost hospitals to local communities after the advent of Medicare, or the end of bandage rolling when peace was declared in 1918 and again in 1945.

The decision to decline a role in the new blood system (which emerged as Canadian Blood Services and Héma-Québec) constituted a transformation all on its own; the subsequent decades produced further transformation, as disaster relief in Canada and abroad quietly emerged as a new flagship endeavour. Surprisingly, the enormous amount of bad press the CRCS received in the course of the Tainted Blood Scandal did not permanently alienate Canadians from the Red Cross. Since the year 2000, tsunamis, hurricanes, and other disasters around the world have prompted Canadians to donate hundreds of millions of dollars to a range of worthy international humanitarian aid organizations like Save the Children, World Vision, CARE, and Oxfam, but the CRCS consistently emerges as the leading recipient of Canadians' disaster relief donations. When Super-Typhoon Haiyan devastated parts of the Philippines on 7 November 2013, the Canadian government immediately donated $30,000 to the CRCS for relief purposes (later increasing this donation substantially); the Ontario government donated $1 million to the Red Cross, and the Alberta government matched $500,000 in Albertan donations to the CRCS. Individual and corporate donations to the CRCS from the Canadian public reached $5.6 million within five days, and exceeded $30 million by mid-December.[19] This generous response was then outdone by the $42 million Canadians donated for southern Alberta flood relief in 2013, and the more than $125 million donated by individuals, corporate partners, and community groups for the victims of wildfires that devastated Fort McMurray, Alberta in May 2016. By 28 June 2016 more than a million individual Canadians had donated to the wildfire relief fund.[20] The relationship between Canadians and their national Red Cross has clearly bounced back from its 1990s nadir, and continues to unfold in intriguing ways.

What prompted this resurgence of public confidence in a supposedly disgraced organization? The long and successful history of Red Cross response to natural disasters throughout the twentieth century is one answer; another is the fact that disaster relief and the BTS were two separate entities, and a loss of confidence in one did not necessarily mean a loss of confidence in the other. A Gallup Poll survey of public attitudes toward the Red Cross in Canada, conducted in 1971 for the Long-Range Planning Committee, suggests a third contributing factor: a resilient CRCS "brand." Of the 711 Canadians interviewed, 88 percent had a favourable impression of the CRCS, and nearly four-fifths based their good opinion on a sense that the CRCS did a lot of good, helped people, and "you never hear anything bad about it."[21] (Roughly half of those holding an unfavourable opinion of the society based it on a bad personal experience or wartime sock-selling rumours.) Both current programs and historical interventions factored into these attitudes: interviewees regarded the Blood Transfusion Service and disaster relief most highly, while those who had lived through the Second World War also valued CRCS wartime work and veteran services. The international Red Cross movement found similar results around the world during its early 1970s assessment exercise. Donald D. Tansley, the study's Canadian director, observed that "actual knowledge of the movement in any significant detail may be limited among most people, but the name 'Red Cross' evokes an image of compassionate help, integrity and impartiality. Red Cross is viewed as an institution that can be trusted and that should continue to function."[22] The Canadian Red Cross Society's reputation nestled comfortably within, and contributed to, that international context of goodwill.

Beginning with the First World War, the CRCS inadvertently forged a malleable Red Cross brand out of its wide range of activities and the powerful meanings attached to them. The Seven Fundamental Principles of the Red Cross movement proclaimed in 1965 – humanity, impartiality, neutrality, independence, voluntary service, unity, and universality – have been important to the organization as an international humanitarian aid agency; closer to home, however, a different if sometimes overlapping set of virtues has animated the history of the CRCS. As the preceding chapters have shown, the positive qualities of mothering, caring, love, life-saving, mercy, patriotism, service, sacrifice, healing, and helping that became associated with the CRCS – qualities compatible with many world religions as well as secular humanism – both shaped its work and helped it adapt to changing circumstances throughout the twentieth century. Perhaps even more powerfully, wordless images like the lovely "Red Cross nurse" with outstretched hand, or the red cross emblem itself, became concise and powerful visual signifiers of both the organization and its positive qualities. By the turn of the twenty-first century, the agency's slogans deliberately capitalized on the Red Cross brand for the benefit of the organization. Accompanied by images including swimming lessons, disaster relief workers, and the red cross emblem, the Canadian Red Cross's "Across the World, Across the Street" and "Anywhere. Anytime." campaigns of the late 1990s and early 2000s (clearly echoing CRCS slogans of the 1950s and 1960s) explicitly presented the broad and ever-changing nature of Red Cross work as *the* defining feature of the agency, and in the process highlighted the fact that the Red Cross had become a brand, rather than a particular service.

Over time it became unnecessary to detail what the Canadian Red Cross actually did because the name and the emblem spoke for themselves. Another CRCS slogan from the late 1990s neatly summarizes the Red Cross brand, stating simply, "When Help is Needed. The Canadian Red Cross."[23] A century of being associated with qualities like caring and helping contributed significantly to the society's ability to survive its late-twentieth-century fall from grace.

The Big Picture: 1885–1970

Many of the activities in which the CRCS and its volunteers participated have faded into the mists of history, but traces of the society's historical contributions linger on the fringes of Canadian life. Experimental techniques pioneered at the Windsor, Ontario Red Cross branch's rehabilitation pool and demonstration nursing school moved into mainstream health care. Booklets of knitting instructions from the First and Second World Wars regularly turn up in attics and at yard sales. Wilberforce, Ontario's former Red Cross outpost hospital is now a community museum and national historic site.[24] Canada's national blood collection system still revolves around the concept of voluntary, unpaid donations provided free of charge to recipients. Meanwhile, the society itself carries on, occasionally celebrating bits of its past, forgetful of many others, and generally getting on with the tricky business of being an active human-

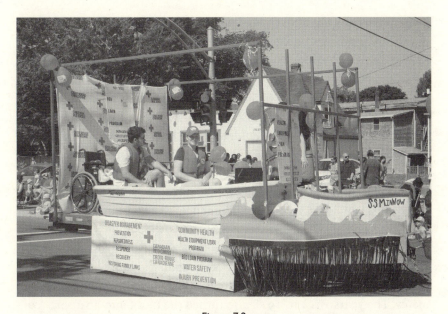

Figure 7.2
Canadian Red Cross float in the Gold Cup and Saucer Parade, Charlottetown,
Prince Edward Island, 21 August 2015. The float decorations emphasize local disaster
management, community health, and water safety efforts – the latter particularly
relevant to an island province.

itarian aid organization at home and abroad. When we step back and assess the first eighty-five years in the history of the Red Cross in Canada, what do we learn?

First, the entire history of the Canadian Red Cross Society is characterized by a tension between renewal and obsolescence. From its first unofficial work in 1885, the Red Cross fought to survive in Canada. Over the ensuing decades it underwent a series of important transformations, periodically expanding or contracting, reorganizing, redirecting its focus, and altering its relationships with governments and other charitable and public health organizations.

From an organizational standpoint, the society's establishment as a branch of the BNAS, temporary growth during the South African War, and reorganization and incorporation in 1909 were important milestones. But in terms of the Red Cross's place in Canadian society, the First World War was the crucial turning point. Had Europe maintained an uneasy peace, the Red Cross might have remained a small, relatively unimportant agency in Canada. Instead, out of the mud and gas and barbed wire of France, Canada won a place on the world stage, and with humble tools like knitting needles, bandages, and index cards, Canadians wove their Red Cross inextricably into the warp and woof of wartime Canada. As ICRC co-founder Henry Dunant wrote in *A Memory of Solferino*, "There is no coldness or indifference in the public when the country's sons are fighting. After all, the blood that is being spilled in battle is the same that runs in the veins of the whole nation."[25] Canadians from coast to coast turned to the CRCS as a conduit for the love and care they wished to lavish on Canada's citizen-soldiers, on Canada itself, and on the wider British Empire. More than any other factor, the crucible of the Great War produced a Canadian Red Cross Society that was truly national in scope, with roots deep in the shared Canadian experience, engaging in a distinctly "maple leaf" version of humanitarian mercy. The years 1914 to 1918 also turned the CRCS into an agency confident enough to take the leading role in Canadian and British Red Cross relief work in Siberia at war's end.

In an echo of the First World War's role in the Western world more broadly, that conflict marked both a "creative moment" and a "last gasp"[26] for the CRCS: it brought the era of well-meaning, self-aggrandizing Dr Ryerson and his Toronto military medical friends to an end, and ushered in the age of efficient, businesslike Mrs Plumptre and a host of public health experts from across Canada. The society's 1918 decision not to fold up until the next war but instead to shift its focus to public health, must rank second only to the First World War on a list of the most significant turning points in the organization's history. Armed with a new peacetime mandate, the society contributed to the surge of Canadian public health work in the 1920s and 1930s, maintained a core of supporters, and became a recognizable and enduring part of peacetime Canadian society. Child and maternal health in a country at peace failed to rouse the same level of public financial support as the cause of sick and wounded citizen-soldiers in a country at war, but the society's interwar public health ventures allowed the organization to survive, even through the Great Depression. As a result, the society's response to the outbreak of the Second World War was all the quicker and more effective, and the transition to peacetime after 1945 all the smoother in turn.

Lessons learned featured heavily in both the Second World War activity of the CRCS and its postwar initiatives. The outbreak of war in September 1939 revived the CRCS as it did the Canadian economy as a whole, filling the society's coffers and imprinting the CRCS on the consciousness of a new generation. In many ways the Second World War marked a return to the older First World War model of the CRCS, but Red Cross leaders' desire to return to familiar channels was quickly thwarted by an interventionist federal government bent on regulating wartime charitable activity. The society had to alter some of its preferred approaches, and unlike some of its earlier transformations, this one was painful: leaders and ordinary volunteers alike resisted change at nearly every turn. Ultimately, however, it proved to be a necessary introduction to the adaptation that would be required of the society in the postwar world.

The society's leaders began postwar planning midway through the Second World War, determined to avoid as many of the troubles it encountered during the interwar period as possible. Circumstances would soon make even such planned changes insufficient. The unforeseen vagaries of the Cold War, youth revolt, and a combination of rising costs, declining revenues, and the growing welfare state made the 1950s and 1960s one extended period of incremental but sweeping change. By the mid-1950s any CRCS illusions about a return to normalcy were overtaken by the challenges of remaining relevant in a rapidly changing Canada. CRCS leaders came to view a Red Cross-run, nationwide, free blood transfusion service as the key to their organization's continued survival in peacetime, and although the CRCS continued many of its now-traditional peacetime activities (with the important addition of swimming and water safety), the blood program came to overshadow all else. At the same time, the evolution of warfare (nuclear and otherwise) over the second half of the twentieth-century removed any likelihood of a return to the kind of large-scale auxiliary medical role the CRCS played in the South African War and the two world wars. Between 1885 and 1970, therefore, circumstances repeatedly conspired to push the CRCS toward obsolescence, making the history of the CRCS one of tension between the old and the new, of soul-searching and angst over what to hold onto and what to relinquish. At each step the society had to adapt, and because it adapted, it survived.

Second, the history of the Canadian Red Cross Society repeatedly demonstrates the truth of historian Wendy Mitchinson's assertion that "health is where the public and private worlds merge."[27] Over the years, the private worlds of sickness and injury were the constant subjects of public appeals by the CRCS and the objects of a wide range of voluntary action under its banner. The Red Cross as an international movement owed its existence to the belief that the health of individual soldiers on the battlefield should be an object of public concern and public action, while Red Cross initiatives in Canada extended that concern to women and children, immigrants, veterans, victims of natural disasters, those engaging in water activities – and even to the metaphorical health of the nation itself. The history of CRCS work in war and peace over the course of the twentieth century also highlights the many ways in which organizations outside the hospital or other traditional health care settings have played a role in reflecting public opinion, pioneering services, and providing health care. Health care in Canada has been a concern and a preoccupation of many citizens, not just health care professionals, and voluntary organizations like the Red Cross have long histories of active participation in the health realm. Notably, through the blood program the CRCS became Canada's flag-bearer in the field of large-scale, private, voluntary sector involvement in the biomedical field – involvement that expanded dramatically in the United States after the Second World War but did not grow to anywhere near the same extent in Canada.[28]

Third, the history of the CRCS provides a valuable window into late-nineteenth- and twentieth-century women's health and welfare work, as well as the roles of twentieth-century children in voluntary organizations. As Charlotte Whitton found in 1939, it can be very difficult to pin down what is at the core of the CRCS, given its wide array of seemingly unrelated activities and intermittent transformations. One vibrant thread running through CRCS history is the presence and work of women. As a national body, the CRCS was never purely a women's organization. Men formed the society as a way to help other men on the battlefields, dominated its national leadership throughout the entire period covered by this book, donated time and money at the grassroots level, and served the society overseas in a variety of conflicts. Significantly, however, it took a direct appeal to women during the South African War to bring the society its first widespread popular support.

Canadian women breathed life into the CRCS at the local level, and much of its wartime activity relating to food, clothing, comforts, and fundraising was considered "women's work." Women's voluntary labour subsequently provided a solid base from which the society branched out into peacetime public health initiatives, and professional nurses and teachers – usually women in this period – provided an ever-increasing support and complement to the unpaid work of volunteers. From 1899 to 1970, the society consistently mobilized women's voluntary labour as a way to fill gaps in the existing systems of health care provision. "Without our women there would be no Red Cross as we know it," wrote former executive committee chairman P.H. Gordon in the late 1960s.[29]

Women responded in vast numbers because the CRCS gave them opportunities to care for distant loved ones, contribute to the betterment of their communities, access the public sphere, engage in health care work whether they were professionally trained or not, and express patriotism and female imperialism. The continuity between the society's appeals to women's maternalism in wartime and during the interwar years argues strongly for the persistence of maternalism in Canada after many women attained suffrage at the federal level in 1918. The CRCS offered women a venue for civic work and a means to access the public sphere but without focusing exclusively on the women-helping-women model that prevailed among many organizations prior to 1914.[30] Moreover, at no point in the organization's history did women's Red Cross involvement disrupt prevailing gender norms. Women were seen as being particularly suited to voluntary Red Cross work either by virtue of their gender or, later in the century, as a result of their professional training. Over the twentieth century the CRCS mobilized and organized women for health-related service because both the organization and prevailing gender norms viewed women as inherently fitted to care.[31]

Children are another common thread in the history of the CRCS, as both objects of and contributors to the society's work. The successful mobilization of young Canadians for Red Cross war work during the First World War led directly to the creation of the Junior Red Cross after the war. Until the social and cultural upheavals of the later 1960s prompted a move to integrate youth into the senior Red Cross, the Junior Red Cross served as a tool for engaging children and youth in community and humanitarian service for others at home and abroad. Its two other simultaneous goals – citizenship training and health education – highlight the fact that after 1918 children and youth were seen as a prime site for improving the health of the nation, both in the sense of raising healthy, productive bodies, and in terms of training engaged, service-oriented, and public-spirited democratic citizens. These goals remained equally important during the Second World War, when democracy battled fascism, and again in the postwar decades, when the Cold War pitted democratic capitalism against communism. From the First World War through the 1970s, Canadian children and youth were both active volunteers and a focus for adult hopes for the world, the country, and the survival of the CRCS.

Fifth, the history of the Canadian Red Cross often mirrors that of Canada itself. As the Long Range Planning Committee recognized in its 1973 report, "Canadian Red Cross is not susceptible to any type of change that would not be equally suited to Canada as a nation."[32] This mirroring tendency appears in the society's sometimes fractious federal organization and occasional regional animosities; in its founding members' Victorian adherence to the values of militarism, imperialism, and particular understandings of women's roles; and in its emergence into official independence as a result of the 1931 Statute of Westminster. It shows up in the long, slow shift over the course of the twentieth century from emulating British Red Cross models to embracing American Red Cross precedents, punctuated by wartime bursts of pride in distinctly Canadian Red Cross accomplishments; it is similarly apparent in the society's affectionate ties to Britain that outlasted Canada's official colonial status. It appears again in the society's post-1945 "discovery" of a world beyond Europe and North America receptive to international aid. These parallels should come as no surprise: in political scientist Michael Barnett's words, all "humanitarianism is a creature of the world it aspires to civilize."[33] Like other humanitarian aid organizations, no matter how visionary, the CRCS has always been composed of individuals influenced to a greater or lesser degree by the world views of their time. Its history therefore highlights some of the shifting attitudes and preoccupations of the country as a whole.

Running alongside this national story is an international one. As Canada's relationship with the wider world has changed, so too has the society's. The Red Cross movement's complicated existence as a transnational movement that attempts to live out its ideals through nationally based organizations has been both a challenge and a strength for the CRCS. The international relationships within the Red Cross movement allowed Canadians to reach behind enemy lines and helped the CRCS fend off a certain amount of state regulation in wartime, but also raised difficult questions over what activity the CRCS could or should legitimately do (raised most articulately and pointedly by Charlotte Whitton early in the Second World War), in light of its Geneva Convention obligations. At its best, the pre-1970 society was inspired by its membership in a global family of Red Cross societies to build bridges of friendship and exchange ideas and expertise – through Junior Red Cross portfolios or adult participation in IRC conferences and governing bodies – and to offer assistance to those suffering from conflict and disaster in other countries. At its most problematic, the transnational bonds of common humanity were submerged in an uncritical Red Cross patriotism that used propaganda steeped in wartime nationalism to finance its humanitarian work. The tension between nationalism and internationalism has waned considerably since the end of the Second World War, but recognizing its existence earlier in the society's history serves as a warning for the future.

Sixth, the society's interwar history highlights certain Canadian-American differences and complicates the prevailing understanding of the Social Gospel movement. There has been a tendency to see the First World War as the endpoint of the massive and multifaceted social reform movement that characterized the prewar period, but this literature focuses primarily on the Social Gospel's urban reform work. By contrast, the history of the CRCS suggests that at least some of the prewar Social Gospellers simply shifted their attention to rural Canada after the war. The society's many provincial forays into outpost hospitals, mobile dental clinics, health literature, Junior Red Cross branches in rural schools, and visits to lighthouses and other remote locations, indicate an active concern with reforming and assisting Canadians outside urban areas.

As seen through the history of the CRCS, the relationship between the state and the voluntary sector emerges as complex, constantly shifting, yet consistently mutually dependent. Above all, the society's relationships with federal and provincial governments support Mariana Valverde's argument that Canada has been historically characterized by a mixed social economy in which services are provided by a combination of private and public bodies. Seemingly neither the wartime nor peacetime Canadian blood systems could be created by a federal government that lacked jurisdiction over health, whereas a popular, well-respected, national voluntary organization was capable of getting the provinces and territories on board. Yet the costs of the blood program forced the voluntary sector to turn to government for financial support. It suited both the state and the CRCS to work in partnership, and the resulting system, in which governments covered an increasing proportion of technical costs while the CRCS covered donor procurement and administered the system, is a quintessential example of the mixed social economy in action. The two world wars and Korean War, as well as interwar CRCS work for veterans, offer further examples: it suited the government to delegate certain tasks to the voluntary sector, benefiting as a result from an engaged citizenry, increased morale, the provision of supplementary goods and services, and the collection of what amounted to "voluntary" taxes. Charitable registration, budget supervision, forced joint campaigns, access to shipping space, and access to military personnel were among the tools the state could use behind the scenes to direct "private" charity and the "voluntary" efforts of citizens into its own preferred channels.

The CRCS also made pragmatic use of its relationship with the state at certain times. Despite its much-vaunted autonomy, the CRCS (like other national Red Cross societies) was not entirely independent. In the early twentieth century, national governments successively brought their Red Cross organizations under some measure of state control: in Canada, this took place in the society's 1909 Act of Incorporation. In addition to gaining the useful ability to hold property and engage in financial transactions like an individual, the CRCS also acquired the responsibility of having its finances reviewed annually by the state, and an "auxiliary" status in wartime. The society was proud of this auxiliary status, using it to maximum effect in order to secure donations and motivate volunteers, and brandishing it as a tacit form of government support when the society's few vocal critics raised objections to some aspect of CRCS work. The society also publicized other indications of government support at every opportunity – from royal visits and royal patronage, to prominent civic elites on the executive, to public statements by politicians, government grants, and government requests for CRCS assistance. These links to public authorities helped bolster the private moral authority upon which the CRCS normally relied. This closely intertwined relationship between state and civil society was perhaps best expressed by Dr Stanbury who described the society in 1957 as simultaneously "a private organization and a public service." It takes a combination of adaptability, determination, and luck to remain a relevant and leading voluntary and charitable organization for more than a hundred years. The CRCS has been just as successful as the Canadian state in using the mixed social economy to its advantage, deliberately inhabiting the muddy no man's land between public and private, in order to advance its goals of engaging citizens in humanitarian work at home and abroad.

The society's struggles during the Great Depression highlight differences in Canadian and American attitudes toward the respective responsibilities of the state and the voluntary sector at a particular moment in time. Faced with equally devastating rates of unemployment and regional droughts, both countries had prominent Red Cross societies and traditions of being disinclined toward state intervention. Yet by the 1930s a shift had clearly taken place in Canada. When the Depression struck, American president Herbert Hoover quickly turned to the American Red Cross to handle relief for sufferers of the southern drought and attempted to get the ARC to take responsibility for all relief work generally. Canadian prime minister R.B. Bennett, on the other hand, refused the pleas of CRCS leaders for his government to help the CRCS play a similar role in Canada, arguing that governments must be responsible for such work. While the Canadian federal government resisted taking on massive relief itself, it did not want the voluntary sector to do so either. The country was shifting from its traditional reliance on voluntary and charitable activity toward a conviction that the state should intervene in social welfare, and the CRCS of the early 1930s found its desire to help thwarted by a particularly ambivalent moment in that shift. Both the ambivalence and the Canadian-American difference appear again in the postwar period. Canadians created a nationwide free blood transfusion system under the banner of the CRCS, then turned to government funding to help cover its costs, creating a mixed voluntary-state system. Americans, on the other hand, created a mixed system where citizens could choose to donate voluntarily to the ARC or sell their blood to a private firm, while recipients of blood paid a fee regardless of the source. Neither country saw the state take full control of blood donation, but the Canadian voluntary-state partnership demonstrates a distinctly different ethos from the American voluntary-private capital alternative, in terms of both state involvement and attitudes toward the commodification of human blood.

Beyond these two examples, the American Red Cross emerges as an occasional foil and more often as an example of what is possible, in the history of the CRCS. The pre-1970 society enviously observed, borrowed from, and piggybacked upon ARC advertising and fundraising techniques; successful ARC disaster relief and water safety programs gave CRCS leaders the courage they needed to expand into those fields in their own time. Instances of cooperation and support abound and yet their histories are, in fact, very different. The ARC's early start in disaster and international relief work, experience of protracted neutrality in both world wars, close ties to the American government and deliberate role in American foreign policy, presence in a Cold War superpower, and exponentially larger population (and funding) base shaped the ARC in directions the CRCS did not follow. More research on the histories of both organizations will undoubtedly enrich the existing portrait of these two friendly, but very different, North American Red Cross societies.

Seventh, although it may appear that the society took a scattershot approach to its peacetime public health work – the decentralized structure in peacetime encouraged this – its seemingly disparate initiatives were united by several common characteristics, including the type of work, its target populations, and its providers. The society largely focused its peacetime efforts on health education and disease prevention rather than dealing with existing sickness and injury, although outpost hospitals, Crippled Children's Hospitals, and the BTS are notable exceptions. At the same time, before 1970 the society provided most of its peacetime care to Canadian civilians in Canada rather than to others abroad. Servicemen-turned-veterans received ongoing Red Cross attention, but ordinary Canadians – in particular women and children – became the principal targets of Red Cross peacetime efforts. Meanwhile, although there was always a place for voluntary labour, professionals and specialists became more and more crucial to the society's ability to fulfill its peacetime mandate as the twentieth century progressed. But above all, the society's peacetime work has been unified by the two common goals motivating it: first, saving lives – whether through disease prevention, blood transfusion, pre-natal care, or POW parcels – and second, caring for the vulnerable – whether that vulnerability arises from youth, natural disaster, war, migration, or living far from health care facilities. This persistent desire to save lives and care for the vulnerable demonstrates that despite the diverse and often pragmatic considerations that motivated its activities, the society's work has always *also* revolved around a nucleus of humanitarianism.

Finally, as any institutional history or volunteer recruitment brochure produced by the CRCS – and even the preface to the final report of the Krever Inquiry – will attest, front-line volunteers have been the heart and soul of the Canadian Red Cross Society since the beginning. Key leaders at the provincial and national levels wielded great power in shaping the organization's policies and directions, and a very few, like Dr Ryerson, Mrs Plumptre, and Dr Stanbury, left the stamp of their personality or vision on the entire organization. But it was millions of ordinary people in communities across Canada who chose, for reasons best known to themselves but explored in this book, to help others by donating their nickels, dimes, and dollars; their pints of blood; their energy and enthusiasm; and their time, talents, and training. Without these ordinary Canadians, much of the story told here would never have come to pass. This is their history as much as it is the history of the organization they worked for or supported. Through the dramatic changes that shaped Canada after 1885, they kept the Canadian Red Cross Society and its humanitarian ideals alive.

NOTES

INTRODUCTION

1 Toronto CRCS, *History Toronto Branch*, 9.

2 See Wilson, "Reciprocal Work Bees"; Ferry, *Uniting in Measures of Common Good*; Sutherland, "Voluntary Societies"; and G. Kealey, *Toronto Workers Respond*.

3 An enormous body of literature examines (a) organizations and how they function, and (b) what is alternately called the "Third Sector," the "Nonprofit Sector," "civil society," and/or "NGOs" (non-governmental organizations). A helpful entry-point is Pugh and Hickson, *Writers on Organizations*. Powell and Clemens, eds, *Private Action and the Public Good* offers a thorough introduction to non-profit organizations, the concept of civil society, and voluntary organizations as a form of civic engagement. Salamon, Sokolowski and Associates, *Global Civil Society* compares the non-profit sector in forty countries, while four linked volumes edited by Banting and Brock and published by the School of Policy Studies at Queen's University (Kingston) survey the contemporary Canadian context: *The Nonprofit Sector in Canada*, *The Nonprofit Sector and Government*, *The Nonprofit Sector in Interesting Times*, and *Delicate Dances*. Campbell, *The Voluntary Non-Profit Sector* is a dated but still helpful survey of major developments in the field.

4 The essays in Weindling, ed., *International Health Organisations* offer case studies of interwar health organizations that pioneered new health services or filled gaps in existing provisions. Weindling argues that "the state as a provider of welfare can be problematic" (1) for reasons of politics and financial expediency, while non-governmental organizations are sometimes able to remedy various deficiencies by working outside that system.

5 Victoria Alexander writes that non-profit organizations are "character-ized by complex goals, multiple constituencies, and fragmented environ-ments" which complicate the working out of their organizational missions. When different constituencies disagree over organizational goals, for example, the organization must somehow manage these fac-tions in order to remain viable. Not all organizations successfully do so. Victoria Alexander, "Environmental Constraints and Organizational Strategies: Complexity, Conflict, and Coping in the Nonprofit Sector," in Powell and Clemens, *Private Action*, 272.

6 Valverde, "The Mixed Social Economy," 33–8.

7 Dunant, *A Memory of Solferino*, 62–3, 115–27.

8 Pictet, *Development and Principles*, 26–30; Moorehead, *Dunant's Dream*, 17–24; Hutchinson, *Champions of Charity*, 26; Best, *Humanity in Warfare*, 129.

9 *Basic Rules of the Geneva Conventions*.

10 Best, *Humanity in Warfare*, 1–2, 132–6. The pre-war effort to build in-ternational connections is surveyed in Iriye, *Cultural Internationalism*.

11 Moorehead, *Dunant's Dream*, 19; Hutchinson, *Champions of Charity*, 344.

12 Barnett, *Empire of Humanity*, 37–40.

13 Best, *Humanity in Warfare*, 142, 151–3.

14 "The Structure and Role of the Red Cross," no pagination. The symbol of a red crescent was first used in Turkey in the nineteenth century. The ICRC and Geneva Conventions subsequently granted it official recogni-tion as an alternate symbol, and today it is used in many countries that object to the traditional association of the cross with Christianity. Effec-tive January 2007, the Red Cross movement adopted a third symbol, a red crystal, for use by countries (notably Israel) that object to both the red cross and the red crescent.

15 Smith, "The Role of Nongovernmental Organizations," 293.

16 Hutchinson, *Champions of Charity*, 282.

17 Joint Committee, *An Agenda for Red Cross*, 47–9.

18 Klein, *No Logo*, 23.

19 Chatelain and Neukomm, "The Story of an Idea."

20 ICRC, "The Fundamental Principles."

21 Hutchinson, "Rethinking the Origins," 557–78. Hutchinson later ex-plicitly discussed this "sacred cow" reputation in the introductory chap-ter of *Champions of Charity*.

22 Boissier, *From Solferino to Tsushima*; Durand, *From Sarajevo to Hi-roshima*; Berry, *War and the Red Cross*; Moorehead, *Dunant's Dream*;

Favez, *The Red Cross and the Holocaust*; Forsythe, *The Humanitarians*; Hutchinson, *Champions of Charity*.

23 The first chapter of Barnett, *Empire of Humanity*, provides a useful overview of this argument as developed throughout the rest of the book.

24 Irwin, *Making the World Safe*; Moser Jones, *American Red Cross from Clara Barton to the New Deal*.

25 Oppenheimer, *The Power of Humanity*; Tennant, *Across the Street, Across the World*; Willis, *Ministering Angels*.

26 Best, *Humanity in Warfare*, 141. Hutchinson notes that "Best's brief but suggestive comments on the history of the Red Cross (pp. 141–50) are worth more to the historian than all the hagiographical works" written about the Red Cross. Hutchinson, "Rethinking the Origins," 559n5.

27 Hutchinson, *Champions of Charity*, 256.

28 Watson, *History Ontario Red Cross*; Gordon, *Fifty Years*; Mitchell and Deacon, 641; Ellis with Dingman, *Face Powder and Gunpowder*; Day, Spence, and Ladouceur, eds, *Women Overseas*; Macleod Moore, *Maple Leaf's Red Cross*.

29 M. Porter, *To All Men*. Details of how Porter sought information and structured his book may be found in the Canadian Red Cross Society National Archive (hereafter CRCNA), box 6, file 6.II, W.S. Stanbury to Friends of Red Cross, [1958?].

30 Sheehan, "The Red Cross and Relief"; Sheehan, "Junior Red Cross in the Schools"; Sheehan, "Junior Red Cross Movement in Saskatchewan."

31 Kapp, "Charles H. Best"; Toxopeus, "1951 Agreement."

32 L. Kealey, "Delivering Health Care"; Elliott, "Keep the Flag Flying"; Elliott, "Blurring the Boundaries of Space"; Elliot, "(Re)constructing the Identity of a Red Cross Outpost Nurse," in Elliot, Stuart, and Toman, *Place and Practice*; and Elliot, "A Negotiated Process," in Rutherdale, *Caregiving on the Periphery*.

33 Quiney, "Bravely and Loyally"; Quiney, "We Must not Neglect Our Duty"; Quiney, "'Suitable Young Women,'" in Elliot, Stuart, and Toman, *Place and Practice*; Polk, "Relief in Siberia"; Baldwin and Poulter, "Mona Wilson"; Vance, "Canadian Relief Agencies"; Pomerleau, "La Société canadienne."

34 Mosby, *Food Will Win the War*, 111–25; Glassford, "Bearing the Burdens"; Glassford, "The Greatest Mother of Them All"; Glassford, "Mobilisées, organisées"; Glassford, "Practical Patriotism."

35 Dunant, *A Memory of Solferino*; Cole-Mackintosh, *A Century of Service*, 14–17; Dulles, *The American Red Cross*, chapter 1.

36 See, for example, Black, *A Cause for Our Times*; Black, *The Children*

and the Nations; Buchanan, "The Truth Will Set You Free"; *Remembering Herbert Hoover*; Sellick, "Responding to Children."

37 Women's First World War voluntary labour is the subject of Pickles, *Female Imperialism*; D. Morton, *Fight or Pay*; and Quiney, "Bravely and Loyally." See also Glassford and Shaw, eds, *A Sisterhood of Suffering and Service*. Key works on women's paid and unpaid labour include Kinnear, *In Subordination*; Parr, *The Gender of Breadwinners*; Pierson, *They're Still Women After All*; Cuthbert Brandt et al., *Canadian Women*, and Baillargeon, *A Brief History*. They offer useful overviews of the shifting roles and perceptions of women and work throughout Canadian and Quebec history. Child labour is explored in Rollings-Magnusson, *Heavy Burdens on Small Shoulders*, and McIntosh, "The Boys in the Nova Scotian Coal Mines."

38 Tillotson, *Contributing Citizens*. Canadian historians have produced a wide literature on the interwar public health movement and its impact on childhood and motherhood, a movement in which voluntary organizations were deeply involved. See, for instance, Comacchio, *Nations Are Built of Babies*; Valverde, *The Age of Light, Soap, and Water*; Sutherland, *Children in English-Canadian Society*; Arnup, *Education for Motherhood*; Dodd, "Advice to Parents."

39 Poulter, "Archives of the British Red Cross," 146.

40 Hutchinson, *Champions of Charity*; Moorehead, *Dunant's Dream*.

41 Cooter, "Medicine and the Goodness of War," 155.

CHAPTER ONE

1 Ryerson, *Looking Backward*, 81.

2 Buchanan, "The Truth Will Set You Free," 575–7.

3 "The Latest – The Midnight Report," *Globe*, 1 September 1864, 2; "Geneva Congress," *Globe*, 11 November 1868, 1.

4 Marquis, *In Armageddon's Shadow*.

5 Oppenheimer, *The Power of Humanity*, 9–15; Tennant, *Across the Street, Across the World*, 23–30.

6 The BNAS was often referred to as the British Red Cross Society. On the American Red Cross expansion, see "Notes from Washington," *Globe*, 24 January 1882, 2. For a Red Cross nurse example, see "In the Name of Charity," *World* (Toronto), 26 November 1885, 1.

7 "A Red Cross Corps," *Globe*, 10 April 1885, 4.

8 Volunteer Surgeon, "A Suggestion," *Montreal Gazette*, 1 April 1885, 8. There is no evidence to prove or disprove this suggestion, but "Volunteer Surgeon" may have been G.S. Ryerson himself. The article has a tone similar to Ryerson's other writings, and his lifelong concern with

military medical provision bordered on obsession. However, anonymity was decidedly not his style. Thomas Roddick is another possibility.

9 Bryce, "Alfred Codd"; Nicholson, *Seventy Years of Service*, 32; "Codd Flag's Storied History," *StarPhoenix*, 13 May 2010. National Red Cross publications rarely mention Codd (although the Saskatchewan organization is quite proud of him), but he is discussed in "The Canadian Red Cross Society," *Despatch* 27, no. 3 (1966): 16; and "The Canadian Red Cross Society," *Service* 38, no. 1 (Spring 1977): 18. In each case, Ryerson and his flag still dominate the narrative.

10 Bergin was a Cornwall, Ontario physician, stockbreeder, railway entrepreneur, and eventually Conservative MP. He was also a member of the militia and in 1885 was appointed surgeon-general. Charles G. Roland, "Bergin, Darby," in *Dictionary of Canadian Biography Online* [hereafter DCB *Online*].

11 Darby Bergin, "Appendix 5 – Report of the Surgeon General," *Sessional Papers*, vol. 19, no. 5, 6 to 6a (1886), 332 states that roughly half of the corps members belonged to the Queen's Own Rifles, while C.F. Winter indicates that all the members were Queen's Own men, in Mackay, ed., "The North-West Rebellion, 1885," 12.

12 "The Red Cross Ambulance Corps," *World* (Toronto), 10 April 1885, 1; "A Red Cross Corps," *Globe*, 10 April 1885, 4; "The Red Cross," *Globe*, 16 April 1885, 6; Nicholson, *Seventy Years of Service*, 32; Bull, "Dr William Nattress," 222b.

13 Nicholson, *Seventy Years of Service*, 32; Nattress, "Field Hospitals"; "Home Again," *Globe*, 21 April 1885, 3; "Poundmaker's Beating," *World* (Toronto), 21 May 1885, 1; Bergin, "Report of the Surgeon General," *Sessional Papers* (1886), 332.

14 D. Morton, *The Last War Drum*, 91–2.

15 Ryerson, *Looking Backward*, 81.

16 The Ryerson Flag is on display inside the national headquarters of the CRCS in Ottawa (occasionally loaned to the Canadian War Museum for special exhibits). The Codd Flag is on display in the Regina office of the Southern Saskatchewan regional office of the CRCS, and was designated as a Provincial Historic Property in 2006.

17 The British commissioner is mentioned in "Aid for the Wounded," *Globe*, 16 October 1896, 7. This article about the founding of a Canadian branch of the BNAS notes that the British Society "sent a commissioner with stores and money to our Northwest rebellion." Unfortunately no relevant records have been located in the BRCS or CRCS archives, or anywhere else.

18 Volunteer Surgeon, "A Suggestion," *Montreal Gazette*, 1 April 1885, 8.

An editorial the following day supported this suggestion, stating that "it is a matter in which ladies can render valuable services." "A Timely Suggestion," *Montreal Gazette*, 2 April 1885, 4.

19 Darby Bergin to Adolphe Caron, 12 April 1885, as quoted in Nicholson, *Canada's Nursing Sisters*, 19. Bergin alludes to this in his "Report of the Surgeon General," *Sessional Papers* (1886), 328.

20 "The Red Cross Ambulance Corps," *World* (Toronto), 10 April 1885, 1; "A Red Cross Corps," *Globe*, 10 April 1885, 4; "The Red Cross," *Globe*, 16 April 1885, 6.

21 "A Red Cross Corps," *Globe*, 10 April 1885, 4; "The Red Cross," *Globe*, 16 April 1885, 6; "Poundmaker's Beating," *World* (Toronto), 21 May 1885, 1. On women's nursing work in the Northwest, see *A Memoir of the Life and Work of Hannah Grier Coome*, 91–5; Domm, "Called to Duty," 15–23; Domm, "From the Streets of Toronto to the Northwest Rebellion: Hannah Grier Coome's Call to Duty," in Rutherdale, *Caregiving on the Periphery*, 109–26. The description of a "Recreation Room" (*A Memoir of the Life and Work of Hannah Grier Coome*, 92) attached to the Anglican sisters' hospital in Moose Jaw, furnished with reading material, games, and tobacco (donated by Toronto ladies) closely resembles the CRCS's provision of comforts and recreation rooms to Canadian Army Medical Corps hospitals during the Great War. On donors to the Red Cross corps, see a series of articles all titled "The Red Cross," *Globe*, 16 April 1885, 6; 1 May 1885, 6; 5 May 1885, 6; 16 May 1885, 14.

22 Bergin, "Report of the Surgeon General," *Sessional Papers* (1886), 327.

23 "The Red Cross," *Globe*, 16 April 1885, 6.

24 Winter, quoted in Mackay, ed., "The North-West Rebellion," 15.

25 D. Morton, *Last War Drum*, ix.

26 Moorehead, *Dunant's Dream*, 61.

27 D. Morton, *Last War Drum*, 31; Ryerson, *Looking Backward*, 94.

28 Bergin, "Report of the Surgeon General," *Sessional Papers* (1886); Nicholson, *Seventy Years of Service*, 35–6.

29 Ryerson, *Looking Backward*, 117.

30 MacDermot, *Sir Thomas Roddick*, 145, 140; Joseph Hanaway, "Roddick, Sir Thomas George," DCB *Online*.

31 On Nattress's textbook, see Lenskyj, "Raising 'Good Vigorous Animals,'" 31; also S. Cook, "Evangelical Moral Reform," 189. On Mason, see Morgan, ed., "Mason, Lt.-Col. James," in *The Canadian Men and Women of the Time* (1898), 609; also Mulvany, *The History of the North-West Rebellion of 1885*, 213.

32 Dembski, "Ryerson, George Ansel Sterling," DCB *Online*; Ryerson, *Looking Backward*, 34.

33 Ryerson, *Looking Backward* – European travels, chapters 3 and 4; militia enlistment, 60. The migration of American students to Europe in the mid-nineteenth century is explored in Rodgers, *Atlantic Crossings*, 76–97.

34 Moorehead, *Dunant's Dream*, 61, 121.

35 Ryerson, *Looking Backward*, chapter 5; Dembski, "Ryerson," DCB *Online*.

36 Ferry, *Uniting in Measures of Common Good*, 288–9. Ferry's study focuses primarily on men; women and voluntary organizations are examined in Strong-Boag, "'Setting the Stage'"; Linda Kealey, "Introduction," in L. Kealey, ed., *A Not Unreasonable Claim*; Nielson, *Private Women and the Public Good*.

37 Ryerson, *Looking Backward*, 94–7; Nicholson, *Seventy Years of Service*, 38–9; CRCNA, George Sterling Ryerson Papers [hereafter Ryerson Papers], file D, "Constitution and By-Laws of the Association of Medical Officers of the Militia of Canada" (Toronto: William Briggs, 1892), 3–5.

38 Cole-Mackintosh, *A Century of Service*, 7–13; Ryerson, *Looking Backward*, 108; Nicholson, *The White Cross in Canada*, 32–3.

39 Ryerson, *Looking Backward*, 117.

40 Cole-Mackintosh, *A Century of Service*, 14–15; Ryerson, *Looking Backward*, 117–18.

41 In return for political services to the then-ruling Conservative Party, Ryerson got himself appointed to a special and hitherto unknown rank, above the heads of senior officers. General Officer Commanding W.J. Gascoigne (a blunt man who did not get along with the Conservative minister of militia) claimed to find such ruthlessness atrocious, and wrote in 1896 that he thought Ryerson (who "openly confessed he did not care how he hurt his comrades to gain his own aggrandisement") "the most selfish, the vainest, the most unprincipled man" he had ever met. British Red Cross Museum and Archive [hereafter BRCMA], Lord Wantage Papers, D/Wan/18/1/18, W.J. Gascoigne to Lord Wantage, 25 October 1896; Dembski, "Ryerson," DCB *Online*.

42 C. Miller, "The Montreal Militia," 57–63.

43 Mulvany, *The History of the North-West Rebellion of 1885*, 437–8; Geo. Maclean Rose, "John George Hodgins," and "Edward H. Smythe," *A Cyclopaedia of Canadian Biography*, 566–7 and 305; Morgan, ed., "Frederick LeMaistre Grasett," "Major John Bayne MacLean," and "Lt.-Col. James Mason," *The Canadian Men and Women of the Time* (1898), 403–4, 706, 609; Paul Adolphus Bator, "Charles

O'Reilly," DCB *Online*; André Sévigny, "Frederick Montizambert," DCB *Online*; "Charles A. Hodgetts: Fundamental to the Advancement of the First Aid Movement in Canada."

44 P.B. Waite, "Sir Charles Hibbert Tupper," Hal J. Guest, "Sir Hugh John Macdonald," and Carolyn E. Gray, "Sir John Morison Gibson," all in DCB *Online*.

45 CRCS, *Report of the Canadian Red Cross Society of Its Operations in the South African War 1899–1902* [hereafter *South African War Report*] (Toronto: CRCS, 1902), 12.

46 Hutchinson, *Champions of Charity*, chapters 3–5.

47 CRCS, *South African War Report*, 12.

48 BRCMA, D/Wan/18/1/16, Charles Hodgetts to J.G. Vokes, 15 October 1896; CRCS, *South African War Report*, 11.

CHAPTER TWO

1 "Toronto's Greeting to the Veterans of Africa," *Globe*, 6 November 1900, 1, 10.

2 BRCMA, D/Wan/18/1/20, Charles Hodgetts to J.G. Vokes, 21 November 1896.

3 Ibid. "Aid for the wounded," *Globe*, 16 October 1896, 7.

4 [untitled], *Toronto Star*, 5 May 1898, 5; "Senor Du Bosc Will Lecture," *Globe*, 2 May 1898, 9.

5 Judd and Surridge, *The Boer War*, 1.

6 B. Porter, *The Lion's Share*, 167–77.

7 C. Miller, *A Knight in Politics*, 113. Miller refers to an assessment made by Jonathan Miller in the "Introduction" to Tabitha Jackson, *The Boer War* (London, UK: Channel Four Books, 1999), 7.

8 Page, *The Boer War and Canadian Imperialism*, 12; Penny, "Australia's Reactions to the Boer War," 97; Krebs, *Gender, Race and the Writing of Empire*, 7.

9 Brown and Cook, *Canada 1896–1921*, 39–41.

10 Lowry, "The Boers were the beginning," 225–6.

11 Brown and Cook, *Canada 1896–1921*, 39–41; Page, *The Boer War and Canadian Imperialism*, 12, 15; Lowry, "The Boers were the beginning," 225–6; Canada raised 8,400 men (versus 6,000 New Zealanders, 16,500 Australians, and 355,750 Britons) and spent £620,000 (versus the £223,000,000 spent by Britain). Britain spent more money in Canada buying food, horses, and equipment than Ottawa did. On the British humanitarian response, see Gill, "Networks of Concern," 827.

12 C. Miller, *Painting the Map Red*, 429; "Red Cross Fund," *Globe*, 20 October 1899, 10.

13 The government initially accepted the offer of socks and underclothing, but later decided the militia would provide these items. Department of Militia and Defence for the Dominion of Canada, "Supplementary Report – Organization, Equipment, Despatch and Service of the Canadian Contingents during the War in South Africa 1899–1900," in "Report of the Major General on the South African Contingents," *Sessional Papers* vol. 35a, no. 12 (1901), 7; "Free insurance," *The Globe*, 23 October 1899, 5.

14 Ryerson, *Looking Backward*, 161; "Red Cross Fund," *The Globe*, 23 October 1899, 12; CRCS, *South African War Report*, 63.

15 "Women of Canada – An Appeal to Them on Behalf of the Red Cross," *The Globe*, 4 January 1900, 5; Rosa Shaw, *Proud Heritage*, 153.

16 CRCNA, box 49, file 49.1, St Catharines' Red Cross Charter, 1900.

17 Evans, *The Canadian Contingents*, 251.

18 CRCS, *South African War Report*, 13–14.

19 Ibid., 48, 60–2, 67–9, 72–6.

20 "Chit Chat," *Globe*, 8 March 1900, 8; "Sir Samuel Leonard Tilley," *DCB Online*. Lady Tilley was born Alice Starr Chipman. She married Leonard Tilley, a close friend of her father's, in October 1867, five years after the death of his first wife of nearly twenty years, and became well known in New Brunswick for her organizational and philanthropic work.

21 CRCS, *South African War Report*, 60, 65–6.

22 Ibid., 79; "Funds for Soldiers," *Montreal Gazette*, 5 January 1900, 1; "General News," *Globe*, 4 January 1900, 1; Miller, *A Knight in Politics*, 292.

23 See, for example, "Red Cross Fund," *Globe*, 27 January 1900, 24.

24 "Patriotic School Children," *Globe*, 29 December 1899, 10; CRCNA, box 52, Kathleen Herman to Dr Stanbury, Memo: "History of Junior Red Cross," 4 September 1958; CRCS, *South African War Report*, 69.

25 "'Maple Leaves' Worked for Red Cross in the South African War," *The Canadian Red Cross Junior* [hereafter CRC *Junior*] (March 1937), 3; "'Maple Leaves' Organized in 1899," CRC *Junior* (November 1937), 2. In 2016 terms, this $341 is worth more than $7,300. Bank of Canada Inflation Calculator, www.bankofcanada.ca.

26 "Chit Chat," *Globe*, 10 March 1900, 21.

27 Maroney, "'The Peaceable Kingdom' Reconsidered," 318–25.

28 Hutchinson, *Champions of Charity*, 256–76.

29 Maroney, "'The Peaceable Kingdom' Reconsidered," 339.

30 Berger, *The Sense of Power*, 5, 9, 259–60.

31 CRCNA, box 49, file 49.1, letter to newspaper editors from James Mason and Charles Hodgetts, 1 March 1900.

32 Gill, "Networks of Concern," 828.

33 Kipling, "The Absent-Minded Beggar," 451.

34 B. Gordon, *The Saturated World*, 108, 123–5, 138; "Chit Chat," *Globe*, 6 February 1900, 9; "A Great Concert," *Globe*, 8 March 1900, 14; "Chit Chat," *Globe*, 5 May 1900, 25.

35 CRCNA, box 49, file 49.1, circular from Newmarket Branch CRCS, 1900 [?].

36 Ryerson, *Looking Backward*, 121; CRCNA, Ryerson Papers, file D, "Resolution of United Empire Loyalists Association," 8 March 1900.

37 Canadian Patriotic Fund Association, "As you are doubtless aware"; Evans, *The Canadian Contingents*, 253.

38 "Welland County's Contribution," "Dufferin County Grants $500," and "Notes," *Globe*, 27 January 1900, 17; "Paris Red Cross Society," *Globe*, 9 January 1900, 4.

39 The importance of an aseptic environment and good nursing in aiding patient recovery prior to the discovery of antibiotics is apparent in the parameters of nursing work before 1940, as discussed in McPherson, *Bedside Matters*, 83–99.

40 See Dr Ryerson's report in the CRCS *South African War Report*, 21–2; see also Appendix XIII of *Report by the Central British Red Cross Committee* (1902), 205. Items shipped or purchased on location included bedding, dishes and cutlery, handkerchiefs, mosquito netting, towels, screens (for the dying), feeding cups, walking sticks and crutches, surgical dressings, basins and jugs, cholera belts, Listerine, sponges, soap, Vaseline, hot-water bottles, rubber sheeting, a wide variety of non-perishable food items (such as arrowroot biscuits, barley, condensed milk and soups, tinned meats and vegetables, chocolate, tea), alcohol (brandy, champagne, whiskey, wine), an array of sleepwear, undergarments, and other clothing, tooth brushes, tobacco, periodicals, books, hymn books, games, and stationery.

41 CRCS, *South African War Report*, 16.

42 Strong-Boag, "Setting the Stage," 95.

43 L. Kealey, *A Not Unreasonable Claim*, 6–8.

44 This was also true of female imperialists' work elsewhere in the British Empire. Bush, *Edwardian Ladies*, 74.

45 Bush, *Edwardian Ladies*, 3; Pickles, *Female Imperialism*, 16–19; de Groot, "'Sex' and 'Race,'" 51.

46 "Supplementary Report – Organization, Equipment, Despatch and Service of the Canadian Contingents during the War in South Africa 1899–1900," in "Report of the Major General on the South African Contingents," *Sessional Papers* (1901), 65.

47 CRCS, *South African War Report*, 47; C. Miller, *Painting the Map Red*, 431. The Bank of Canada's inflation calculator only goes back to 1914. The purchasing power of $82,379.39 in 1914 dollars is equivalent to $1,765,545.96 in 2016 dollars, so its value in 1899–1902 dollars would be even higher. In 2016 the CPFA's $340,000 raised would be worth more than $7.3 million, and the British Red Cross's £178,950 would be roughly equivalent to $25.5 million Canadian. These calculations were made using tools on the following websites: The Bank of Canada, Inflation Calculator www.bankofcanada.ca; The National Archives (UK), Currency Converter www.nationalarchives.gov.uk/currency/; OANDA, Historical Exchange Rates www.oanda.com/currency/historical-rates/.

48 Ryerson, *Looking Backward*, chapters 17 and 18.

49 D. Morton, "Colonel Otter," 108; Sutphen, "Striving to Be Separate?" 58.

50 CRCS, *South African War Report*, 17–25; *Report of the Central British Red Cross Committee* (1902), 15–16.

51 Excerpts in CRCS, *South African War Report*: John Furley to Colonel Ryerson, 4 July 1900, 31; Field Marshal Roberts to the Secretary of State for War, 10 September 1901, 30–1; Lt-General Methuen to Lt-General Lord Kitchener, Chief of Staff, 29 March 1900, 30.

52 CRCS, *South African War Report*, 33–6.

53 Baughan, "Every Citizen of Empire," 125–9; Alexander, "The Girl Guide Movement," 37–63.

54 BRCMA, D/Wan/15/4/29, Charles Hodgetts to J.G. Vokes, 3 July 1900.

55 CRCS, *South African War Report*, 23.

56 CRCNA, box 49, file 49.1, circular from Newmarket Branch CRCS, 1900 [?]; Ryerson, *Looking Backward*, 170; Heath, *A War with a Silver Lining*, 41; Gill, "Networks of Concern," 828, 830.

57 "Work during the War," *Globe*, 23 July 1902, 4; CRCS, *South African War Report*, Georgina F. Pope to Col Ryerson, 23 January 1901, 33 and W.G. Lane to Col. Ryerson, [n.d.], 32.

58 Carman Miller summarizes Otter's attitude toward Ryerson in *Painting the Map Red*, 430; Miller believes the evidence for this assessment appeared in Otter's diaries or letters to his wife, but I have been unable to locate the exact source. Miller's research has led him to see Ryerson as

"very much a one-man operation" and he suspects that due to Ryerson's opinionated self-importance "he may not have always won friends in his efforts to influence people." Carman Miller, email messages to author, 8 April 2010 and 19 April 2010. This assessment, which mirrors my own, is supported by statements made by the British General Officer Commanding the Canadian militia, W.J. Gascoigne, in 1896, with regard to Ryerson's appointment to a special rank, above the heads of senior officers. (See chapter 1, note 41.) As a militia man, Colonel Otter would have been aware of Ryerson's actions, which Gascoigne wrote were "at one time in every bodys [sic] mouth." BRCMA, D/Wan/18/1/18, W.J. Gascoigne to Lord Wantage, 25 October 1896; C. Miller, *A Knight in Politics*, 98.

59 Mair, "W. Burdett-Coutts (Westminster)," 35.

60 W.L. Ashmead Bartlett Burdett-Coutts, "Our Wars and Our Wounded," *Times* (London), 29 June 1900, 14, and 30 June 1900, 16; "A Mass of Evidence," *Montreal Gazette*, 29 August 1900, 1; "Ryerson's Report," *Montreal Gazette*, 30 August 1900, 1; "Dr Ryerson's Flat Denial," *Globe*, 29 August 1900, 5; McKenzie Porter, *To All Men*, 35; BRCMA, D/Wan/15/9/23, G.S. Ryerson to Lord Wantage, 25 July 1900.

61 "Mr Burdett-Coutts and the Wounded," *Times* (London) 19 January 1900, 7; C. Miller, *Painting the Map Red*, 82–3; C. Miller, *A Knight in Politics*, 157–8.

62 "Money for the Third Contingent," *Globe*, 6 January 1902, 10; "They Sail away To-day," *Globe*, 14 January 1902, 5; *Report by the Central British Red Cross Committee* (1902), 17–20; C. Miller, *A Knight in Politics*, 154.

63 Dunant, *A Memory of Solferino*, 117.

64 CRCS, *Annual Report 1912* (Toronto: CRCS, 1913), 12.

65 *Report by the Central British Red Cross Committee* (1902), 2, 61.

66 CRCNA, Ryerson Papers, file T-U-V, Charles Hodgetts to Central Council members, 19 November 1900; "Red Cross Work," *Globe*, 16 November 1900, 12.

67 Ryerson, *The Soldier and the Surgeon*.

68 Carman Miller, "Borden, Sir Frederick William," DCB *Online*; Roland, "Bergin, Darby," DCB *Online*; C. Miller, *A Knight in Politics*, 19, 74–5, 77, 122, 145 (quotation), 189, 210–12, 292.

69 Nicholson, *Seventy Years of Service*, 56–60; C. Miller, *A Knight in Politics*, 201–2.

70 "Canadian Red Cross," *Globe*, 16 May 1907, 5.

71 C. Miller, *A Knight in Politics*, 197–8; quotation by Desmond Morton, in C. Miller, *A Knight in Politics*, 197.

72 Hutchinson, *Champions of Charity*, 151.

73 Ibid., 231–3; Moser Jones, *The American Red Cross*, chapter 6. Moser Jones unpacks the class, gender, and generational conflicts between the two women that turned a leadership struggle into an all-out internal war, but notes that the basic clash was between Barton's aid-first-and-accounting-after-(if at all) approach, and Boardman's Progressive-era agenda to bring better management (particularly financial accountability) to the venerable ARC (98, 106–8).

74 Hutchinson, *Champions of Charity*, 248–50.

75 Eight prominent Torontonians signed the petition, many of them long-time CRCS supporters, militia members, and/or medical professionals: Ontario lieutenant governor Col John M. Gibson, entrepreneur Col Sir Henry Pellatt, Col George A. Sweny, Col G.S. Ryerson, Lt-Col James Mason, bank manager D.R. Wilkie, Dr Charles A. Hodgetts, and lawyer John T. Small, K.C.

76 Library and Archives Canada [hereafter LAC], Department of the Secretary of State, RG 6, vol. 138, file 945, "Petition of the Canadian Red Cross Society for an Act of Incorporation," 27 March 1909.

77 House of Commons, *Official Report of Debates* (1909), 4988, 5487, 6068, 7087.

78 Page, *The Boer War and Canadian Imperialism*, 22; Brown and Cook, *Canada 1896–1921*, 166–7.

79 "An Act to Incorporate the Canadian Red Cross Society," *Statutes of Canada* (8–9 Edward VII ch. 68, 1909), 98.

80 The incorporated men included prominent public figures such as Ontario lieutenant governor John Morrison Gibson, Toronto entrepreneur Henry Pellatt, Montreal surgeon Thomas Roddick, and public health officer Frederick Montizambert, as well as long-term Red Cross supporters such as G.S. Ryerson, George Sweny, James Mason, and Charles Hodgetts. Of the thirty-two men, nine had political careers (municipal, provincial, or federal), six were physicians or surgeons, three practised law, one was an entrepreneur, and three are unknown. Twelve were militia officers. Sixteen lived in Toronto, three in Montreal, two in Ottawa and Winnipeg respectively, and one each in Fredericton, Hamilton, Saint John, Victoria, and the small Ontario towns of Belleville, St Thomas, and Ingersoll. The sixteen incorporated women were all married, and none lived in the same community. They lived in Alberta (Edmonton), Manitoba (Brandon), Ontario (Toronto, Hamilton, London, Brampton, Newmarket, Bradford), and New Brunswick (Saint John, Rothesay, Dorchester, Moncton, Sussex, Sackville). The Ontario and New Brunswick predominance makes it likely that these women had been active branch-level leaders during the

South African War, since these two provinces were most active in Red Cross work during the conflict.

81 Biographical details from the *Census of Canada*, 1911 (Gooderham, Robertson) and *Census of Canada*, 1891 (Nordheimer). All three women were in their late forties or early fifties, and Robertson and Nordheimer were among the sixteen women originally incorporated in 1909. Florence Robertson was the wife of a prosperous Newmarket barrister, while Mary Gooderham was the American-born wife of a Toronto distillery baron, and Edith Nordheimer was the wife of a leading Toronto piano and sheet music manufacturer. The Robertsons did not have any live-in servants, but Gooderham and Nordheimer each oversaw live-in household staffs of five or six, a clear indication of their prosperity.

82 CRCS, *Annual Report 1912*, 10–11. In order to familiarize Canadians and others with the society, copies were sent to CRCS members, the military establishment, Parliament, newspaper editors, public libraries, the British royal family, the BRCS, and other national Red Cross societies.

83 CRCNA, Executive Committee Archived Minute Book [hereafter ECAMB] 1, Executive Committee [hereafter EC] meeting 11 June 1914. In contrast, the ARC sent Prime Minister Sir Wilfrid Laurier $1,000 from its International Relief Fund when fire devastated the northern Ontario towns of Porcupine and Cochrane in 1911. "American Red Cross Offer Accepted," *Globe*, 18 July 1911, 2.

84 Hutchinson, *Champions of Charity*, 247.

85 CRCS, *Annual Report 1910* (Toronto: CRCS, 1911), 12–13.

86 CRCNA, ECAMB 1, EC meetings 16 April 1912 and 12 October 1912. The executive referred these inquiries to hospitals and the St John Ambulance Association respectively.

87 CRCS, *Annual Report 1910*, 15–17; *Annual Report 1911* (Toronto: CRCS, 1912), 12; *Annual Report 1912*, 14.

88 Ryerson, *The Soldier and the Surgeon*, 11–12; CRCNA, ECAMB 1, EC meetings 16 April 1912, 21 November 1912, 22 January 1913, and 11 June 1914; Nicholson, *White Cross*, 47.

89 "Notes and Comments," *Globe*, 9 November 1909, 6.

90 CRCNA, ECAMB 1, EC meeting 16 February 1912. The British law was titled the "Geneva Convention Act, 1911" and it came into force in Canada on 1 May 1912. LAC, Department of National Health and Welfare, RG 29, vol. 861, file 20–C–46 (part 1), notice re: Geneva Convention Act, 1911.

91 *The Red Cross School of Nursing*. The school geared its training toward

home nursing, but also offered specialized courses for women seeking outside employment as private duty nurses or nurses for physicians.

92	CRCS, *Annual Report 1911*, 13–17. See also CRCNA, ECAMB 1, EC meetings 20 September 1911, 12 December 1911, 29 December 1911, and 16 February 1912.

93	"Toronto's Greeting," 1, 10–11; "Burckhardt Gets His Medal," *Waterford Star* (Ontario), 22 November 1900,

CHAPTER THREE

1	CRCS Vancouver Branch, *The Queen's Tea Party*; Bank of Canada Inflation Calculator, www.bankofcanada.ca.

2	CRCNA, Ryerson Papers, file "R"; CRCNA, ECAMB 2, EC meeting 28 December 1915, 65.

3	CRCNA, ECAMB 1, EC meetings 7 August 1914, 65, and 21 August 1914, 68; CRCS, *Annual Report 1914* (Toronto: CRCS, 1915), 22; McKenzie Porter, *To All Men*, 51.

4	Money: CRCS, *Annual Report 1914* (Toronto: CRCS, 1915), 20; advertisements: "For Humanity's Sake" advertisement, *Globe*, 8 October 1914, 3; "Work of the Red Cross in Times of War," *Globe*, 28 September 1914, 4; "'Ware of the Bogus Collectors," *Globe*, 29 September 1914, 7; editorial, *Globe*, 1 October 1914, 4.

5	*The War Charities Act, 1917*, 1–2; CRCS, *What the CRCS Is Doing in the Great War*, 12.

6	M. Porter, *To All Men*, 37–8; CRCS, *Annual Report 1914*, 11–12; CRCS, *What the CRCS Is Doing in the Great War*, 11; CRCS, *Annual Report 1912*, 3–6. For details and examples of provincial organization and branch creation, see Glassford, "Marching as to War," chapter 3.

7	CRCNA, ECAMB 1, EC meeting 3 September 1914, 73, and two EC meetings 24 September 1914, 82, 84; "A Survey of Sixteen Months' Work at Headquarters," *Bulletin* (January 1916): 16.

8	CRCS, *Annual Report 1914*, 30; CRCNA, ECAMB 3, EC meeting 30 May 1916, 32.

9	"Col Jeffrey Burland Will Serve Red Cross," *Globe*, 29 September 1914, 6; CRCNA, *Annual Report 1914*, 26; Macleod Moore, *The Maple Leaf's Red Cross*, 30–3, 153–4, 156; Quebec Division, "In Memoriam Lieut-Colonel David Law," *Annual Report 1923* (Montreal: CRCS, 1924), [no pagination].

10	CRCNA, ECAMB 1, EC meeting 19 February 1915, 162, and 30 March 1915, 179–80; Ryerson Papers, file "C," letter of introduction from H.E. Harcourt Vernon, 31 March 1915.

11 Estimations of the value of CRCS money and goods received during the war have varied. No consolidated wartime financial statement appeared after 1918 as it did after 1945, so authoritative figures are difficult to come by, but we know that the CRCS received $9,073,485.56 in cash donations for its work and that it helped raise a further $6,250,000 for the BRCS in Canada. Both figures are routinely included in later estimates of CRCS wartime receipts (money and goods combined). The most commonly cited figure today is the $35,000,000 in money and goods which was included in an unofficial 1950 survey of CRCS history and published in McKenzie Porter's 1960 history. A 1938 CRCS pamphlet sets the figure at $30,000,000, while a 1934 pamphlet sets it at $22,000,000. Subtracting the CRCS and BRCS cash, a $35,000,000 total would mean just under $20,000,000 worth of goods, $30,000,000 would mean a little over $14,500,000 worth of goods, and $22,000,000 a little over $6,500,000 worth of goods. In 1917 Adelaide Plumptre conjectured that the value of goods sent overseas up to that point might be $14,000,000, and the federal government gave a figure of $13,500,000 worth of goods in 1919, so the $6,500,000 seems unlikely. CRCNA, box 6, file 6.II, "A Brief History of the Canadian Red Cross Society, 1885–1950," 3; M. Porter, *To All Men*, 53; CRCS, "Historical Review of the Red Cross," (Toronto: CRCS, 1938), 6; Ontario Division, "Historical Review of the Canadian Red Cross Society," 5; Adelaide Plumptre, "Canada's Love-Gifts," in *Canada in the Great World War*, vol. 2, 218; *Canada's Part in the Great War*, 43.

12 Quebec Division, *Annual Report 1922* (Montreal: CRCS, 1923), 25; Macleod Moore, *The Maple Leaf's Red Cross*, 52–6; *Bulletin* (February 1918): 41.

13 CRCNA, ECAMB 1, EC meeting 19 February 1915, 162; EC meeting 30 March 1915, 179–80; CRCNA, ECAMB 2, EC meeting 28 December 1915, 65; CRCNA, Ryerson Papers, file "C," letter of introduction from H.E. Harcourt Vernon, 31 March 1915; Macleod Moore, *The Maple Leaf's Red Cross*, 33; Ryerson, *Looking Backward*, 122. See also Oppenheimer, "The Best P.M. for the Empire in War," 108–24.

14 CRCNA, Book of Record: Honorary Counsellors, Canadian Red Cross Society, 1930–64, "Mr H. Milburne"; CRCNA, ECAMB 3, EC meeting 1 May 1917, 156; "A Survey of Sixteen Months' Work at Headquarters," *Bulletin* (January 1916): 17–18.

15 CRCS, *What the CRCS Is Doing in the Great War*, 7; CRCNA, ECAMB 1, EC meetings 29 November 1914, 114–15, and 26 February 1915, 165; *Bulletin* (January 1916): 7–8.

16 Ryerson, *Looking Backward*, chapter 21; CRCS Commissioner's Reports for week ending 8 May 1915, *Bulletin* (June 1915): 10; Moorehead, *Dunant's Dream*, 208.

17 CRCNA, ECAMB 1, EC meetings 30 September 1914, 88, and 29 November 1914, 114–15; CRCNA, box 5, file 5.I, "Report to the Tenth International Red Cross," 1, 12.

18 Nicholson, *White Cross*, 39, 56; Countess Mountbatten of Burma, "Joining Forces," in *I Owe My Life*, 19; CRCNA, ECAMB 1, EC meeting 22 December 1914, 129; ECAMB 4, EC meeting 10 June 1918, 58; Quiney, "Assistant Angels," 57–8; "Is Organized for Province," *Globe*, 22 December 1910, 8.

19 CRCNA, ECAMB 1, EC meeting 8 September 1914, 77.

20 Ibid., 77–8. The 1909 Act of Incorporation limited the number of people on the executive committee to ten, so the three new members (two women, one man) could not join as full members of the committee.

21 City of Toronto Archives (CTA), Information File on Elected Officials: Adelaide Plumptre, "Mrs Adelaide Plumptre Served City and Nation," 4 September 1948, and "An Interesting Canadian ... Mrs Plumptre;" LAC, R.B. Bennett Papers, MG 26K, vol. 947, reel M3175, G. Howard Ferguson to R.B. Bennett, 22 May 1935, 598646.

22 CRCNA, ECAMB 1, EC meeting 6 October 1914, 92. S. Morton summarizes the ethos of Progressives in *Wisdom, Justice, and Charity*, 83–4. The wide social impact of scientific management can be seen in the example of interwar childrearing advice. See Comacchio, *Nations Are Built of Babies*, chapter 6.

23 CRCNA, box 3, Alberta WWI scrapbook (marbled cover), clippings: "Provincial Red Cross Will Facilitate Work," 1 October 1914, and "Splendid Work Done by Local Red Cross Outlined at Meeting," 14 October 1914.

24 CRCS, *Annual Report 1917* (Toronto: CRCS, 1918), 5–6; Glassford, "Marching as to War," 277.

25 On Canadian women's paid labour during the Great War, see Sangster, "Mobilizing Women for War," in D. Mackenzie, ed., *Canada and the First World War;* Ramkhalawansingh, "Women during the Great War"; Street, "Bankers and Bomb Makers"; and Street, "Patriotic, not Permanent: Attitudes towards Women Being Bankers and Making Bombs," in Glassford and Shaw, *A Sisterhood of Suffering and Service*, 148–70. For the broader context of women's labour in this period, see L. Kealey, *Enlisting Women for the Cause*.

26 Easton McLeod, *In Good Hands*, 24, 35–6; M. Porter, *To All Men*, 66;

Macleod Moore, *The Maple Leaf's Red Cross*, 15. Holmes-Orr quotation: editorial, *The Canadian Red Cross Junior* (March 1938), 3. On girls' work during the Great War, see Alexander, "An Honour and a Burden," in Glassford and Shaw, *A Sisterhood of Suffering and Service*, 173–94. The Australian and Canadian Red Cross societies each independently began more widespread and concerted attempts to enlist children's voluntary labour in 1916. On Australia, see Campbell, "thousands of tiny fingers," 186–7.

27 Montgomery, *Rilla of Ingleside*, 52–3. Historical and literary elements of *Rilla* are discussed in Edwards and Litster, "The End of Canadian Innocence," 31–46; Tector, "A Righteous War," 72–86; Young, "L.M. Montgomery's *Rilla of Ingleside*," 95–122; A. McKenzie, "Women at War," 83–108.

28 Macleod Moore, *The Maple Leaf's Red Cross*, 14–15.

29 Aboriginal examples: "Patriotic Indians," *Bulletin* (November 1915): 3; McClung, *The Stream Runs Fast*, 160; CRCNA, box 3, Alberta WWI scrapbook (green cover with red cross), clipping "Blackfoot Indians Give to Red Cross," 9 January 1917. Saskatchewan branch honorary secretary P.H. Gordon stated in 1917 that the province's aboriginal population participated in the Red Cross "in proportion to their numbers and means in a manner that might well be emulated by their white brothers." Saskatchewan Division CRCS, *Red Cross in Saskatchewan*, 4. Chinese example: R. Rutherdale, *Hometown Horizons*, 107.

30 R. Rutherdale, *Hometown Horizons*, 90, 94.

31 CRCS, *Annual Report 1918*, 126–7; R. Rutherdale, *Hometown Horizons*, 210, 301.

32 CRCNA, ECAMB 1, EC meetings 30 October 1914, 101, and 22 January 1915, 140; CRCNA, ECAMB 4, Central Council [hereafter CC] meeting 7 May 1918, 35; D. Morton, *Fight or Pay*, 175.

33 CRCNA, box 5, file 5.I, "Report to the Tenth Annual International Red Cross Conference on the War Activities of the Canadian Red Cross Society," 6. The exact figures are as follows: Ontario $3,737,994.11; Saskatchewan $1,746,404.30; Manitoba $965,371.72; United States $609,816.76; Quebec $491,071.53; British Columbia $469,468.63; Alberta $486,253.06; Nova Scotia $398,166.68; New Brunswick $66,107.11; Yukon $31,147.14; Prince Edward Island $51,362.90; Cuba $20,000; other $321.62; total $9,073,485.56.

34 An Act to amend An Act to incorporate The Canadian Red Cross Society, *Statutes of Canada* (6–7 George V, ch. 58, 1916); House of Commons, *Debates* (1916), 1325. The 1915 Central Council contained three

Montrealers (Sir H. Montgu Allan, Lt-Col A.E. Labelle, and Lt-Col H.B. Yates, MD) and an Edmontonian, J.H. McDougall) in addition to its twenty Ontarians. In 1916 the council was augmented by a further nine official provincial representatives, and by 1918 provinces other than Ontario had three or four representatives each. Alberta: MP R.B. Bennett, Premier Charles Stewart, Judge J.A. Jackson, Miss Mary Pinkham; British Columbia: Lieutenant Governor Sir Frank S. Barnard, Judge F. McB. Young, F.W. Jones; Manitoba: George F. Galt, Mrs R.C. Osborne, M.F. Christie, J.C. Waugh; New Brunswick: Lady Tilley, Brig-Gen H.H. McLean, Clarence B. Allan; Nova Scotia: Mrs William Dennis, Mrs Charles Archibald, J.L. Hetherington, H.E. Mahon; Ontario: Dr James W. Robertson; PEI: Sir Louis H. Davies, Dr S.R. Jenkins, Theodore Ross; Quebec: W.R. Miller, Mrs Ernest Stuart, Mrs Colin A. Sewell, Lady Drummond; Saskatchewan: A.B. Perry, Lieutenant Governor R.S. Lake, Judge R. Rimmer, D.H. McDonald. CRCS, *Annual Report 1914*, 5; CRCS, *Annual Report 1915*, 2; CRCS, *Annual Report 1917*, 5–6.

35 "The Rose of No Man's Land," in Corfield, *To Alleviate Suffering*, 8; Plumptre, "Canada's Love-Gifts," vol. 2, 196–7.

36 CRCNA, ECAMB 1, EC meeting 12 March 1915, 171; ECAMB 2, EC meeting 23 April 1915, 5–7; CRCS, *Annual Report 1915* (Toronto: CRCS, 1916), 5–7; CRCS, *Annual Report 1916*, 49; Mann, *Margaret Macdonald*, 89; CRCS, *Annual Report 1918* (Toronto: CRCS, 1919), 72. Margaret Macfarlane, a CRCS nurse who served in Malta, is profiled in Barron Norris, *Sister Heroines*, 152–5; see also 82–5. For a few details of nursing work in the Ogden home, see Munn Smith, "Marion Moodie," 14. For photos of Gregory's 1919 train journey, and a transcript of her 1920s Port Nursery work diary, see "Bertha Gregory: Port Nurse Diary; Saint John, NB 1920–22," https://berthagregory. wordpress.com/home.

37 Quiney, "Assistant Angels," 64; Quiney, "Borrowed Halos," 93.

38 CRCNA, ECAMB 3, EC meeting 8 May 1917, 161; CRCS, *Annual Report 1915*, 42, 51–2; CRCS *Annual Report 1916* (Toronto: CRCS, 1917), 50.

39 Macleod Moore, *The Maple Leaf's Red Cross*, 95–7.

40 Adami, *War Story of the Canadian Army Medical Corps*, vol. 1, 87–96.

41 Macleod Moore, *The Maple Leaf's Red Cross*, 90–100; LAC, Department of Militia and Defence, RG 9, vol. 3511, files 19-1-130 and 10-11-23; Mann, *Margaret Macdonald*, 130–3; Reznick, *Healing the Nation*, 43, 45–6. The Joinville-le-Pont hospital was presented by Prime Minister Borden to the people of France in a ceremony on 3 July 1918, as a symbol of the friendship between France and Canada.

42 Macleod Moore, *The Maple Leaf's Red Cross*, 90–1; Reznick, *Healing the Nation*, 43; LAC, Anne E. Ross Papers, MG 30 E446, Anne E. Ross, "Narrative of World War I Nursing Service," 9.

43 Bruce, *Back the Attack*, 6, 9, 29, 41. CRCNA, ECAMB 3, EC meetings 5 December 1916, 87–8, and 30 January 1917, 111; LAC, RG 9, vol. 3493, file 12–1–1 (part 1), CRCS Commissioner to DMS Canadian Contingents, 27 October 1916; Macleod Moore, *The Maple Leaf's Red Cross*, 214, 219. The inquiry showed Hodgetts to be guilty of poor administration at Cliveden, but not of criminal activity. For the context and wider significance of Bruce's report, see D. Morton, *A Peculiar Kind of Politics*, 86–7, 94–5, and D. Morton, *When Your Number's Up*, 203–4.

44 "Lady Grace Julia Drummond," unpaginated; "Drummond, Sir George Alexander," DCB; Vance, *Objects of Concern*, 34.

45 CRCS, *Annual Report 1912*, 11–12; Carr, *A Story of the Canadian Red Cross Information Bureau*, 8–9; "Information Department," *Bulletin* (June 1916): 7. The bureau was Lady Drummond's idea. Hodgetts gave her a free hand to develop it as she wished, and she channelled much of her own wealth into it.

46 Carrie E. Holman, "Canadian Red Cross Information Bureau," in *Canada in the Great World War*, vol. 2, 223, 228; "Report of the Information Bureau," *Bulletin* (December 1917–January 1918): 20; Schneider, "The British Red Cross Wounded and Missing," 297–8.

47 The ICRC's POW services are explored at "Prisoners of the First World War, The ICRC Archives," www.grandeguerre.icrc.org, and "1914–1918 War: International Prisoners of War Agency," www.icrc.org.

48 D. Morton, *Silent Battle*, 52; Moorehead, *Dunant's Dream*, 182–4; Carrie E. Holman, "Canadian Red Cross Information Bureau," in *Canada in the Great World War*, vol. 2, 223–4; Vance, *Objects of Concern*, 26, 34–6.

49 Vance, *Objects of Concern*, 54; D. Morton, *Silent Battle*, 50; Letter from a POW, *Bulletin* (September 1915): 21; LAC, Nina Cohen Papers, MG 30 C152, vol. 2, file: "Correspondence and 3 speeches: RC Society Activities, Sydney NS, 1943–1946," T.R. Richard to Mrs Harry Cohen, 5 March 1943; CRCNA, box 3, Alberta WWI scrapbook (green cover with red cross), clipping, "REMEMBER," March 1918. The 1917 "Serve by Giving" campaign, for example, stated that it cost 35 cents to feed a Canadian in captivity, and asked "In what way can a Canadian spend 35 cents better than in providing necessary, nourishing food for our Canadian brothers daily suffering for us?" Red Cross advertisement, *Globe*, 13 January 1917, 7.

50 Vance, *Objects of Concern*, 25, 39, 42–55.

51 CRCNA, ECAMB 3, EC meeting 5 February 1918, 269; CRCNA, ECAMB 4, EC meeting 11 October 1918, 134; Macleod Moore, *The Maple Leaf's Red Cross*, 191–206.

52 "We Had Our British Flag with Us Too," *Bulletin* (April 1916): 1; CRCNA, ECAMB 3, EC meetings 25 July 1916, 58, 3 November 1916, 77, and 8 June 1917, 170; ECAMB 4, EC meetings 10 June 1918, 57, and 16 September 1918, 106. This marriage of practical and symbolic support was similarly evident in July 1916, when the BRCS donated £25,000 to the CRCS "so that they might build [recreation] huts and have an inscription bearing the name of the Canadian Red Cross Society placed upon them." CRCNA, ECAMB 3, EC meeting 25 July 1916, 52.

53 CRCS, *South African War Report*, 15.

54 CRCNA, box 5, file 5.I, "Report to the Tenth International Red Cross Conference on the War Activities of the Canadian Red Cross Society" (1921), 6; Bank of Canada Inflation Calculator, www.bankofcanada.ca. Because the cumulative CRCS figures do not account for steep inflation during the war itself (which makes $9,000,000 in 1914 worth $13,000,000 by 1918) I have calculated the $9,000,000 as from 1916, to average the difference.

55 Many examples may be found in Morris, ed., *The Canadian Patriotic Fund*. See also "$333 in Town of 1,400," *Globe*, 24 August 1914, 3.

56 Montgomery, *Selected Journals*, 197; Maroney, "The Great Adventure," 79–82; Canadian War Museum, "PROPAGANDA: Canadian Wartime Propaganda," First World War CRCS poster, "If You Cannot Give a Life"; Hutchinson, *Champions of Charity*, 56.

57 These campaigns are discussed in greater detail in Glassford, "Marching as to War," 233–9.

58 CRCNA, ECAMB 4, EC meetings 25 March 1918, 1–2, and 7 May 1918, 37.

59 Glenbow Museum and Archives [hereafter GMA], Canadian Red Cross Society, Alberta-Northwest Territories Division, M8228/16, Alberta-NWT Division Minutes, Sub-Executive meeting 6 June 1918, 93; Hutchinson, "The Nagler Case," 182, 186–7; Hutchinson, *Champions of Charity*, quotation on 256, also see 268–75.

60 GMA, M8228/16, Alberta-NWT Division minutes, Sub-Executive meeting 6 June 1918, 95.

61 CRCS, *Annual Report 1917*, 97–8.

62 Hotson, "Sphagnum from Bog to Bandage," 212; "Nature's Dressings for the World's Wounded," *Bulletin* (November 1918): 9–11; "Sphagnum

Moss Committee Has Had a Ton of Moss," *Bulletin* (December 1918–January 1919): 47–8; Riegler, "Sphagnum Moss," 38. The best quality sphagnum can absorb up to twenty-two times its weight in water and even the poorest quality is more absorbent than cotton.

63 D. Morton, *Fight or Pay*, 155; CRCS, *Annual Report 1918*, 63; CRCNA, ECAMB 4, EC meetings 10 June 1918, 53, and 20 August 1918, 97.

64 Mrs Elaine Nelson, quoted in Read, *The Great War and Canadian Society*, 152, 186.

65 CRCNA, ECAMB 1, EC meeting 28 September 1914, 85.

66 CRCS, *Annual Report 1914*, 26; "Canadian Women's Societies: What Is Being Done the Length and Breadth of Canada," *Everywoman's World* (April 1915), 18; Lucy Swanton Doyle, "Canadian Women Help the Empire: 'What Could Women Do in Time of War?'" *Everywoman's World* (November 1914), 32; Fallis, "World War I Knitting"; Wilde, "Freshettes, Farmerettes and Feminine Fortitude," in Glassford and Shaw, *A Sisterhood of Suffering and Service*, 75–97; CRCNA, D. Geneva Lent, "Alberta Red Cross in Peace and War (1914–1947)," unpublished manuscript (1947), 4.

67 Ward, "Empire and the Everyday," 274; D. Morton, *When Your Number's Up*, 139; Brittain, *Testament of Youth*, 100; "Supply Department," *Bulletin* (April 1916): 10–11.

68 Nova Scotia Division, *Nova Scotia Red Cross during the Great War*, 8.

69 Quoted in Mainville, *Till the Boys Come Home*, 79.

70 LAC, Sophie Hoerner Papers, MG 30 E290, Sophie Hoerner to Mollie, 22 August 1915; Macleod Moore, *The Maple Leaf's Red Cross*, 53, 63.

71 LAC, MG 30 E290, Sophie Hoerner to Mollie, 22 August 1915.

72 Reznick, *Healing the Nation*, 81, 83–7.

73 Quoted in Mainville, *Till the Boys Come Home*, 82.

74 CRCNA, box 3, Alberta WWI scrapbook (green with red cross on cover), clippings: "Women Responsible for Reduction of French Supplies," January 1917; "20,950 Articles Shipped from Supplies," 17 March 1917. Efforts to coerce co-eds into war work, and co-eds' subtle forms of resistance, are the focus of Quiney, "We Must not Neglect Our Duty," 71–94.

75 For example, "Not a Single Box or Bale Lost," *Bulletin* (September 1915): 18; "False Reports. Germans at Work?" *Bulletin* (October 1915): 5; "Does the Red Cross Neglect the Canadian Military Hospitals in England?" *Bulletin* (November 1915): 7; "Do Prisoners of War Get Their Parcels?" *Bulletin* (December 1915): 6; CRCNA, box 3, Alberta WWI scrapbook (marbled cover), clipping, "Red Cross Notes," 8 January

1916; Duley, "The Unquiet Knitters of Newfoundland," in Glassford and Shaw, *A Sisterhood of Suffering and Service*, 62–4. In both Newfoundland and Canada the rumours reached their height in 1916.

76 Adut, *On Scandal*, 27–8.

77 LAC, RG 9, vol. 3493, file 12–1–1 (part 1), correspondence between DMS Canadian Contingents and CRCNA Commissioner, October 1915–September 1916; CRCNA, ECAMB 1, EC meeting 25 September 1914, 86; ECAMB 4, CC meeting 17 September 1918, 121; "The Quest of the Sold Socks," *Bulletin* (November 1915): 8. By September 1918 Noel Marshall warned Central Council that many officers feared they could not afford to work for free much longer.

78 CRCNA, box 3, Alberta WWI scrapbook (marbled cover), clipping, "Help Must Be Given Red Cross by Everyone," December 1916; Macleod Moore, *The Maple Leaf's Red Cross*, 36. National Headquarters did receive word from the federal government in October 1916 that German agents from the United States might attempt to infiltrate CRCS activities "with sinister intent." CRCNA, ECAMB 3, EC meeting 17 October 1916, 72.

79 The American Red Cross, for example, held responsibility for the welfare of *all* American soldiers, not simply the sick and wounded. "Our American Friends," *Bulletin* (October 1917): 4.

80 Bloch, trans. Holoka, "Reflections of a Historian," 3.

81 Quoted in D. Morton, *Fight or Pay*, 189. On returned soldiers, war weariness, and the war's financial demands, see Maroney, "The Great Adventure," 90; Maclean Miller, *Our Glory and Our Grief*, 134; Brown and Cook, *Canada 1896–1921*, 231–3.

82 *Bulletin* (July 1916): 4.

83 CRCNA, box 3, Alberta WWI scrapbook (marbled cover), clipping, "Passive Red Cross Members Become Active," 12 August 1915.

84 Beynon, *Aleta Dey*, 167–9.

85 Julia Drummond, "Foreword" to Carr, *A Story of the CRC Information Bureau*, 4; Clements, *The Work of the CRCS in New Brunswick*, 3–4; Marlene Epp, quoted in Marr, "Paying 'the price of war,'" 273; McClung, *The Next of Kin*, 239–40.

86 Fussell, *The Great War and Modern Society*, 21–2; Vance, *Death So Noble*, 36.

87 CRCNA, box 3, Alberta WWI scrapbook (marbled cover), clipping, "Medicine Hat Does Much Work for Red Cross," 5 May 1915.

88 Plumptre, "Canada's Love-Gifts," in *Canada in the Great War* vol. 2, 198, 200; Reznick, *Healing the Nation*, 3.

89 Editorial, *Globe*, 9 October 1914, 4; "Go to Front or Knit: The Motto in Bradford," *Globe*, 2 October 1914, 9; Hutchinson, *Champions of Charity*, 352–4.

90 See, for example, "Royal City's Send-off," *Globe*, 20 August 1914, 3, and "Ten Thousand Pounds for British Red Cross," *Globe*, 26 September 1914, 21, versus Mary Macleod Moore's 1919 book relating the CRCS's overseas activities entitled *The Maple Leaf's Red Cross*.

91 Plumptre, "Canada's Love-Gifts," in *Canada in the Great War* vol. 2, 196; Vance, *Death So Noble*, 136.

92 Dr Ryerson described the CRCS as "the avenue through which flows the practical sympathy of the friends at home." Ryerson, *Looking Backward*, 210.

93 Montgomery, *Rilla of Ingleside*, 234; Scates, "The Unknown Sock Knitter," 39–40.

94 "Thanks to the Information Department," *Bulletin* (June 1916): 29.

95 Ibid., 31, 35; E. Schneider, "The British Red Cross Missing and Wounded," 296–7; Winter, *Sites of Memory*, 29–30.

96 Macleod Moore, *The Maple Leaf's Red Cross*, 70; Glassford, "The Greatest Mother in the World," 219–32; Darracott and Loftus, *First World War Posters*, 28.

97 Macphail, *Official History of the Canadian Forces – Medical Services*, 342; Prentice et al., *Canadian Women: A History*, 2nd ed., 231; Glassford, "Marching as to War," 269–72.

98 "The Canadian Red Cross," *New Glasgow Enterprise*, 8 December 1918, 12.

99 "They Drown the Conversation," *Bulletin* (October 1916): 6–7.

100 Szychter, "The War Work of Women," 8; Brittain, *Testament of Youth*, 101; Montgomery, *Selected Journals*, 174; Lawrence, "Red Cross at Halifax, a Sketch," in Clements, *The Work of the CRCS in New Brunswick*, 46–7.

101 D. Mackenzie, "Eastern Approaches," in D. Mackenzie, *Canada and the First World War*, 365.

102 Nova Scotia Branch, *Annual Report 1917–18* (Halifax: CRCS, 1918), 3; Nova Scotia Division, *Nova Scotia Red Cross during the Great War*, 62, 66; GMA, M8228/16, Alberta-NWT Division Minutes 1916–19, Sub-Executive meeting 10 December 1917, 59; MacDonald, *Curse of the Narrows*, 113.

103 MacDonald, *Curse of the Narrows*, 169–71.

104 Ibid., 187, 223, 235; Nova Scotia branch, *Annual Report 1917–18*, 3–4;

Nova Scotia branch, *Nova Scotia Red Cross during the Great War*, 64–6.

105 See Isitt, *From Victoria to Vladivostok*. Chapters 1 to 3 cover the geopolitical context and Canada's reasons for intervention; CRCS work in Siberia is discussed on 121–2 and 163.

106 Polk, "The CRC and Relief in Siberia," 25–30.

107 Ibid., 71, 184–90.

108 R. Rutherdale, *Hometown Horizons*; Anderson, *Imagined Communities*.

CHAPTER FOUR

1 "Junior Red Cross in a Log School," CRC *Junior* 18, no. 4 (April 1939): 2.

2 CRCNA, box 5, file 5.1, "Report to the Tenth International Red Cross Conference," 14–15.

3 CRCNA, ECAMB 4, EC meeting 19 November 1918, 163, 167.

4 This was also the case for the ARC, where membership declined and fundraising campaigns faced diminishing returns for several consecutive years after the war. Moser Jones, *The American Red Cross*, 175. The Australian Red Cross saw a similar contraction in its volunteer workforce. Oppenheimer, *The Power of Humanity*, 56.

5 CRCS, *Annual Report 1912*, 12.

6 "The Duchess of Connaught's Canadian Red Cross Endowment Fund," *Bulletin* (June 1916): 3–4.

7 CRCNA, ECAMB 3, CC meeting 5 February 1918, 268; CRCNA, Ryerson Papers, file "W," memorandum signed by G.S. Ryerson, 5 February 1918.

8 CRCNA, ECAMB 3, Annual Meeting, 6 February 1918, 276; CRCS *Annual Report 1917*, 54–5.

9 Davison, *Proposed Plan*, 6. The LRCS headquartered itself in Paris near the League of Nations and facilitated cooperation between national Red Cross societies, while providing public health information, study facilities, demonstration materials, and expert advisers. *The League of Red Cross Societies*, 1.

10 Durand, *From Sarajevo to Hiroshima*, 152–6.

11 *Proceedings of the Medical Conference ... Cannes*, 13–17.

12 Durand, *From Sarajevo to Hiroshima*, 155–6; Moorehead, *Dunant's Dream*, 258–65.

13 CRCNA, ECAMB 4, CC meeting 26 November 1918, 180–93.

14 CRCNA, ECAMB 4, EC meeting 21 January 1919, 207.

15 LAC, Robert Laird Borden Papers, MG 26H, vol. 248, reel C-4418, Norman Sommerville to Sir Thomas White, 15 April 1919, 139208; CRCNA, ECAMB 4, EC meeting 15 April 1919, 286.

16 LAC, MG 26H, vol. 248, reel C-4418, memorandum and correspondence re: proposed CRCS charter amendment, April–May 1919, 139220–9.

17 An Act to amend An Act to incorporate The Canadian Red Cross Society, *Statutes of Canada* (9–10 George V, ch. 101, 1919), 61.

18 Charles-Edward Amory Winslow was the founding chair of public health in the Yale University medical school, a position he held from 1915 to 1945. His illustrious career included serving as president of the American Public Health Association and editor of the *American Journal of Public Health*. Winslow's innovative and influential approach to public health included seeing the field as a mutable social science that emphasized international cooperation and preventive approaches. Winslow also served as a member of the American Red Cross's mission to Siberia in the aftermath of the Russian Revolution, and directed the League of Red Cross Societies' public health department. Atwater, "C.-E. A. Winslow," 1065–70; Yale School of Public Health, "Who Was C.-E. A. Winslow?"

19 CRCNA, ECAMB 5, EC meeting, 2 September 1919, 34. On Adelaide Plumptre's involvement with the National Council of Women, see Griffiths, *The Splendid Vision,* 148. The NCWC's "Women's Platform," which Plumptre helped draft, focused on many of the same issues as the CRCS's peace policy. Griffiths, *The Splendid Vision,* 139.

20 CRCNA, box 49, file 49.5, CRCS, "National Peace Policy."

21 On Nova Scotia: Nova Scotia Division, *Annual Report 1921* (Halifax: CRCS, 1922), 9. On PEI: Baldwin, "Amy MacMahon," 20–7; Baldwin, "Volunteers in Action," 121–47. On Quebec: Quebec Division, *Annual Report 1922,* 9. The Quebec Division executive committee noted that many other agencies were already engaged in public health work and felt that war funds should be used to help veterans. On Alberta: Jones: *Empire of Dust,* 113, 123; Cormack, *The Red Cross Lady*. Conquest's popular radio program ran from the early 1920s until the mid-1950s.

22 Jones, *Influenza 1918,* 18; CRCS, *Annual Report 1918,* 72. On the origins and spread of the epidemic, official responses, its impact on Canadian public health measures, and the class and gender dynamics of the epidemic, see Jones, *Influenza 1918*; Humphries, *The Last Plague*; Fahrni and Jones, *Epidemic Encounters*.

23 CRCNA, Lent, "Alberta Red Cross," 31–4; Nova Scotia Division, *Annual Report 1917–18,* 6–7; Clements, *The Work of the CRCS in New Brunswick,* 7–8; Windsor-Essex County CRC Branch, Lori Collins, "Seventy Years of Service," unpublished manuscript (1988), 1–2.

24 CRCS, *Annual Report 1919* (Toronto: CRCS, 1920), 1; CRCS, *Annual Report 1920* (Toronto: CRCS, 1921), 20–4; GMA, M8228/225, "Summary of addresses delivered ... by Jas. W. Robertson," 5.

25 An Act respecting The Canadian Red Cross Society, *Statutes of Canada* (12–13 George V, ch. 13, 1922), 61. The existing Ontario-based Central Council was augmented by one member per province during the war. Provincial representation expanded further after the war, and by 1922 thirty of the fifty Central Council members were from outside Ontario. To determine national representativeness I compiled a list of executive committee members as reported in the CRCS annual reports for 1919, 1924, 1929, 1934, and 1939, and sought biographical details in contemporary volumes of Greene, ed., *Who's Who* (1920, 1931, 1946). Places of residence were found for sixty of the seventy individuals listed. Twenty-nine members (41 percent) were from Ontario; twenty of the Ontarians (70 percent) lived in Toronto.

26 CRCS, *Annual Report 1920*, 25; CRCS, *Annual Report 1924* (Toronto: CRCS, 1925), 16.

27 CRCS, *Annual Report 1919*, i.

28 Margaret Macmillan, "Canada and the Peace Settlements," in D. Mackenzie, *Canada and the First World War*, 385.

29 "Reconnaissance de la Croix-Rouge canadienne," 835–6; CRCNA, ECAMB 8, CC meeting 25 April 1928, "38–16 International Red Cross Conference," 96.

30 CRCNA, ECAMB 8, EC "meeting 13 January 1930, "264–4 British Empire Red Cross Conference," 235; CRCNA, ECAMB 8, EC meeting 19 September 1930, "266–7 Report on British Empire Red Cross Conference," 277–98. On the Belgian IRC conference, see CRCNA, ECAMB 8, EC meeting 19 September 1930, "266–12 International Red Cross Conference."

31 For instance, see MacNaughton, "Promoting Clean Water"; and Burnett, "Race, Disease, and Public Violence."

32 Valverde, *Light, Soap, and Water*, 17.

33 Winslow, "Suggestions," 490. See note 18 for biographical details about Winslow.

34 GMA, M8228/224, "Nation Builders. Are You One?" cover page.

35 CRCNA, box 49, file 49.5; Robertson, "Peace-Time Policy and Health Program," 4; Routley, "Radio Talk Prepared for the Canadian Social Hygiene Council," 281.

36 GMA, M8228/226, "The Story of the Red Cross," 13–14.

37 Nova Scotia Division, *Annual Report 1923* (Halifax: CRCS, 1924), 30;
   CRCNA, box 11, file 11.II, "Still Serving: The Red Cross in Pictures,"
   back cover.

38 Winslow, "Suggestions," 489–90; CRCNA, box 49, file 49.5, "Join This
   Great Crusade" pamphlet, front cover; Vance, *Death So Noble,* 38–9.
   The popularity of the crusader motif sprang from the crusader's role as
   a "soldier for Christ," which fit well with the themes of sacrifice and redemption prevalent in Canadians' popular conceptions of the Great War.

39 Tillotson, *Contributing Citizens,* 75–6. It seems the American Red Cross
   did not need to "de-feminize" its image in quite the same way, perhaps
   because it already had a long history of action-oriented American and
   foreign disaster relief work behind it (and more underway as the peace
   treaty was signed in 1919) to balance the "Greatest Mother" image. See
   Moser Jones, *The American Red Cross,* chapters 10–13, and Irwin,
   Making the World Safe, chapters 5–6.

40 R. Cook, *The Regenerators,* 4, 176, 217; Allen, *The Social Passion,* 3–4;
   Nova Scotia Archives and Records Management [hereafter NSARM],
   Canadian Red Cross Society, Nova Scotia Division, MG 20, vol. 1366,
   #5, "The Red Cross in Nova Scotia," 5 December 1926.

41 Allen, *The Social Passion,* 19; Christie and Gauvreau, *A Full-Orbed
   Christianity,* xi–xiv. Christie and Gauvreau argue that 1900 to 1940
   marked the highpoint for Christian leadership in social welfare and social policymaking, and challenge the secularization thesis advanced by
   Ramsay Cook and others for this period. Although not a Christian organization as such, the CRCS demonstrates the persistence of Christian
   ideology in one area of health work.

42 GMA, M8228/224, "An Interpretation of Red Cross," 12.

43 Vance, *Death So Noble,* 258, 220; Brown and Cook, *Canada 1896–
   1921,* 303.

44 NSARM, MG 20, vol. 1366, #5, "The Red Cross in Nova Scotia,"
   5 December 1926.

45 Comacchio, *Nations Are Built of Babies,* chapters 1 and 2; N. Sutherland, *Children in English-Canadian Society,* 84.

46 GMA, M8228/225, "Summary of Addresses delivered … by Jas. W.
   Robertson," 10; Hasian Jr., *The Rhetoric of Eugenics,* 76.

47 See, for instance, Arnup, "Educating Mothers," 190–210; Arnup, *Edu-
   cation for Motherhood*; Baillargeon, "Care of Mothers and Infants," in
   Dodd and Gorham, *Caring and Curing*; Dodd, "Advice to Parents";
   Dodd, "Helen MacMurchy," in Dodd and Gorham, *Caring and Curing.*

48 Nova Scotia Division, *Annual Report 1928* (Halifax: CRCS, 1929), 21;

NSARM, MG 20, vol. 1366, #3, "Christmas at the Seaport Nursery Halifax, N.S."

49 Strong-Boag, *The New Day Recalled*, 145.

50 McClung, *In Times Like These*, 156, 141.

51 See, for example, CRCNA, box 3, Alberta scrapbook (green), clipping, "When Strife Will Cease; What Is Peace?" *Albertan*, 12 September 1925; GMA, M8228/224, "Onward Alberta!" 4.

52 Sheehan, "Junior Red Cross in Saskatchewan," 68–9.

53 CRCS, *Annual Report 1919*, 17. Agnes (Mrs William) Dennis was an active suffragist and reformer in Halifax. Her husband was a prominent Conservative Senator and publisher of the *Halifax Herald*. S. Morton, *Wisdom, Justice, and Charity*, 112.

54 CRCNA, ECAMB 4, EC meeting 10 December 1918, 172; CRCNA, ECAMB 4, EC meeting 6 May 1919, 290–1; LAC MG 26H, vol. 248, reel C–4418, resolutions opposing extension of the CRCS, March/April 1919, 139205, 139207, 139213–14; Elliott, "Keep the Flag Flying," 10, 38–48; GMA, M8228/224, "An Interpretation of the Red Cross – An Address by Mrs C.B. Waagen" (Calgary: CRCS, 1926), 7.

55 GMA, M8228/225, "The Crusade for Good Health: Summary of Addresses Delivered in Ontario by Jas. W. Robertson" (Toronto: CRCS, 1921?), 9–10.

56 Social worker Charlotte Whitton would later become mayor of Ottawa.

57 LAC, Canadian Council on Social Development, MG 28 I10, vol. 178, file 178–6, Charlotte Whitton to Maryn G. Emerson, 10 November 1938; Marjorie Bradford to George F. Davison, 12 May 1939; Davidson to Bradford, 18 May 1939.

58 CRCS, *Annual Report 1920*, 22, 25; GMA, M8228/225, "Summary of addresses delivered ... by Jas. W. Robertson," 10.

59 McCuaig, "'From Social Reform to Social Service," 495; Feldberg, *Disease and Class*, 88–9, 104, 107, 120; Junior Red Cross "Rules of the Health Game" poster (circa 1925) reproduced in Sheehan, "Junior Red Cross in Saskatchewan," 66. See also Minnett and Poutanen, "Swatting Flies for Health."

60 CRCNA, ECAMB 5, EC meetings 6 January 1920 and 30 January 1920, 75–6, 81; CC meeting 22–23 October 1920, 175.

61 Quebec Division, *Annual Report 1922*, 21; Quebec Division, *Annual Report 1924* (Montreal: CRCS, 1925), 12, 14.

62 Sheehan, "Junior Red Cross in the Schools," 255.

63 On attitudes toward and treatment of "crippled children" in this period, see Hanes, "Linking Mental Defect."

64 CRCNA, box 3, Alberta scrapbook (green), newspaper clipping "Circle of Young Canada: Dominion Day Messages from Seven National Organizations Shaping Citizens of Tomorrow," 27 July 1925; LAC, RG 29, vol. 861, file 20–C–46 (part 1), chart: "Canadian Red Cross Society: Activities of Provincial Divisions for the year 1922"; CRCNA, box 1, file 1.I, "The Canadian Red Cross Society 1914 – and After," 8. An additional 1,000 branches with 35,000 members existed in the neighbouring Dominion of Newfoundland, run as a division of the Canadian Junior Red Cross.

65 Pier 21 Museum, Halifax, "The Volunteers" display, July 2005; Iacovetta, *Gatekeepers*, 290.

66 Quebec Division, *Annual Report 1921* (Montreal: CRCS, 1922), 14; Nova Scotia Division, *Annual Report 1922* (Halifax: CRCS, 1923), 19–20; NSARM, MG 20, vol. 1366, #3, CRCS-Nova Scotia Division Policy Book, "Seaport Nursery Stories"; CRCNA, box 49, file 49.5, Vivian Tremaine, "A Busy Day in the Red Cross Nursery."

67 CRCNA, ECAMB 8, EC meeting 17 November 1927, "251–12 British Empire Settlement Scheme," 44; GMA, M8228/17, Alberta NWT Division minutes, 1920–22, Report of Alberta Division Annual Meeting, 21–22 January 1921, 187.

68 Quotation: "Red Cross and Immigration," *Advocate* (Carr, Alberta), 16 October 1925; "Red Cross Carries Relief to Settlers in Isolated Districts," *Journal* (Edmonton), 25 September 1925.

69 L. Kealey, "Delivering Health Care," 183, 187–8. The broader history of nursing work in non-traditional Canadian settings is explored in the essays found in Rutherdale, *Caregiving on the Periphery*.

70 Comacchio Abeele, "The Mothers of the Land Must Suffer," 8; NSARM, MG 20, vol. 1366, #700, Laurier C. Grant, "Guysborough Hospital: How a Community Filled a Need"; Warder, *Fifty Years of Service*; Quebec Division, *Annual Report 1928* (Montreal: CRCS, 1929), 11, 17; CRCNA, box 24, file 24.V, Noel Robinson, "Florence Nightingale of the Wilds"; Elliott, "Keep the Flag Flying," ii.

71 L. Kealey, "Delivering Health Care," 186.

72 Massie, "Ruth Dulmage Shewchuk," 37. LeRoy Miller, *Mustard Plasters and Handcars* offers an interesting memoir of outpost nursing, but Elliott, "Keep the Flag Flying" is by far the most in-depth study of Red Cross outposts and their nurses. Elliott's study is limited to Ontario, but Linda Kealey offers a similarly rigorous New Brunswick comparison in "Delivering Health Care," 183–98. Quotation, L. Kealey, "Delivering Health Care," 183.

73 LAC, RG 29, vol. 861, file 10–C–46 (part 1), chart, "Canadian Red Cross Society: Activities of Provincial Divisions for the Year 1922"; CRCNA, box 49, file 49.5, James W. Robertson, "Peace-Time Policy and Health Program of the Red Cross in Canada," 6. On the enrolment of nurses, see, for example, CRCNA, box 1, file 1.I, "Voluntary Enrolment of Registered Nurses for Service in War and Disaster"; GMA, M8228/16, Alberta-NWT Division minutes, Sub-Executive meeting 13 July 1919, 141.

74 Morton and Wright, *Winning the Second Battle*, 64; House of Commons, *Debates* (1924), 2682; CRCNA, box 1, file 1.V, "Outline of Principles for Provision of Sheltered Employment," 1923, 9–11; Struthers, "How Much Is Enough?" 65.

75 CRCNA, box 5, file 5.II, CRCS, "Co-operation with Governmental Bodies," 1938, 2.

76 Winslow, "Suggestions," 493; Nova Scotia Division, *Annual Report 1929* (Halifax: CRCS, 1930), 33.

77 Glassford, "Mobilisées, organisées," 73–7.

78 CRCNA, ECAMB 10, CC meeting 31 March 1938, "49–19 XVIIth International Red Cross Conference," 40. See Glassford, "Marching as to War," 282–3 for details of CRCS interest and attendance at international conferences in the 1930s.

79 Alberta Division flirted with bankruptcy and had to apply for large grants from National Headquarters in the early 1930s. See for example, CRCNA, ECAMB 9, Sub-Executive meeting 24 January 1933, "281–3 Alberta Division," 160–2.

80 For example, Quebec Division's 1938 budget amounted to just over half that of its 1933–34 budget. Quebec Division, *Annual Report 1937* (Montreal: CRCS, 1938). On divisional tensions, see LAC, MG 26K, vol. 968, reel M3184, Mary Waagen to Adelaide Plumptre, 0613670–1, and Egbert, Duggan, and Pinkham to Norman Sommerville, 20 April 1932, 0613678–95.

81 Quebec Division, *Annual Report 1928*, 10–11; Quebec Division, *Annual Report 1930* (Montreal: CRCS, 1931), 10, 15–16; LAC, MG 26K, vol. 304, reel M1045, Adelaide Plumptre to R.B. Bennett, 20 and 24 April 1931, 204213, 204215–17, and "Report of Red Cross Hostels, Toronto Branch CRCS, 1930–31," 204233; CRCNA, ECAMB 9, CC meeting 6 April 1933, 177.

82 Sheehan, "Red Cross and Relief," 277–98. As an indicator of the scale of CRCS clothing relief efforts, in the winter of 1931–32 the Saskatchewan Division distributed 23,529 new pairs of leather boots and 21,799 suits of underwear among the thirty different types of items

it provided to destitute citizens on behalf of the provincial government. LAC, MG 26K, vol. 968, reel M3184, W.F. Marshall to J.T.M. Anderson, 8 April 1932, 0613684.

83 Sheehan, "Red Cross and Relief," 291.

84 LAC, MG 26 K, vol. 304, reel M1045, correspondence between Mary Waagen, D.M. Duggan, Norman Sommerville, and R.B. Bennett, December 1930–January 1931, 204146–51, 204156–61, 204165–79.

85 Congress gave the ARC 80 million bushels of wheat and 500,000 bales of cotton to provide food and clothing to impoverished Americans. LAC, MG 26K, vol. 304, reel M1045, John A. Cooper to R.B. Bennett and Bennett to Cooper, both 14 November 1932, 0613750–1.

86 On the loss of branches: Quebec Division, *Annual Report 1932* (Montreal: CRCS, 1933), 22–3. On unemployment: *Report of the Royal Commission on Dominion-Provincial Relations Book 1*, 150. On Saskatchewan and Alberta anxieties: CRCNA, ECAMB 9, Sub-Executive meeting 21 September 1933, "284–9 Situation in Saskatchewan Division," and "284–10 Finances of Alberta Division," 219–22.

87 Ontario Division's financial buoyancy was due to the very active Toronto branch, which made large contributions to divisional funds as well as covering its own program expenses. Toronto Branch CRCS, *History Toronto Branch*, 31–3. In 1950 Central Council heard statements at its annual meeting such as "Ontario kept Red Cross alive during the period between the wars." CRCNA, ECAMB IV (new series [hereafter ns]), CC meeting 2–4 May 1950, 5317. Early in the Second World War, discussions regarding a greater unification of the Red Cross across Canada often referred to the struggles of provinces outside of Central Canada after the mid-1920s. CRCNA, Nationalization Documents, "Report of the Special Committee Appointed to Consider the Re-Organization or Unification of Services of the Red Cross," 3–4 December 1942, and EC meeting 28 June 1943, "Observations on the Advantages to be Gained by Closer Unification of the Organization of the Canadian Red Cross Society," 1942.

88 Thompson and Seager, *Canada 1922–1939*, 28–37, 75, 330; Grauer, *Public Health*, 32–5. The interwar concern with infant mortality is discussed in Dodd, "Advice to Parents."

89 Tillotson, *Contributing Citizens*, 81.

90 *Report of the Royal Commission on Dominion-Provincial Relations Book 2*, 33–4.

91 Grauer, *Public Health*, 63a, 55, 52.

CHAPTER FIVE

1 CRCNA, Julia Drummond, inscription in Carr, *A Story of the Canadian
Red Cross Information Bureau*, front page; CRCNA, box 49, file 49.3
"Lady Drummond – Correspondence," Norman Sommerville to Lady
Julia Drummond, 17 September 1939.

2 *Canada Year Book 1945*, 101; CRCS, *Annual Report 1945* (Toronto:
CRCS, 1946), 25; Feasby, ed., *Official History of the Canadian Medical
Services 1939–1945*, 1: 527; Bank of Canada Inflation Calculator,
www.bankofcanada.ca. Of adults over the age of nineteen, 28.8 percent
were members, meaning they had made at least a one dollar campaign
contribution or were registered volunteers, while 28.4 percent of youth
between the ages of five and nineteen were Junior Red Cross members.

3 The first chapter, about the period between 1939 and1945, in McKenzie
Porter's 1960 CRCS history *To All Men* is titled "The Greatest Challenge," echoing a similar slant in the broader historiography and social
memory of Second World War Canada, as Jeffrey Keshen notes in *Saints,
Sinners, and Soldiers*, 3. Mona Wilson considered her CRCS service in
wartime Newfoundland to be the pinnacle of her many achievements.
Baldwin and Poulter, "Mona Wilson," 281–311.

4 Granatstein, *Canada's War*, 19; Granatstein and Neary, *The Good Fight*,
6; Slater with Bryce, *War Finance and Reconstruction*, 27–8.

5 LAC, RG 44, vol. 5, file "Canadian Red Cross Society," memo for J.L.
Ilsley, 31 April 1942.

6 All citations from *Globe & Mail*, September 1939: "Toronto Poles Reaffirm Their Loyalty to Fatherland and British Empire," 2 September;
"Red Cross Put on War Basis across Canada," 4 September; "Ready to
Volunteer for Service during War," 5 September; "Notes and Comments," 6 September; "Private Funds Can Help," 7 September; "Wood-
stock Red Cross," "Lambton Registration," "Red Cross Committee
Leader," and "Red Cross Classes Open at Y.W.C.A. Next Week," 8 September; "Citizens Organize for Red Cross Work," and Bride Broder,
"Red Cross Society Is Ready," 11 September; "Reopen Headquarters for
Red Cross Supplies," 12 September; "Junior League Takes New Duties,"
13 September.

7 CRCS, *Annual Report 1939* (Toronto: CRCS, 1940), 15; CRCNA, ECAMB
1 (ns), 55th Sub-Executive meeting, held 20 November 1939, 128–9 and
52nd Sub-Executive meeting, held 23 October 1939, 88–9. The agreement with SJAA was established in October 1939.

8 "Flag of Mercy" full-page ad, *Globe & Mail*, 13 November 1939; CRCS,
Annual Report 1939 (Toronto: CRCS, 1940), 14.

9 Tillotson, *Contributing Citizens*, 1–3; Walker, "Over the Top," 14–15; CRCS, *Annual Report 1939*, 14; "War Council Is Organized by Red Cross," *Globe & Mail*, 13 September 1939.

10 McCullough, *Origin and History*, 92–3; LAC, MG 26K, vol. 969, M3185, Sir Edward Peacock to R.B. Bennett, 21 October 1940, p. 0614327; LAC, RG 44, vol. 16, file "Canadian Red Cross Society, 1941–42," P.H. Gordon to T.C. Davis, 21 January 1941.

11 LAC, Canadian Council on Social Development, MG 28 I10, vol. 178, file 178–7, Edward Reid to Charlotte Whitton, 27 February 1941.

12 I use sociologist Max Weber's distinction between "power" as the ability to force people to obey regardless of their resistance, and "authority," in which those receiving orders voluntarily obey them. Pugh and Hickson, *Writers on Organizations*, 3.

13 Desmond Morton, "Supporting Soldiers' Wives and Families in the Great War: What Was Transformed?" in Glassford and Shaw, *A Sisterhood of Suffering and Service*, 214.

14 This figure is from the 1944 peak of voluntary registrations. LAC, RG 44, vol. 11, History of the Voluntary and Auxiliary Services Division, cited in Mosby, *Food Will Win the War*, 111; Keshen, *Saints, Sinners, and Soldiers*, especially 25–7; Durflinger, *Fighting from Home*, especially 109–16; Granatstein and Neary, *The Good Fight*, 9–10.

15 Valverde, "The Mixed Social Economy," 38.

16 *War Charities Act, 1939*, Statutes of Canada, 1939 (3–4 George VI, ch. 10, 1939); LAC, Department of National War Services, RG 44, vol. 39, file "CRC (1939–1941)," Norman Sommerville to W.G. Gunn, 22 May 1940; LAC, RG 44, vol. 57, file "CUARF-RC Relations Jan. 1947 vol. 12," Application for Registration of a War Charities Fund under the War Charities Act, 1939. For a Canadian-Australian comparison, see Oppenheimer, "Control of Wartime Patriotic Funds," 77–9; Oppenheimer, "Controlling Civilian Volunteering," 27–50.

17 On this transition, see T. Cook, *Warlords*, chapter 13.

18 Tillotson, *Contributing Citizens*, 2–5, 42–4.

19 LAC, RG 44, vol. 5, file "Canadian War Services Fund," James Murdoch to J.T. Thorson, 23 March 1942 (including press release).

20 LAC, RG 44, vol. 16, file "CRCS (1941–1942)," P.H. Gordon to T.C. Davis, 2 April 1942 and 8 April 1942.

21 One example is LAC, RG 44, vol. 16, file "Canadian Red Cross Society (1941–1942)," P.H. Gordon to T.C. Davis, 15 October 1941.

22 LAC, RG 44, vol. 16, file "CRCS (1941–1942)," George B. Webster to J.T. Thoroson [sic], 11 October 1941.

23 LAC, RG 44, vol. 16, file "CRCS (1941–1942)," P.H. Gordon to T.C. Davis, 15 October 1941; LAC, RG 44, vol. 5, file "Canadian Red Cross Society," 13 April 1942.

24 LAC, MG 28 I10, vol. 178, file 178-7, memo of 4 December 1945. Information about EC and CC members drawn from CRCS, *Annual Report 1940*, 5.

25 LAC, RG 44, vol. 16, file "CRCS (1941–1942)," T.C. Davis to P.H. Gordon, 27 February 1942; LAC, MG 26K, vol. 969, M3185, P.H. Gordon to R.B. Bennett, 17 February 1942, p. 0614668; LAC, RG 44, vol. 1, P.C. 3439 (April 1943), and related correspondence, January-May 1943; CRCNA, Nationalization documents, "Report of the Special Committee Appointed to Consider the Re-Organization of Unification of Services of the Red Cross," 3–4 December 1942; McCullough, *Origins and History*, 98–9. National Headquarters would not move to Ottawa until 1987.

26 LAC, RG 44, vol. 16, file "Canadian Red Cross Society & Canadian War Services Fund," transcript of address, [undated, 1943?].

27 LAC, RG 44, vol. 5, file "Canadian Red Cross Society," article by J.T. Thorson (attached to letter, J.A. Hume to Adelaide Plumptre), 25 July 1941; Hutchinson, *Champions of Charity*, part two.

28 Vance, *Maple Leaf Empire*, 153–6, 161–3; LAC, RG 44, vol. 16, file "Canadian Red Cross Society (1941–1942)," P.H. Gordon to T.C. Davis, 25 August 1941 and 29 August 1941.

29 Thompson, *Ethnic Minorities*, 14; Caccia, *Managing the Canadian Mosaic*, 29–36; LAC, RG 44, vol. 17, file "Russian Relief Fund – Canadian Red Cross Society," T.C. Davis to Jas. Y. Murdoch, 1 November 1941; T.C. Davis to J.T. Thorson, 4 November 1941; T.C. Davis to P.H. Gordon, 13 June 1942; and P.H. Gordon to T.C. Davis, 4 November 1941; LAC, RG 44, vol. 5, file "Canadian Red Cross Society," T.C. Davis to P.H. Gordon, 7 November 1941.

30 LAC, RG 44, vol. 17, file "Russian Relief Fund – Canadian Red Cross Society," T.C. Davis to Norman A. Robertson, 18 June 1942; vol. 1, file "Canadian Red Cross," P.H. Gordon to L.R. LaFlèche, 13 February 1943; L.R. LaFlèche to N.A. Robertson, 27 February 1943. For details of the CRCS campaign, see Walker, "Over the Top," 46–52.

31 Walker, "Over the Top," 82–90; LAC, RG 44, vol. 65, "Proceeding of meeting of representatives of Canadian organizations interested in relief to peoples of allied nations, with the Minister of National War Services, to consider a unified appeal to the Canadian people," 29 October 1943; LAC, RG 44, accession 85–86/S37, Box 7, file "Canadian Red Cross, vol. 2," secret memo to N.A. Robertson, 29 October 1943.

32 LAC, RG 44, vol. 15, file "Canadian Red Cross (1943–1944)," Margaret
    Gould to C.H. Payne, 6 March 1944; C.H. Payne to Margaret Gould, 9
    March 1944; LAC, RG 44, vol. 2, file "Canadian Red Cross," L.R.
    LaFlèche to R.P. Jellet, 4 October 1944; P.L. Browne to L.R. LaFlèche, 2
    December 1944.

33 LAC, RG 44, vol. 2, file "CRCS part 3," "Memorandum submitted to the
    Department by Dr Lawrence J. Burpee as an indication of the situation
    in the present negotiations of that organization with the CRCS, from the
    point of view of CUARF," 28 November 1944; and vol. 55, file "CUARF-
    Red Cross Relationship (Memoranda re:)," Lawrence J. Burpee to P.L.
    Browne, 13 November 1944. Off-hand comments by CRCS leaders and
    draft terms of agreement support Burpee's assessment. Dr Burpee was a
    historian, librarian, and archivist in Ottawa.

34 LAC, RG 44, vol. 2, file "Canadian Red Cross," P.L. Browne to L.R.
    LaFlèche, 1 December 1944 (quotation); LAC, RG 44, vol. 55, file
    "CUARF-R.C. Relations," draft press release [undated]. UNRRA was an
    organization created to help Allied governments in the war zones solve
    their relief problems, funded by other Allied governments. On Canada's
    involvement with UNRRA, see Armstrong Reid and Murray, *Armies of
    Peace*.

35 Walker, "Over the Top," 90.

36 Quebec Division, *Annual Report 1940* (Montreal: CRCS, 1941), 14–18;
    Auger and Lamothe, *De la poêle à frire*, 109–11; Durflinger, *Fighting
    from Home*, 111.

37 Quebec Division, *Annual Report 1939* (Montreal: CRCS, 1940), 2;
    CRCNA, box 7, file 7.II, J.M. Rodrigue Villeneuve to "Mr President," 27
    October 1941; Quebec Division, *Annual Report 1941* (Montreal: CRCS,
    1942), 52; LAC, RG 44, vol. 23, file "Meeting Held Oct. 16, 1940,"
    "Proceedings of NWS Conference on Coordination of Appeals for War
    Charities Purposes, 16 October 1940," 40; Auger and Lamothe, *De la
    poêle à frire*, 110.

38 Both quotations, CRCNA, box 11, file 11.II, "Red Cross Sunday, Septem-
    ber 22nd 1940."

39 CRCNA, box 12, green scrapbook, "Red Cross Sunday, November 12,
    1939."

40 Centre for Mennonite Brethren Studies, Cornelius F. Klassen fonds, file
    21, A.H. Unruh to Victor Sifton, 29 November 1939; Toews, *Alternative
    Service in Canada*, 109; Epp, *Mennonite Women in Canada*, 213–14.

41 LAC, Mrs Martin Wolff, MG 0-A30, vol. 7, file "Mrs Martin Wolff: Red
    Cross 1939–1940," Saidye Bronfman to "Madame President," 19 Sep-

tember 1939; Saidye Bronfman to "Friend," 17 October 1939; "Jewish Women Are Active in Local Red Cross Branch," *Montreal Daily Star*, 29 February 1940; R. Rutherdale, *Hometown Horizons*, 106–7, 118.

42 Saskatchewan Division, *Annual Report 1943* (Regina: CRCS, 1944), 59–72.

43 CRCNA, box 11, file 11.II, "The Red Cross needs $9,000,000 NOW," [1942?].

44 CRCNA, box 7, file 7.X, "Canadian Red Cross Emergency Call," 23 September 1940; LAC, RG 44, vol. 16, file "Canadian Red Cross Society & Canadian War Services Fund," transcript of address, [undated, 1943?].

45 For example, CRCNA, box 12, green scrapbook, "Red Cross Sunday November 12, 1939," and scrapbook with no cover, clipping "Every Dollar You Give Will Help Save Lives, Relieve Suffering," *Albertan*, 23 November 1939; box 11, file 11.II, "A Challenge to Canadians!" speakers' manual, 1940, and "The Red Cross Needs $9,000,000 NOW," [1942?]; LAC, MG 28 I10, vol. 178, file 178–7, "Give" pamphlet, March 1945. Descriptions of "the kindly Red Cross nurse in her clean white uniform" also appeared in advertising text, such as CRCNA, box 12, scrapbook with no cover, clipping "Thank God for the Red Cross! ... say Great War Veterans," 15 November 1939.

46 LAC, MG 28 I10, vol. 178, file 178–7, "Give" pamphlet, March 1945.

47 CRCNA, box 11, file 11.II, "The Red Cross needs $9,000,000 NOW," [1942?]; "A Challenge to Canadians!" speakers' manual, 1940, 19.

48 CRCNA, box 12, green scrapbook, clipping "Red Cross Work" [1940?]; box 15, file 15.I, Report of National Women's War Work Committee 1939–1946.

49 Smart, *By Grand Central Station*, 70.

50 Caccia, *Managing the Canadian Mosaic*, 141.

51 CRCS, "Statistical Highlights of Various Red Cross Services in Canada and Britain," *Annual Report 1944* (Toronto: CRCS, 1945), 158; Glassford, "Practical Patriotism ," 219–42; Myers and Poutanen, "Cadets, Curfews," 367–98; Keshen, *Saints, Sinners and Soldiers*, 202–3; CRCS, "Report of the Junior Red Cross for the School Year 1940–41," *Annual Report 1941* (Toronto: CRCS, 1942), 52; Dominion Bureau of Statistics, "Table 5: Population by Age Groups and Sex, Census of 1941, with Estimates (as at June 1), 1942–49," *Canadian Year Book 1951*, 125.

52 *Lux Glebana* 1941, p. 17, quoted in Hamelin, "A Sense of Purpose," 36; Scates, "The Unknown Sock Knitter," 29–49; Nowlan, "Junior Red Cross Volunteer Knitting," 64.

53 LAC, MG 28 I10, vol. 178, file 178–6, correspondence between Charlotte

Whitton and Jean Browne, 25 September to 18 November 1939; file 178–7, Charlotte Whitton to Philip Fisher, 6 January 1940, and Charlotte Whitton to Blair M. Clerk, 15 October 1941.

54 LAC, MG 28 I10, vol. 178, file 178–7, Philip Fisher to Charlotte Whitton, 3 January 1940.

55 LAC, MG 28 I10, vol. 178, file 178–6, Jean Browne to Charlotte Whitton, 14 November 1939; file 178–7, correspondence and clippings; LAC RG 44, vol. 15, file "Canadian Red Cross Society (1941–1942)," J.J. Leddy to C.L. Burton, 26 March 1941.

56 CRCNA, box 7, file 7.II, "Memorandum Used by Mr Sommerville" and file 7.III, "Soldier Comforts"; box 9, blue duotang, "CRCS: Field Comforts." The French and German Red Crosses reportedly also gave comforts to combatants.

57 CRCNA, box 9, blue duotang, Victor Sifton to Norman Sommerville, 13 January 1940; Norman Sommerville to Victor Sifton, 17 January 1940.

58 Hutchinson, *Champions of Charity*, 1.

59 Shaw, "The Peoples' Papers," 20–1.

60 GMA, M8228/175, "Red Cross Big Shots Should Disclose Salaries," *Hush*, 8 March 1941.

61 LAC, RG 44, vol. 16, file "Canadian Red Cross Society (1941–1942)," K. Duncan to T.C. Davis, 11 December 1941, with attached RCMP file; P.H. Gordon to T.C. Davis, 24 December 1941; Bourrie, *The Fog of War*, 10, 51.

62 LAC, RG 44, vol. 16, file "Canadian Red Cross Society (1941–1942)," K. Duncan to T.C. Davis, 24 December 1941; P.H. Gordon to T.C. Davis, 16 January and 5 February 1942.

63 LAC, RG 44, vol. 17, file "Red Cross POW Parcels," P.H. Gordon to T.C. Davis, 27 May 1942. For examples of CRCS efforts to combat rumours, see "Red Cross Policy," *Despatch* (January 1940): 3; CRCNA, box 12, green scrapbook, clipping "Red Cross Work" [undated, 1940?].

64 LAC, RG 44, vol. 16, file "Canadian Red Cross Society (1941–1942)," K. Duncan to T.C. Davis, 11 December 1941, with attached RCMP file; CRCNA, box 7, file 7.III, "$100 for a Headline," *The Canadian Veteran*, 30 September 1940 and 28 February 1941.

65 GMA, M8228/175, H.C. Hilton, letter to the editor, *Calgary Herald*, 21 October 1961; E.P. Foster to H.C. Hilton, 23 October 1961; H.J. McDonald to H.C. Hilton, 22 October 1961.

66 CRCNA, ECAMB III (ns), minutes of 422nd EC meeting, 5 September 1945, H.G. Donaldson, "Report on Visit to the Channel Islands," 3453–4.

67 CRCNA, box 47, clippings file, "Red Cross Funds not Spent in Enemy

Country," undated; LAC, RG 24, Department of National Defence, C–1–a, vol. 29, reel C–5368, correspondence between Adelaide Plumptre and L.N. Streight, 7 and 10 June 1943; LAC, RG 44, vol. 17, file "Red Cross POW Parcels," T.C. Davis to L.N. Streight, 16 April 1944.

68 LAC, MG 28 I10, vol. 178, file 178-6, Norman Sommerville to Charlotte Whitton, 21 November 1939.

69 LAC, MG 28 I10, vol. 178, file 178–6, Charlotte Whitton to Norman Sommerville, 24 November 1939 (2 letters).

70 LAC, MG 26K, vol. 969, M3185, Adelaide Plumptre to R.B. Bennett, 8 June 1940, p. 0614227; LAC, MG 28 I10, vol. 178, file 178-6, Norman Sommerville to Charlotte Whitton, 28 November 1939.

71 CRCNA, box 12, green scrapbook, clipping "Travelling Salesmen Plan Red Cross Unit," September 1939; clipping "Boy Scouts Will Repeat Services of Great War," September 1939; clipping "Red Cross on All Fronts Keeps up Effective Fight," [undated] (small branch fundraising in Alberta); clipping "Help Red Cross," spring 1940 (Cree contributions).

72 Thomas and Dawson, *My Grandmother's Wartime Diary*, 27.

73 CRCNA, box 12, green scrapbook, clipping "Letters to the Editor – Why Red Cross Needs Money," 1940.

74 Walker, "Over the Top."

75 LAC, RG 44, vol. 57, file "CUARF-RC Relations Jan. 1947 vol. 12," CRCS application for registration under the War Charities Act, 10 October 1939; LAC, Vida Peene, MG 31–D26, vol. 2, file 2–9, "Red Cross War Campaign Publicity from National Headquarters," November 1939.

76 Walker, "Over the Top," 21–2.

77 Ibid., 24–5; LAC, RG 44, vol. 16, file "Canadian Red Cross Society (1941–1942)," P.H. Gordon to T.C. Davis, 1 April 1942. No copy of the film has been located, but still photos of the Queen with CRCS comforts have survived.

78 Walker, "Over the Top," 45–6, 53, and chapters 3–4. Conversion, Bank of Canada inflation calculator, www.bankofcanada.ca.

79 Walker, "Over the Top," 66–7, 72–3.

80 LAC, RG 44, vol. 16, file "Canadian Red Cross Society (1941–1942)," T.C. Davis to P.H. Gordon, 21 February 1942.

81 Glassford, "Practical Patriotism," 229, 234–5. That $3,000,000 is equivalent to over $40,000,000 today. Bank of Canada inflation calculator, www.bankofcanada.ca.

82 Spencer, *Lipstick and High Heels*, 173–6; Bruce, *Back the Attack*, 1.

83 Bruce, *Back the Attack*, 22; CRCNA, box 12, green scrapbook, clipping "Busy Fingers Knit Sox for Soldiers," 25 September 1939; CRCNA,

box 15, file 15.I, Report of the National Women's Work Committee 1939–1946; "More than 700 ... " photo caption, *Harvester World* 35, 1 (January 1944), 9; CRCNA, box 15, file 15.I, "A Message from Mrs McEachren," *Courier*, 25 April 1946; Pierson, *They're Still Women after All*, 35–7, 41; Keshen, *Saints, Sinners and Soldiers*, 146–8.

84 CRCNA, box 15, file 15.1, Clara McEachren, "National Women's War Work Committee, 1939–1946," 4.

85 Keshen, *Saints, Sinners and Soldiers*, 146.

86 CRCNA, box 15, file 15.1, *Globe & Mail* clipping, 24 May [year?]; file 15.3, "Application for Registration of a War Charities Fund under the War Charities Act, 1939"; membership record book; file 15.2, circular letter, 29 January 1946. Parrsboro, Nova Scotia branch had its own workroom and committees, plus four outlying auxiliaries. NSARM, MG 20, vol. 3553, file #9, Parrsboro Red Cross Society Branch Annual Report, 1941.

87 CRCNA, box 15, file 15.2, "Red Cross Prayer"; Doreen Blain to Alix Downey, 28 April 1942 and 11 May 1942; file 15.4, minutes of special meeting, 6 May 1942.

88 CRCNA, box 15, file 15.2, postcard to members, 26 June 1944; file 15.4, "CH&RA Financial Statement and Annual Report 1941," and workroom reports 1940–45.

89 CRCNA, box 14, file 14.I, "They Walk by a Light," *Courier*, 13 June 1944, 1; box 15, file 15.1, Norma Coleman to Mrs Bate, 9 June 1944; box 12, scrapbook with no cover, Gregory Clark, "Women Accomplish Miracle," *Hardisty World*, 16 October 1941.

90 CRCNA, box 15, file 15.4, McEachren, "National Women's War Work Committee 1939–1946."

91 LAC, Nina Cohen, R2590–O–9–E, vol. 5, file "Personal Documents: Cohen Family, including family tree, biography."

92 LAC, R2590–O–9–E, vol. 5, file "Correspondence: Red Cross War Service," Bernard to Nina Cohen, 22 October 1942; LAC, R2590–2–3–E, vol. 1, file "Correspondence: Red Cross Society, servicemen to Mrs Cohen, Jan.–March 1943," Ernest Bartlett to Nina Cohen, 26 November 1942.

93 CRCNA, box 14, file 14.I, untitled speech given at Harbord Collegiate, 15 November 1945; instruction package "Red Cross Lodge, Christie Street Hospital."

94 Mosby, *Food Will Win the War*, 111–25. See chapter 3 on food and the mobilization of Canadian women more broadly.

95 Smith and Wakewich, "Beauty and the Helldivers," 71–107.

96 LAC, RG 44, accession 85–86/S37, box 7, file "Canadian Red Cross – Photographs"; Vance, *Objects of Concern*, 151.

97 Mosby, *Food Will Win the War*, 125, 113.

98 Stevenson, *Canada's Greatest Wartime Muddle*, 27–8 (regulations), chapter 9 (ineffectiveness); LAC, RG 44, vol. 15, file "Canadian Red Cross Society (1941–1942)," and vol. 16, file "Canadian Red Cross Society (1941–42)," correspondence between P.H. Gordon, T.C. Davis, and Mrs Rex Eaton, 6 August to 29 September 1942.

99 CRCNA, ECAMB III (ns), minutes of 400th meeting 12 January 1944, 238–9.

100 Whitton, *Canadian Women*, 55.

101 See, for example, Pierson, *They're Still Women after All*; Toman, *An Officer and a Lady*, chapter 3; Keshen, *Saints, Sinners, and Soldiers*, chapters 6 and 7; Smith and Wakewich, "Beauty and the Helldivers."

102 Keshen, *Saints, Sinners, and Soldiers*, 148.

103 Stevenson, *Canada's Greatest Wartime Muddle*, 149.

104 CRCNA, box 12, brown scrapbook, clipping "Drop Is Recorded in Red Cross Work," [likely January 1944]. Ruth Fleming was a fifty-two-year-old Anglo-Montrealer, married to coal merchant Andrew Fleming.

105 CRCNA, box 7, file 7.V, "Canadian Red Cross Society: Medical Services for the Armed Forces in World War II," July 1948, 2.

106 Quoted in Bruce, *Back the Attack*, 30.

107 CRCNA, box 15, file 15.4, "Notes on the third conference of representatives of women's organizations co-operating with the Canadian Red Cross Society," 20 November 1940; box 12, green scrapbook, clipping "Red Cross Plans New Motor Unit," July 1940. On women's non-traditional roles in wartime, particularly women in the military, see Pierson, *They're Still Women after All*.

108 CRCNA, box 15, file 15.4, "Notes on the third conference of representatives of women's organizations co-operating with the Canadian Red Cross Society," 20 November 1940.

109 Wade, "Joan Kennedy," 408–9; Keshen, *Saints, Sinners, and Soldiers*, 175-6; CRCNA, box 11, file 11.II, "The Red Cross needs $9,000,000 NOW," [1942?].

110 Shirley Walker, "Red Cross Corps Members Walk Memory Lane Tonight," *Windsor Star*, 24 June 1966.

111 Pierson, *They're Still Women after All*, 99.

112 "Red Cross Corps Members Get Chevrons," *Windsor Daily Star*, 25 February 1943; Pierson, *They're Still Women after All*, 129. On the importance of uniforms, see Toman, *An Officer and a Lady*, 103–10.

113 CRCS, *Annual Report 1945*, 172; Auger and Lamothe, *De la poêle à frire*, 112.

114 Avery, *The Science of War*; on medical science specifically, see Eggleston, *Scientists at War*, chapter 10.

115 W. Schneider, "Blood Transfusion," 188; Kapp, "Charles H. Best," 29–36; Eggleston, *Scientists at War*, 240–2; Stewart and Stewart, *Phoenix*, chapters 9 and 10. On therapeutic blood use in Canada before 1945, see Toman, "Crossing the Technological Line," chapter 2. On plasma versus serum, and the Australian experience, see Cortiula, "Collecting Blood for Battle"; Cortiula, "Serum and the Soluvac."

116 Kapp, "Charles H. Best," 36–9; W. Schneider, "Blood Transfusion," 199–200; *Blood Transfusion: A Red Cross Service*.

117 Kapp, "Charles H. Best," 39–40; Dr J.T. Phair, "Report of the National Blood Donor Service," *Annual Report 1940* (Toronto: CRCS, 1941), 32–4. Further centres for full or partial processing were established in other provinces later in the war. Dr J.T. Phair, "Report of the National Blood Donor Service," *Annual Report 1943* (Toronto: CRCS, 1944), 88–9.

118 Dr J.T. Phair, "Report of the National Blood Donor Service," *Annual Report 1942* (Toronto: CRCS, 1943), 81–3; Dr J.T. Phair, "Report of the National Blood Donor Service," *Annual Report 1944*, 89; Dr J.T. Phair, "Report of the National Blood Donor Service," *Annual Report 1945*, 100.

119 Phair, 1942 Report, 83; Phair, 1944 Report, 92.

120 Phair, 1945 Report, 100; CRCS, *Annual Report 1945*, 165; LAC, RG 44, vol. 16, file "Canadian Red Cross Society (1941–42)," P.H. Gordon to T.C. Davis, 10 April 1942; Kapp, "Charles H. Best," 38 (quotation), 41.

121 "Summary of Reports Submitted by the Acting Overseas Commissioner from the Various Departments of the Overseas Office," in CRCS, *Annual Report 1940*, 45–9.

122 CRCS, *Annual Report 1940*, 45; CRCS, *Annual Report 1945*, 42–3, 46; CRCNA, box 15, file 15.I, Report of National Women's War Work Committee 1939–1946.

123 On tensions in ICRC relationships with belligerent countries, see Crossland, "Expansion, Suspicion," 381–92.

124 P.H. Gordon felt that "as long as we had [Bennett] at the Head of our present London Committee, we really had no worries about what was going on in Britain." LAC, MG 26K, reel no. M3185, vol. 969, P.H. Gordon to R.B. Bennett, 1 December 1941, 0614629. On difficulties with the committee, see LAC, MG 26K, reel no. M3185, vol. 969, R.B.

Bennett correspondence with CRCS National Headquarters, 1940–41, 0614221–3, 0614281–4, 0614267, 0614275, 0614277, 0614317, 0614329.

125 LAC, MG 26K, reel no. M3185, vol. 969, R.B. Bennett correspondence with CRCS National Headquarters, 1940–41, 0614356, 0614367–8, 0614558–9, 0614580–5, 0614595–6, 0614602–5, 0614607–9, 0614612–13, 0614617–19, 0614621–2.

126 LAC, MG 26K, reel no. M3185, vol. 969, P.H. Gordon to R.B. Bennett, 1 December 1941, 614629, 16 May 1945, 0614828–9, and 31 December 1942, 0614800–2; Col. Scott to Jackson Dodds, 27 August 1942, 0614778; LAC, RG 44, vol. 16, file "Canadian Red Cross Society (1941–1942)," P.H. Gordon to T.C. Davis, 14 August 1942.

127 Nicholson, *Seventy Years of Service*, 145.

128 Many CRCS reports about the war years proudly state that the CRCS was the only agency in Britain with the necessary supplies to respond to the civilian need when the Battle of Britain began – as if that had been the plan all along, instead of a convenient accident resulting from the lack of military need for supplies to that point.

129 CRCNA, box 17, file 17.I, Department of Health for Scotland to F.W. Routley, 30 August 1941; Miss Hunter to General Price, 19 October 1943; F.W. Routley to W.S. Woods, 6 February 1946.

130 Nicholson, *Canada's Nursing Sisters*, 126.

131 Toman, "Officers and Ladies," 185–6, 191.

132 Vance, *Maple Leaf Empire*, 170; CRCNA, box 11, file 11.II, "The Red Cross needs $9,000,000 NOW," [1942?]; LAC, MG 26K, reel M3185, vol. 968, R.B. Bennett to Lord Astor, 6 June 1946, 0614021; Feasby, *Official History*, 527.

133 LAC, MG 26K, reel no. M3184, vol. 968, draft agreement between Lord Astor, the King, the CRCS, and the National Trust, 7 May 1940, 0613786; CRCNA, box 7, file 7.V, "Canadian Red Cross Society: Medical Services for the Armed Forces in World War II," July 1948, 9; Bennett quotations, LAC, MG 26K, reel no. 3184, vol. 968, speech at the opening of Cliveden Hospital, 0613642–3.

134 CRCS, *Annual Report 1945*, 173. Renamed "Canadian Red Cross Memorial Hospital," Taplow served Britain's National Health Service for forty years. Abandoned and increasingly derelict after 1985, it was a favourite creepy spot for locals to explore. In 2013 it had its own Wikipedia page and a popular "shrine" website: www.crcmh.com. It was demolished in 2006 and replaced by luxury homes.

135 CRCNA, box 7, file 7.V, "Canadian Red Cross Society: Medical Services for the Armed Forces in World War II," July 1948, 4.

136 McCullough, *Origins and History*, 81–90; CRCS, *Annual Report 1945*, 49, 105–6.

137 Vance, *Maple Leaf Empire*, 170.

138 Mona Wilson, "Report of Assistant Commissioner in Newfoundland," in CRCS, *Annual Report 1945*, 51–2; CRCNA, box 7, file 7.V, "Canadian Red Cross Society: Medical Services for the Armed Forces in World War II," July 1948, 8. See also Baldwin and Poulter, "Mona Wilson"; Baldwin, *She Answered Every Call*.

139 Pierson, *They're Still Women after All*, 103–13; quotation on 113.

140 Feasby, *Official History*, 527; Toman, *An Officer and a Lady*, chapter 3; Pierson, *They're Still Women after All*, chapter 4. Work, adventure, and pride mingle in Corps memoirs: MacDonald Cooper, *Wartime Letters Home*; Day, Spence, and Ladouceur, *Women Overseas*; Ellis with Dingman, *Face Powder and Gunpowder*; Mitchell and Deacon, 641. See also Historica Canada, The Memory Project, WWII section, interviews with Lois Cooper, Miriam Mitchell, and Kay Ruddick, www.thememoryproject.com.

141 Friedland, *Restoring the Spirit*, chapters 7 and 11; "Summary of Reports Submitted by the Acting Overseas Commission from the Various Departments of the Overseas Office," in CRCS, *Annual Report 1940*, 49; Nicholson, *Canada's Nursing Sisters*, 204–5.

142 Pomerleau, "La Société canadienne," 186.

143 CRCNA, box 12, brown scrapbook, clippings "Red Cross Bureau to Answer Queries on War Prisoners" and "Mrs H.P. Plumptre Heads Red Cross Bureau"; McCullough, *Origins and History*, 82–90; Vance, *Objects of Concern*, 99–111.

144 Vance, *Objects of Concern*, 112–25, quotation on 125. See also Vance, "Canadian Relief Agencies," 133–47.

145 Vance, "The Trouble with Allies," 81; LAC, RG 44, vol. 1, file "British Red Cross," Minutes of Meeting with British and Canadian Red Cross, Attachment 1 "Canadian Red Cross Society Activities in Connection with Prisoners of War," 20 September 1943; LAC, MG 26K (Bennett Papers) reel no. M3185, vol. 969, P.H. Gordon to R.B. Bennett, 13 July 1942, 0614754–6.

146 Vance, *Objects of Concern*, 154–5; Feasby, *Official History*, 529; LAC, RG 44, vol. 15, file "Canadian Red Cross (1943–1944)," Minutes of Inter-Departmental Committee Red Cross Prisoner-of-War Program, 18 February 1944; Memo from L.R. LaFlèche to C.H. Payne, 14 February

1944; LAC, RG 44, vol. 1, file "British Red Cross," W.L. Mackenzie King to L.R. LaFlèche, 26 November 1943.

147 Roy et al., *Mutual Hostages*, 68–70.

148 Vance, *Objects of Concern*, 183–202; Roland, "Allied POWs," 83–99. One such relief plan is found in LAC, RG 44, vol. 2, file "Canadian Red Cross," Minutes of Meeting with Representatives of CRCS Re: POW Parcels for Far East, 7 December 1943.

149 Vance, *Objects of Concern*, 205–15; Bruce, *Back the Attack*, 20, 139.

150 CRCNA, box 8, file I, transcript of interviews with prisoners of war, 28 July 1989; Vance, *Objects of Concern*, 156, 147–49.

151 Tisdall, "Canadian Red Cross Food Parcels," 77–8; Tisdall, "Further Report," 135–8; Tisdall et al., "Final Report," 279–86.

152 Total cost of CRCS food parcels: $46,069,676.40. CRCS, *Annual Report 1945* (Toronto: CRCS, 1946), 165, 168; Vance, *Objects of Concern*, 149.

153 Feasby, *Official History*, 529.

154 CRCNA, box 8, file 8.VI, A.L. Cochrane to E.J. King, 22 September 1948; Tisdall et al., "Final Report," 4; CRCNA, box 8, file I, transcript of interviews with prisoners of war, 28 July 1989; box 8, file 8.VI, Harry Crease, "The Unforgettable Klim Tin," unpublished manuscript, 1982.

155 CRCNA, box 8, file 8.VI, transcript from CRCS 1945 radio campaign; Mosby, *Food Will Win the War*, 11, 6.

CHAPTER SIX

1 *Despatch* 13, no. 3 (1952); "Tactics of Red Chinese Disrupt First Session," *Globe & Mail*, 28 July 1952, 1–2.

2 "Address by Dr F.W. Routley, National Commissioner of the CRCS at the Annual Meeting of the Alberta Division, Palliser Hotel, Calgary, 1 March 1946," Alberta Division, *Annual Report 1945* (Calgary: CRCS, 1946), G14–G17.

3 "Report of the Nomination Committee," Quebec Division CRCS, *Annual Report 1946* (Montreal: CRCS, 1946), 13–14.

4 CRCNA, Archived Minutes of Commissioners' Meetings 1942–1947 [hereafter AMCM], meeting 1–2 November 1946, 9, 3.

5 CRCNA, Postwar Planning Committee 1943–45 [hereafter PPC], meeting 24 September 1943.

6 CRCNA, PPC, meetings 11 January 1944, 29 March 1944, 5 September 1944, 2 October 1944.

7 CRCNA, PPC, meetings 30 October 1944, 16 January 1945, 30 April 1945. Only 11 of 1,470 branches had their own building in 1948. CRCS, *Annual Report 1948* (Toronto: CRCS, 1949), 52, 189.

8 LAC, MG 28 I10, vol. 178, file #1278–7, Philip S. Fisher to Nora Lee (with enclosure), 18 October 1945. Rosemount was the then-anglicized name for today's Rosemont district.

9 Membership and branch numbers compiled from national CRCS annual reports, 1945–70.

10 CRCS, *Annual Report 1964* (Toronto: CRCS, 1965), 159; *Canada Year Book 1967*, 195.

11 Membership and branch numbers compiled from national CRCS annual reports, 1945–70.

12 On Red Cross work in Newfoundland, see Duley, "The Unquiet Knitters of Newfoundland," 60–1; Baldwin and Poulter, "Mona Wilson," 281–311; Newfoundland Branch British Red Cross Society, *First Annual Report* (St John's: NL Branch BRCS, 1949); Newfoundland Division, *Annual Report 1950* (St John's: CRCS, 1951). On health conditions and nutrition work in Newfoundland, see Connor, "Medicine Is Here to Stay," 129–51; L. Kealey, "Historical Perspectives on Nutrition," 177–90; Overton, "Brown Flour and Beriberi," 14–20.

13 Fred W. Routley, "Report of the National Commissioner," CRCS, *Annual Report 1944*, 21; CRCNA, ECAMB IV (ns), CC meeting 26–27 October 1948, 4664.

14 CRCNA, ECAMB IV (ns), CC meeting 26–27 October 1948, remarks by Fred W. Routley, 4707.

15 Ibid., 4677; NSARM, MG 20, vol. 1366, item #7s, "Charles L. Illsley to retire," c. 1975.

16 J.T. Phair, "Report of the Acting National Commissioner," CRCS, *Annual Report 1962* (Toronto: CRCS, 1963), 19.

17 National officers and committee members compiled from national CRCS annual reports, 1945–70. This person usually served as honorary secretary.

18 National officers and committee members compiled from national CRCS annual reports, 1945–70.

19 National officers and committee members compiled from national CRCS annual reports, 1945–70.

20 Pierson, *They're Still Women after All*, 215–20; Strong-Boag, "Home Dreams," 471–505; Stephen, *Pick One Intelligent Girl*, chapter 4. The suggestion of women joining other organizations comes from Linda Kealey, conversation with the author, October 2015.

21 This period is examined in Cuthbert Brandt et al., *Canadian Women: A History*, 3rd ed., 384–95.

22 National officers and committee members compiled from national CRCS annual reports, 1945–1970.

23 Honorary members and counsellors compiled from national CRCS annual reports, 1930–70.

24 Keough and Campbell, *Gender History*, 238–9; provincial officers and committee chairs compiled from provincial summaries in national CRCS reports, 1945–70. Arsenault first joined the PEI CRCS as a secretary in 1927. Her work with the CRCS and other organizations was recognized with the Order of Canada in 1977. "Plaque Pays Tribute to Iphigenie Arsenault's 70 Years with Canadian Red Cross," *Guardian* (Charlottetown), 3 June 2008.

25 CRCNA, ECAMB IV (ns), EC meeting 4 October 1949, 5020–21.

26 Revenue, expense, and campaign details compiled from CRCS annual reports, 1945–70. Dr Stanbury first appealed for government funding for the BTS in 1956. CRCS financial records and the records of the Ontario Hospitals Commission are both somewhat opaque on this issue, but it appears that provincial governments began contributing to the technical costs of the BTS sometime in 1957–58, and the federal government by 1959, at which point the figure was pegged at 30 percent of technical costs. AO, RG 10–221–1–64, and RG 10–2222–0–2.

27 "Join the Red Cross for 1946," *Despatch* 7, no. 2 (1946): cover; "The Work of Mercy Never Ends," *Despatch* 8, no. 2 (1947): back cover; "The Work of Mercy Never Ends," *Despatch* 9, no. 2 (1948): back cover; "The Work of Mercy Never Ends," *Despatch* 10, no. 2 (1949): 16; "All Eyes on March," *Despatch* 10, no. 1 (1949): 3; Creighton, *The Forked Road*, 78.

28 CRCNA, ECAMB V (ns), CC meeting 23–24 November 1953, 6616.

29 Tillotson, *Contributing Citizens*, 190–1; "People Help People," *Despatch* 15, no. 1 (1954): 2–3; campaign letter from D. Bruce Shaw, *Despatch* 18, no. 1 (1957): 6; campaign letter from C.D. Shepard, *Despatch* 19, no. 1 (1958): 6.

30 "People Help People"; Shaw campaign letter (1957), 6.

31 Shepard campaign letter (1958), 6; "It Is Your Red Cross," *Despatch* 19, no. 1 (1958): 2; "Remember" *Despatch* 18, no. 1 (1957): 16; "We'll Be Home … for Christmas!" *Despatch* 14, no. 4 (1953): 2–3.

32 [untitled], *Despatch* 28, no. 1 (1967): 9; "You Are Not Alone," *Despatch* 21, no. 1 (1960): 12; Kenneth J. Farthing, "A Good Investment," *Despatch* 28, no. 1 (1967): 2; "In This Centennial Year" *Despatch* 28, no. 1 (1967): 15.

33 "Red Cross Basic Principles," *Despatch* 27, no. 3 (1966): 24.

34 World Vision Canada, "About Our History," 2013,
    www.worldvision.ca; CARE, "History of CARE," 2013, www.care.org;
    Oxfam Canada, "Introduction to Oxfam – History," 2014, www.
    oxfam.ca.

35 Canadian Cancer Society, "Fighting since 1938 – Our History," 2014,
    www.cancer.ca; The Arthritis Society, "Our History," 2014, www.
    arthritis.ca; Heart and Stroke Foundation of Canada, "National
    History," 2014, www.heartandstroke.com; Canadian Diabetes
    Association, "History," 2014, www.diabetes.ca.

36 Putnam, *Bowling Alone*, 16–18.

37 Tillotson, *Contributing Citizens*, 129–33.

38 CRCNA, ECAMB IV (ns), CC meeting 26–27 October 1948, 4687; EC
    meeting 4 October 1949, 5029–30; EC meeting 16 January 1951, 5541–
    4; ECAMB V (ns), CC meeting 2–3 May 1955, 6977–86. For a wider con-
    text, see Tillotson, *Contributing Citizens*, 192–200.

39 Tillotson, *Contributing Citizens*, 196–9. As Tillotson notes, the Red
    Cross came in for criticism in a *Maclean's* article for putting self-interest
    ahead of fundraising cooperation.

40 CRCNA, ECAMB V (ns), CC meeting 2–3 May 1955, 6977–86; ECAMB VI
    (ns), EC meeting 30 April–2 May 1956, "87–13 Federated Fundraising";
    Tillotson, *Contributing Citizens*, 201.

41 Hutchinson, *Champions of Charity*, 1.

42 Archives of Ontario [hereafter AO], Ontario Hospital Services Commis-
    sion, RG 10–221–1–64, CRCS, "Submission to Advisory Committee on
    Hospital Insurance and Diagnostic Services," 7 April 1965, 4; Hutchin-
    son, *Champions of Charity*, 1.

43 CRCS, *Annual Report 1969* (Toronto: CRCS, 1970), 57–61.

44 Neary, *On to Civvy Street*, chapters 6 and 7; Creighton, *The Forked
    Road*, 116. See also Granatstein and Neary, *The Veterans Charter*.

45 CRCNA, box 24, file 24.II, M.G. Graves, "Red Cross to Relinquish Con-
    trol of Hospital after 35 Years of Service to Crippled Children," *The
    Volunteer* 8, no. 2 (1957): 1; CRCS, *Annual Report 1970* (Toronto:
    CRCS, 1971), 66–7.

46 Junior membership numbers compiled from CRCS annual reports 1945–
    70; Clarke, "Keep Communism Out," 93–119; Helleiner, "The Right
    Kind of Children," 143–52; Thorn, "Healthy Activity and Worthwhile
    Ideas," 327–59.

47 CRCS, *Annual Report 1939*, 12; CRCS, *Annual Report 1940*, 42–3;

CRCS, *Annual Report 1941*, 82–4; CRCS, *Annual Report 1942*, 84–5; CRCS, *Annual Report 1943*, 92; CRCS, *Annual Report 1944*, 110; CRCS, *Annual Report 1947* (Toronto: CRCS, 1948), 33, 141–2; CRCS, *Annual Report 1948*, 136–8.

48 CRCS, *Annual Report 1950* (Toronto: CRCS, 1951), 73–4, 133; CRCS, *Annual Report 1954* (Toronto: CRCS, 1955), 61; CRCS, *Annual Report 1956* (Toronto: CRCS, 1957), 65–6; CRCS, *Annual Report 1958* (Toronto: CRCS, 1959), 66–7; Jim Gifford, *Hurricane Hazel*, 84; Manitoba Division CRCS, *Call 320*. See also Robinson and Cruikshank, "Hurricane Hazel."

49 CRCS, *Annual Report 1962*, 63; CRCS, *Annual Report 1963* (Toronto: CRCS, 1964), 68; CRCS, *Annual Report 1965* (Toronto: CRCS, 1966), 64.

50 Kevin G. Jones, "Sport in Canada, 1900–1920," in *Proceedings of the First Canadian Symposium*, 47–8; Bouchier and Cruikshank, "Abandoning Nature," 315–37; Cruikshank and Bouchier, "Dirty Spaces," 59–76; Kossuth, "Dangerous Waters," 800–2.

51 Quebec Division, "Water Safety," *Annual Report 1962* (Montreal: CRCS, 1963), 29; E. Harvey Doney, "Water Wings for Canada," *Despatch* 8, no. 3 (1947): 11; "Two Sides of the Picture," *Despatch* 9, no. 4 (1948): 5.

52 Lifesaving Society, "Lifesaving Society Chronological Timelines," www.lifesaving.ca.

53 CRCNA, ECAMB III (ns), EC meeting 1 May 1945, 3289–90; Harvey Doney, "All Provinces Organized for 1946 'Learn to Swim' Campaign," *Despatch* 7, no. 4 (1946): 6.

54 Berridge, "The Development of the Red Cross Water Safety Service," 15.

55 "Beginners and Experts Swim Safely with the Red Cross," *Despatch* 9, no. 4 (1948): 7; Doney, "Water Wings," 11, 13; CRCNA, ECAMB IV (ns), EC meeting 16 January 1951, 5525; "Unique Red Cross Radio Program Teaches Children How to Swim," *Despatch* 8, no. 7 (1947): 11. For examples of swimming and water safety publicity images, see "Red Cross Guards Canadian Lives," *Despatch* 9, no. 2 (1948): [no pagination].

56 CRCNA, ECAMB IV (ns), CC meeting 2–4 May 1951, 5603–5; ECAMB VI (ns), CC meeting 19–20 November 1956, "88–20 Proposal that a Charge Be Made for Water Safety Badges"; ECAMB VII (ns), CC meeting, 19–20 November 1962, 22–8.

57 CRCNA, ECAMB VII (ns), EC meeting 27 September 1963, 15–20; ECAMB VIII (ns), CC meeting 6–7 May 1968, "Proposed Joint Programmes of Instruction between Canadian Red Cross Society Water Safety Service

and Royal Life Saving Society"; ECAMB IX (ns), CC meeting 24–25 November 1969, 114–18, "Proposed Agreement between the Canadian Red Cross Society and the Royal Life Saving Society;" Mavis E. Berridge, "The Development of the Royal Life Saving Society and the Red Cross Water Safety Service in Canada to 1954," in *Proceedings of the First Canadian Symposium*, 183.

58   "Stanbury, William Stuart," in *The Canadian Who's Who* (1958–1960), 1050–1; "The War Years," *Despatch* 24, no. 3 (1963): 8; Stanbury, *Origin, Development and Future*, 1; CRCNA, "Documents Presented for Consideration by the National Officers Committee January 17, 1953," "Blood Transfusion Service (The history of the Programme told through summaries of, and extracts from, minutes of Central Council and the National Executive Committee)," 1–2, 6–7.

59   CRCS, *Annual Report 1945*, 100, 103; Stanbury, *Survey of Blood Transfusion Facilities*. See also Stanbury, *Origin, Development and Future*, 1–2.

60   Titmuss, *The Gift Relationship*, chapter 7; "The history of blood transfusion," www.redcross.org.uk; *Blood Transfusion: A Red Cross Service*, 7, 13.

61   Immanuel Kant, quoted in Rabinow, "Artificiality and Enlightenment," 91–111.

62   CRCS, *Annual Report 1945*, 101.

63   CRCNA, AMCM, meeting 5–6 October 1948, 11.

64   Stanbury, *Origin, Development and Future*, 2.

65   Ibid., 4.

66   CRCNA, box 29, file 29.I, Stuart Stanbury to J.M. Fortin, 19 October 1956. The "40 cents" figure can be found for example in CRCNA, box 29, file 29.II, press release re: Ontario grant for BTS expansion, 8 August 1957.

67   Stanbury, *Origin, Development and Future*, 3–4; W. Stuart Stanbury, "Report of the National Commissioner," CRCS *Annual Report 1961* (Toronto: CRCS, 1962), 19.

68   AO, RG 10–222–0–2, meetings 22 April, 29 April, and 12 August 1959; RG 10–222–0–3, meeting 27 January 1960; CRCNA, "Documents Presented for Consideration," 13–22.

69   Already in 1948 Dr Stanbury "explained that major surgery was being done today that was not even thought of five years ago" and told his CRCS colleagues that the society would be "required to supply more, and not less blood in the future." CRCNA, AMCM, meeting 5–6 October 1948, 11; CRCNA, ECAMB IV (ns), CC meeting 2–4 May 1950, 5216.

70   AO, RG 10–222–0–1, meeting 11 July 1957.

71 CRCNA, box 29, file 29.II, "Brief to Central Council from Ontario Division," 26 October 1956.

72 AO, RG 10–221–1–64, and RG 10–222–0–2.

73 CRCNA, "Documents Presented for Consideration," 14.

74 AO, RG 10–221–1–64, clipping "$50,000 Grant Will Expand Blood Banks," c. 1958; CRCNA, "Documents Presented for Consideration," 19.

75 AO, RG 10–222–0–259, copy of Central Council resolution; Stanbury, *Origin, Development and Future*, 7, 17–25. Although the American comparison was made (13.6 per thousand) it was not entirely valid because of all the competitor blood banks; AO, RG 10–222–0–259, W.S. Stanbury to Ian Urquhart, 10 April 1961; RG 10–222–0–2, meetings held 8 April 1959, 19 April 1961, 26 April 1961.

76 AO, RG 10–221–1–64, E.P. McGavin, handwritten rough notes and notes attached to drafts, c. 1957–58; "Report of a Meeting Held on Friday, April 17, 1959"; E.P. McGavin to J.B. Neilson, 10 April 1961; E.P. McGavin to J.B. Neilson, 12 February 1962; E.A.D. Boyd, "Study of Red Cross Blood Utilization in Active Treatment Hospitals 1962–1963," 1 October 1964.

77 AO, RG 10–221–1–64, CRCS, "Submission to Advisory Committee on Hospital Insurance and Diagnostic Services," 7 April 1965, 3; E.P. McGavin to J.B. Neilson and Commissioners, 4 May 1965; E.P. McGavin to S.W. Martin, 1 May 1967.

78 CRCNA, "Documents Presented for Consideration," 19–21, 14; CRCNA, box 30, file 30.II, Dan H. Young to Stuart Stanbury, 19 January 1958.

79 CRCNA, "Documents Presented for Consideration," 20.

80 CRCNA, AMCM, meeting 16 May 1949, 6; CRCNA, "Documents Presented for Consideration," 15.

81 Examples from the *Guardian* (Charlottetown): "A MOTHER may die unless YOU give blood," 15 October 1948, 3; "You ... Can Save A Life"; 16 October 1948, 9; "BLOOD IS LIFE," 18 October 1948, 14; "YES – I will be a BLOOD DONOR," 21 October 1948, 9; "The case of the 7 strangers," 25 February 1948, 11; "Twelve Very Little Ones," 9 March 1948, 12; "BLOOD IS LIFE," 18 October 1948, 14; "Coming Our Way Soon," 9 October 1948, 5. Also see CRCNA, AMCM, meeting 16 May 1949, 6; "You Can Save Lives," *Despatch* 12, no. 3 (1951): 16; "Your Blood Saves Lives," *Despatch* 17, no. 3 (1956): 16; "Your Blood the Gift of Life," *Despatch* 26, no. 3 (1965): 3.

82 CRCNA, AMCM, meeting 10–11 September 1956, 3.

83 "No Price Tag on Blood," *Despatch* 13, no. 2 (1952): 15; Stanbury, *Origin, Development and Future*, 6.

84 W. Stuart Stanbury, "Report of the National Commissioner," CRCS *Annual Report 1961*, 31–2.

85 CRCS, *The Role of One Voluntary Organization*, iv–viii.

86 L.J. Harnum, "Commissioner's Report," Newfoundland Division, *Annual Report 1950* (St John's: CRCS, 1951), 17–18.

87 Armstrong Reid and Murray, *Armies of Peace*; Reinisch, "Auntie UNRRA at the Crossroads," 70–97; Salvatici, "'Help the People," 428–51.

88 CRCNA, box 11, crested scrapbook, Monique Nicol letter, 6 November 1946; booklet "Merci à la Croix-rouge Canadienne: Arbre de Noël 1946 – Maisoncelles-Pelvey, Calvados." Author's translations: title: "Thank you to the Canadian Red Cross: Christmas Tree 1946"; quotation: "Long live Canada I love canada and my pretty pink dress, and my sweater. I send big kisses and I say thank-you [sic]." For British recipients' responses, see CRCNA, box 17, file 17.II, "Britain News – Thank You for Food." Also see LAC, RG 44, vol. 15, file "Canadian Red Cross (1946–)," Clara McEachren to Mrs Tilley and Mrs Coleman, 12 June 1946.

89 Military and civilian inquiry branches merged in 1946; the inquiry service merged with the family reunion program around 1970 to become Tracing and Reunion. By 2011 it had been renamed Restoring Family Links. McCullough, *Origin and History*, 114, 125.

90 GMA, M8228, file #25, minutes of Executive Committee Meeting of Alberta Division, 25 October 1946, 5; LAC, RG 44, vol. 49, file "CRCS General (1947)," Undersecretary of External Affairs to Colonel Browne, 30 September 1947, and "Needs for Medical and Food Relief in India and Pakistan," 3 October 1947; Fred W. Routley, "Report of the National Commissioner," *Annual Report 1947* (Toronto: CRCS, 1948), 34–5.

91 Barnett, *Empire of Humanity*, part 3. The motivations of present-day government-funded humanitarian aid are examined in Fielding, "The Dynamics of Humanitarian Aid Decisions," 536–64.

92 Both quotations from *Despatch* 24, no. 3 (1963): "In Other Lands," 14; "A Great Humanitarian," 2.

93 Glassford, "Practical Patriotism," 236–7; Brookfield, *Cold War Comforts*, 5–6; Women's Work statistics compiled from CRCS annual reports, 1945–70.

94 Margaret Wilson, "International Work," CRCS *Annual Report 1961*, 74–7; W. Stuart Stanbury, "Report of the National Director," CRCS *Annual Report 1960* (Toronto: CRCS, 1961), 32.

95 J.T. Phair, "Report of the Acting National Commissioner," CRCS *Annual Report 1962*, 27; A.E. Wrinch, "Report of the National Commissioner," CRCS *Annual Report 1965*, 29–30.

96 Margaret Wilson, "International Work," in CRCS *Annual Report 1968* (Toronto: CRCS, 1969), 71; CRCS *Annual Report 1969*, 65. CIDA granted the CRCS $55,000 in emergency relief money in 1968, and $13,000 for development work in 1969.

97 Holmes, *The Shaping of the Peace*, 84.

98 H. Mackenzie, "Mapping Canada's World," 39–44; Bothwell, Drummond, and English, *Canada since 1945*, 13–14, 61–73, 87; Creighton, *The Forked Road*, chapter 7; Holmes, *The Shaping of the Peace*, 99–104; W. Stuart Stanbury, "Report of the National Commissioner," CRCS *Annual Report 1952* (Toronto: CRCS, 1953), 23; Barnett, *Empire of Humanity*, 108.

99 Bothwell, *The Big Chill*, 1–2; Barnett, *Empire of Humanity*, part 3; Brookfield, *Cold War Comforts*, chapters 4 and 5; Morrison, *Aid and Ebb Tide*, 28–9.

100 W. Stuart Stanbury, "Report of the National Commissioner," in CRCS *Annual Report 1953* (Toronto: CRCS, 1954), 33; CRCS *Annual Report 1955* (Toronto: CRCS, 1956), 30–1. Dr Stanbury pioneered the delicate work of brokering reunions between individuals in Eastern European countries and their next-of-kin in Canada. An argument similar to his about basic needs and ideologies informed the influential 1946 documentary "Seeds of Destiny," directed by David Miller for the US Army. See Kahn Atkins, "Seeds of Destiny," 25–33.

101 W. Stuart Stanbury, "Report of the National Commissioner," CRCS *Annual Report 1956*, 26.

102 Margaret Wilson, "International Work," in CRCS *Annual Report 1966* (Toronto: CRCS, 1967), 70–3; CRCS *Annual Report 1967* (Toronto: CRCS, 1968), 62–9; CRCS *Annual Report 1968*, 70; and CRCS *Annual Report 1969*, 68.

103 Fred W. Routley, "Report of the National Commissioner," *Annual Report 1946* (Toronto: CRCS, 1947), 32; "On the Cover," *Despatch* (November 1948): 2; International Red Cross and Red Crescent Movement, "John MacAulay 1959–65," 1999, www.redcross.int/en/history/not_macaulay.asp.

104 W.S. Stanbury, "Report of the National Commissioner," CRCS *Annual Report 1953*, 35.

105 Ibid., 31; CRCS *Annual Report 1956*, 30; CRCS *Annual Report 1959* (Toronto: CRCS, 1960), 29; CRCS *Annual Report 1960*, 29–31; and CRCS *Annual Report 1961*, 29–30. Also A.E. Wrinch, "Report of the National Commissioner," CRCS *Annual Report 1966*, 27.

106 Desgrandchamps, "Organising the Unpredictable," 1409–16.

107 A.E. Wrinch, "Report of the National Commissioner," in CRCS *Annual Report 1968*, 28; and CRCS *Annual Report 1969*, 15. The ICRC's approach sparked the 1971 creation of Médecins Sans Frontières (Doctors Without Borders), an aid organization that eschewed apolitical neutrality in order to prioritize the rights of sufferers.

108 W. Stuart Stanbury, "Report of the National Commissioner," CRCS *Annual Report 1951* (Toronto: CRCS, 1952), 21–2.

109 CRCNA, ECAMB V (ns), EC meeting 27 March 1952, Margaret E. Wilson, "Report to presidents of Dr Stanbury's statement re: Red Cross workers for Japan."

110 W. Stuart Stanbury, "Report of the National Commissioner," CRCS *Annual Report 1952* (Toronto: CRCS, 1953), 19–20. See memoirs of Dorothea Powell Wiens, Florence Bell, and Jacqueline Robitaille Van Campen in Day, Spence, and Ladouceur, *Women Overseas*, 343–67.

111 CRCNA, Archives Box 20, file 20.III, "Letter from Member of Canadian Red Cross Welfare Team to Friend in Canada"; Stanbury, "Report," CRCS *Annual Report 1952*, 19–20.

112 Eayrs, *In Defence of Canada*, 319, 337.

113 CRCNA, OCC, "The Role of the Red Cross in Civil Defence," March 1951.

114 Toxopeus, "1951 Agreement," chapters 7 and 8.

115 Ibid., 10–11 and chapter 9.

116 Burtch, *Give Me Shelter*, 1–4.

117 Ibid., 119.

118 Brookfield, *Cold War Comforts*, 23, 27–9, 35.

119 Ibid., 222.

120 Soares, "Very Correct Adversaries," 1536–53; Walter H. Waggoner, "U.S. to Limit Role in Red Cross Talks," *New York Times*, 19 July 1952, 2; "The Red Cross," *Times* (London), 26 July 1952, 5.

121 "Tactics of Red Chinese Disrupt First Session," *Globe & Mail*, 28 July 1952, 1–2; "Charge Children Held but Russ again Beaten at Red Cross Meeting," *Globe & Mail*, 26 July 1952, 1; Fred Nossal, "Germ Warfare Waged Red Delegates Insist," *Globe & Mail*, 28 July 1952, 1; "Conflict in Red Cross Goal of Communists, U.S. Delegate Charges," *Globe & Mail*, 31 July 1952, 1–2.

122 "What Went Before," *Despatch* 13, no. 3 (1952): 4–5; "The Conference in Retrospect," *Despatch* 13, no. 3 (1952): 3; "It Is Still Humanitarian," *Globe & Mail*, 7 August 1952, 6; Fred Nossal, "Communists Beaten in Voting but Achieve Propaganda Goal," *Globe & Mail*, 9 August 1952, 1–2; Favez, *The Red Cross and the Holocaust*.

123 ICRC, "The Fundamental Principles," www.icrc.org.

124 Barnett, *Empire of Humanity*, 105, 107–8; Tillotson, *Contributing Citizens*, 44.

125 CRCNA, ECAMB V (ns), CC meeting 4–6 May 1953, 6349–51.

126 CRCNA, ECAMB V (ns), CC meeting 24–26 November 1952, 6189; CRCNA, ECAMB IV (ns), CC meeting 26–27 October 1948, 4676–7.

127 CRCNA, ECAMB VI (ns), EC meeting 21 March 1958, "457–6 Preliminary Report of Programme Evaluation Committee"; CC meeting 34–36 November 1958, "92–9 Report of the Programme Evaluation Committee."

128 CRCNA, National Sub-Executive Committee Archived Minutes, vol. 1 (1967–1972), National Officers Meeting 26 June 1967, 6–7; CRCS, *And Who Is My Stranger*; A.E. Wrinch, "Report of the National Commissioner," CRCS *Annual Report 1970* (Toronto: CRCS, 1971), 30.

129 Brookfield, *Cold War Comforts*, 222, 145.

130 CRCNA, ECAMB V (ns), "Study of Volunteer Services Progress Report to Central Council," 23–24 November 1953, 6619.

131 Paul V. Dansereau, "Junior Red Cross," Quebec Division, *Annual Report 1962*, 33–4; Gerald Bronfman, "President's Address," Quebec Division, *Annual Report 1964* (Montreal: CRCS, 1965), 10–12.

132 "Junior Red Cross Week," *News of Red Cross* 10, no. 5 (1962), 3–4; CRCS, *And Who Is My Stranger*, 40; Ormston, "A Community Approach," 75; Bronfman, "President's Address," Quebec Division, *Annual Report 1964*, 10–12; J.P.C. Gauthier, "Red Cross Youth," Quebec Division, *Annual Report 1966* (Montreal: CRCS, 1967), 38.

133 Henderson, *Making the Scene*, 16.

134 GMA, M8228/201, "Junior Red Cross Gets New Name," *The Volunteer* 16, no. 3 (1966): 6; Trepanier, "Building Boys, Building Canada," 242; CRCNA, Archived Minutes of National Officers' Meetings [hereafter AMNOM], vol. 7 (1964–66), meeting 16 September 1966, 13; AMNOM, vol. 6 (1962–64), meeting 29 October 1964, 6; AMNOM, vol. 7 (1964–66), meeting 18 July 1966, 11g. See also CRCNA, AMCM, meeting 10 May 1967, 5–6; Granatstein, *Canada 1957–1967*, 301–3.

135 CRCNA, AMCM, meeting 10 May 1967, 6; Ian McKay, "Sarnia in the Sixties," 26; Compton Brouwer, *Canada's Global Villagers*; Marshall and Sterparn, "Oxfam Aid to Canada's First Nations," 298–344.

136 NSARM, MG 20, vol. 1369, item #96h, "Minutes of a Meeting of Divisional Chairmen – Volunteer Registration and Orientation Services Committee," 24 September 1969, 4–6.

137 Myers, "Blistered and Bleeding," 247; CRCNA, ECAMB vol. VIII (ns), CC meeting 25–26 November 1968, attachment to CC minute 112–12(b), "Address by Mr Michael Worsoff: Youth Blood Programme."

CONCLUSION

1 GMA, M8228/209, Lloyd Liggett, "Some Chicken – Some Neck!" *Action*
   5, no. 1 (1974), inside front cover.
2 CRCNA, National Sub-Executive Committee Archived Minutes, vol. 1,
   Minutes of National Officers Meeting, 26 June 1967, 6–7. The ICRC
   and LRCS created a Joint Committee for Reappraisal of the Role of the
   Red Cross, whose study and final report were directed by Canadian
   Donald D. Tansley, who was at that time executive vice-president for
   CIDA. Joint Committee, *An Agenda for Red Cross*.
3 NSARM, MG20 vol. 1366, #7ff, Ken Miller, "Self-sufficiency aim of commissioner."
4 CRCS, *And Who Is My Stranger*, vii, 2, 4–5.
5 Ibid., 27–50.
6 GMA, M8228/205, H.C. Hilton, "Where from Here?" *Action* 1, no. 1
   (1970); LAC MG28 I10 (Canadian Council on Social Development
   fonds), vol. 179, file 179–1 "CRCS: Relationship with Funds 1966–
   1971," Henry E. Stegmayer to Henry Stubbins, 12 March 1970.
   Stegmayer was executive director of the United Fund of Greater Saint
   John (NB), and Stubbins the executive secretary of the Community
   Funds and Councils of Canada.
7 Ann Oakley and John Ashton, eds, "Editor's Introduction" to Titmuss,
   The Gift Relationship, 5–8.
8 Titmuss, *The Gift Relationship*, 58–9 (questions), 279, 292, 311.
9 Skocpol, *Diminished Democracy*, 153–4; Barnett, Empire of Humanity,
   219, 105.
10 Skocpol, *Diminished Democracy*, 135–43, 153–4; NSARM, MG20, vol.
   1368, item #60, "Radical surgery is needed!" *nova scotia red cross
   newsnewsnews* 2 (October 1973). The Cancer Society, Mental Health
   Association, and Canadian Arthritis and Rheumatism Society are identified as "worthy organizations" competing with the CRCS for Canadians'
   time and money.
11 CRCNA, box 30, file 30.II, "Red Cross 'Bled' by Donor Service Past President of Group Charges," *Calgary Herald* clipping, 28 February 1958.
12 André Picard, "Tainted-blood Compensation Incomplete as Deadline
   Nears," *Globe and Mail*, 29 June 2010, www.theglobeandmail.com.
13 No-fault compensation was a key recommendation of the Krever Inquiry.
   Final Report by the Commission of Inquiry into Canada's Blood System,
   vol. 3 (Ottawa: 1997), chapter 39. On the 2001 ruling, see Supreme
   Court of Canada, Walker Estate *v.* York Finch General Hospital.
14 Feldman, "Blood Justice," 652.

15 Duffin, review of *Tainted*, 229–31.

16 Krever Inquiry, *Final Report*; Picard, *The Gift of Death*; Dean, "Broken Promises"; Paterson, "Tainted Blood, Tainted Knowledge"; Vallée, "Naissance et développement."

17 Oppenheimer, *The Power of Humanity*, 226–30.

18 CRCS, "Toward a Renewed Canadian Red Cross"; CRCS, "Partnering to Build a Resilient Civil Society." The "somewhat demoralized" assessment springs from my time working at a local branch both immediately pre- and post- BTS relinquishment.

19 CBC TV news *The National*, 11 November 2013; "Barrie Groups Collecting Money Food and Clothing for Stricken Philippines," *Barrie Examiner*, 12 November 2013, www.thebarrieexaminer.com; Gina Holmes, "Infographic: An update on Red Cross response in the Philippines," Red Cross Talks blog, 19 December 2013, www.redcross.ca.

20 CBC Radio Two, CBC Radio News, 4 June 2014; CRCS, "Alberta Floods One Year Progress Report," 4 June 2014, 8, www.redcross.ca; CRCS, "Alberta Fires One Month Donor Update," 2 June 2016, 3, www.redcross.ca; CBC News Edmonton, "One million Canadians have donated to Red Cross campaign for Fort McMurray fire victims," 28 June 2016, www.cbc.ca.

21 "Appendix D: A Study on Public Attitudes towards the Canadian Red Cross Society" (Gallup Poll for CRCS, September 1971), in CRCS, *And Who Is My Stranger*, 112–13.

22 Joint Committee, *An Agenda for Red Cross*, 44.

23 Author's personal collection, CRC posters, and other advertising material, 1997–2014. Significantly, these campaigns followed in the wake of the Tainted Blood Scandal.

24 Red Cross Outpost Historic House Museum, www.redcrossoutpost.org.

25 Dunant, *A Memory of Solferino*, 127.

26 David MacKenzie, "Introduction: Myth, Memory, and the Transformation of Canadian Society," in D. Mackenzie, *Canada and the First World War*, 13.

27 Mitchinson, *The Nature of Their Bodies*, 7.

28 Feldberg et al., "Comparative Perspectives," 21–2.

29 P.H. Gordon, *Fifty Years*, 97.

30 Compton Brouwer discusses this shift in *Modern Women Modernizing Men*, 3–4.

31 I develop this argument in "Mobilisées, organisées," 59–78.

32 CRCS, *And Who Is My Stranger*, 24.

33 Barnett, *Empire of Humanity*, 9.

BIBLIOGRAPHY

ARCHIVAL SOURCES

Archives of Ontario, Toronto
  John Boyd Fonds
  Ontario Hospitals Commission Records

British Red Cross Museum and Archive, London, England
  Lord Wantage Papers

Canadian Red Cross National Archive, Ottawa
  Archived Minutes of Commissioners' Meetings
  Archived Minutes of National Officers' Meetings
  Executive Committee and Central Council Archived Minute Books
  George Sterling Ryerson Papers
  Lent, D. Geneva. "Alberta Red Cross in Peace and War (1914–1947)"
    Unpublished manuscript, 1947
  National Annual Reports
  National Sub-Executive Committee Archived Minutes
  Nationalization Documents
  Numbered archival boxes, 1899–present
  Overseas Club Collection
  Photograph Collection
  Postwar Planning Committee Minutes
  Provincial Annual Reports
  Red Cross Periodical Collection

Canadian War Museum, Ottawa
  Wartime Propaganda

Centre for Mennonite Brethren Studies, Winnipeg
  Cornelius F. Klassen Fonds

City of Toronto Archives
Information File on Elected Officials: Adelaide Plumptre

Glenbow Museum and Archives, Calgary
Canadian Red Cross Society, Alberta-Northwest Territories Division Fonds

Library and Archives Canada, Ottawa
Government Documents
Department of Militia and Defence
Department of National Defence
Department of National Health and Welfare
Department of National War Services
Department of the Secretary of State
Personal and Association Papers
Anne E. Ross
Canadian Council on Social Development
Canadian Red Cross Society
Mrs Martin Wolff
Nina Cohen
R.B. Bennett
Robert Laird Borden
Sophie Hoerner
Vida Peene
William Lyon Mackenzie King

McCord Museum, Montreal
Photograph Collection

Nova Scotia Archives and Records Management, Halifax
Canadian Red Cross Society, Nova Scotia Division Fonds

Pier 21 Museum, Halifax
Permanent Exhibition – "The Volunteers"

Prince Edward Island Public Archives and Record Office, Charlottetown
Mona Wilson Papers

Robertson Library Special Collections, University of Prince Edward Island,
Charlottetown
Georgina Fane Pope Photograph Album

Windsor-Essex County Branch CRCS, Windsor, Ontario
Collins, Lori. "Seventy Years of Service: A History of the Windsor Branch
of the Canadian Red Cross Society 1918–1988." Unpublished manuscript,
1988

PUBLISHED SOURCES

Canadian Red Cross Periodicals

Action
Bulletin
The Canadian Red Cross
The Canadian Red Cross Junior
The Courier
Despatch
nova scotia red cross newsnewsnews
Service
The Volunteer

Other Periodicals and News Media

The Albertan, Calgary
Barrie Examiner, Ontario
Calgary Herald
CBC Radio news
CBC TV news *The National*
Everywoman's World
The Globe, Toronto
The Globe and Mail, Toronto
The Guardian, Charlottetown
Hardisty World, Alberta
Harvester World
Montreal Daily Star
Montreal Gazette
New Glasgow Enterprise, Nova Scotia
New York Times
The StarPhoenix, Saskatoon
The Times, London
Waterford Star, Ontario
Windsor Daily Star, Ontario
The World, Toronto

Government Documents

Canada. *Canada Year Book*
– *Census of Canada*
– *Statutes of Canada*
House of Commons. *Official Record of Debates*
– *Sessional Papers*
Supreme Court of Canada, Walker Estate *v.* York Finch General Hospital, 2001
SCC 23

ARTICLES, BOOKS, THESES, WEBSITES

Adami, J. George. *War Story of the Canadian Army Medical Corps*, vol. 1, *The First Contingent*. Toronto: Musson Book Co. for the Canadian War Records Office 1918

Adut, Ari. *On Scandal: Moral Disturbances in Society, Politics, and Art*. Cambridge: Cambridge University Press 2008

Alexander, Kristine. "The Girl Guide Movement and Imperial Internationalism during the 1920s and 1930s." *Journal of the History of Childhood and Youth* 2, no. 1 (2009): 37–63

– "An Honour and a Burden: Canadian Girls and the Great War," in Glassford and Shaw, *A Sisterhood of Suffering and Service*, 173–94

Alexander, Victoria. "Environmental Constraints and Organizational Strategies: Complexity, Conflict, and Coping in the Nonprofit Sector," in Powell and Clemens, *Private Action*, 272–90

Allen, Richard. *The Social Passion: Religion and Social Reform in Canada 1914–28*. Toronto: University of Toronto Press 1971

Anderson, Benedict. *Imagined Communities: Reflections on the Rise and Spread of Nationalism*. London: Verso 1991

Armstrong Reid, Susan, and David Murray. *Armies of Peace: Canada and the UNRRA Years*. Toronto: University of Toronto Press 2008

Arnup, Katherine. "Educating Mothers: Government Advice for Women in the Interwar Years." In *Delivering Motherhood: Maternal Ideologies and Practices in the 19th and 20th Centuries*, edited by Katherine Arnup, Andrée Lévesque, and Ruth Roach Pierson, 190–210. London: Routledge 1990

– *Education for Motherhood: Advice for Mothers in Twentieth-Century Canada*. Toronto: University of Toronto 1994

The Arthritis Society. "Our History." 2014 www.arthritis.ca

Atwater, Reginald M. "C.-E.A. Winslow: An Appreciation of a Great Statesman." *American Journal of Public Health* 47, no. 9 (1957): 1065–70

Auger, Geneviève, and Raymonde Lamothe. *De la poêle à frire à la ligne de feu: La vie quotidienne des québécoises pendant la guerre '39–'45*. Montreal: Boréal Express 1981

Avery, Donald H. *The Science of War: Canadian Scientists and Allied Military Technology during the Second World War*. Toronto: University of Toronto Press 1998

Baillargeon, Denyse. *A Brief History of Women in Quebec*. Translated by W. Donald Wilson. Waterloo: Wilfrid Laurier University Press 2014

– "Care of Mothers and Infants in Montreal between the Wars: The Visiting Nurses of Metropolitan Life, Les Gouttes de lait, and Assistance maternelle," translated by Susan Joss, in Dodd and Gorham, *Caring and Curing*, 163–81

Baldwin, Douglas O. "Amy MacMahon and the Struggle for Public Health." *The Island Magazine* 34 (1993): 20–7

- *She Answered Every Call: The Life of Public Health Nurse Mona Gordon Wilson (1894–1981)*. Charlottetown: Indigo Press 1997
- "Volunteers in Action: The Establishment of Government Health Care on Prince Edward Island, 1900–1931." *Acadiensis* 19 (spring 1990): 121–47
- and Gillian Poulter. "Mona Wilson and the Canadian Red Cross in Newfoundland, 1940–1945." *Newfoundland and Labrador Studies* 20 (2005): 281–311
Banting, Keith G., and Kathy L. Brock, eds. *Delicate Dances: Public Policy and the Nonprofit Sector*. Kingston: School of Policy Studies at Queen's University 2003
- eds. *The Nonprofit Sector and Government in a New Century*. Kingston: School of Policy Studies at Queen's University 2001
- eds. *The Nonprofit Sector in Canada: Roles and Relationships*. Kingston: School of Policy Studies at Queen's University 2000
- eds. *The Nonprofit Sector in Interesting Times: Case Studies in a Changing Sector*. Kingston: School of Policy Studies at Queen's University 2003
Barnett, Michael. *Empire of Humanity: A History of Humanitarianism*. Ithaca, NY: Cornell University Press 2011
Barron Norris, Marjorie. *Sister Heroines: The Roseate Glow of Wartime Nursing 1914–1918*. Calgary: Bunker to Bunker 2002
Basic Rules of the Geneva Conventions and Their Additional Protocols. Geneva: ICRC 1987
Baughan, Emily. "'Every Citizen of Empire Implored to Save the Children!' Empire, Internationalism and the Save the Children Fund in Inter-War Britain." *Historical Research* 86, no. 231 (2013): 116–37
Berger, Carl. *The Sense of Power: Studies in the Ideas of Canadian Imperialism 1867–1914*. Toronto: University of Toronto Press 1970
Berridge, Mavis E. "The Development of the Red Cross Water Safety Service and the Royal Life Saving Society in Canada." Master's thesis, University of Wisconsin 1966
- "The Development of the Royal Life Saving Society and the Red Cross Water Safety Service in Canada to 1954," in *Proceedings of the First Canadian Symposium on the History of Sport and Physical Education*, 173–86
Berry, Nicholas. *War and the Red Cross: The Unspoken Mission*. New York: St. Martin's Press 1997
"Bertha Gregory: Port Nurse Diary; Saint John, NB 1920–22." Transcribed by Alyssa Allen. 2011 http://berthagregory.wordpress.com/home
Best, Geoffrey. *Humanity in Warfare: The Modern History of the International Law of Armed Conflicts*. London: Weidenfeld and Nicolson 1980
Beynon, Francis Marion. *Aleta Dey* [1919]. London: Virago 1988
Black, Maggie. *A Cause for Our Times: Oxfam, the First 50 Years*. London: Oxfam Publishing 1992
- *The Children and the Nations: Growing up together in the Postwar World*. New York: UNICEF 1987

Bloch, Marc. "Reflections of a Historian on the False News of the War,"
    [1921] trans. James P. Holoka. *Michigan War Studies Review* 2013–051
    (July 2013): 1–11
Blood Transfusion: A Red Cross Service. Paris: LRCS 1934
Boissier, Pierre. *From Solferino to Tsushima: History of the International
    Committee of the Red Cross*. Geneva: Henry Dunant Institute 1985
Bothwell, Robert. *The Big Chill: Canada and the Cold War*. Toronto: Irwin
    Publishing 1998
– Ian Drummond, and John English. *Canada since 1945: Power, Politics, and
    Provincialism*. Rev. ed. Toronto: University of Toronto Press 1989
Bouchier, Nancy B., and Ken Cruikshank. "Abandoning Nature: Swimming
    Pools and Clean, Healthy Recreation in Hamilton, Ontario, c. 1930s–
    1950s." *Canadian Bulletin of Medical History* 28, no. 2 (2011): 315–37
Bourrie, Mark. *The Fog of War: Censorship of Canada's Media in World War
    Two*. Vancouver: Douglas & McIntyre 2011
British Red Cross. 2014 www.redcross.org.uk
Brittain, Vera. *Testament of Youth: An Autobiographical Study of the Years
    1900–1925* [1933]. London: Penguin 1994
Brookfield, Tarah. *Cold War Comforts: Canadian Women, Child Safety, and
    Global Insecurity*. Waterloo: Wilfrid Laurier University Press 2012
Brown, Robert Craig, and Ramsay Cook. *Canada 1896–1921: A Nation
    Transformed*. Toronto: McClelland & Stewart 1974
Bruce, Jean. *Back the Attack: Canadian Women during the Second World War
    – At Home and Abroad*. Toronto: Macmillan 1985
Bryce, George. "Alfred Codd, 1843–1916." In *A History of Manitoba: Its
    Resources and People*. Toronto: The Canadian History Company 1906.
    Manitoba Historical Society www.mhs.mb.ca/docs/people/codd_a.shtml
Buchanan, Tom. "'The Truth Will Set You Free': The Making of Amnesty In-
    ternational." *Journal of Contemporary History* 37, no. 4 (2002): 575–97
Bull, William Perkins. "Dr William Nattress." In *From Medicine Man to
    Medical Man: A Record of a Century and a Half of Progress in Health and
    Sanitation as Exemplified by Developments in Peel*. Toronto: The Perkins
    Bull Foundation, George J. McLeod Ltd 1934
Burnett, Kristin. "Race, Disease, and Public Violence: Smallpox and the
    (Un)Making of Calgary's Chinatown, 1892." *Social History of Medicine* 25,
    no. 2 (2012): 362–79
Burtch, Andrew. *Give Me Shelter: The Failure of Canada's Cold War Civil
    Defence*. Vancouver: UBC Press 2012
Bush, Julia. *Edwardian Ladies and Imperial Power*. London: Leicester Univer-
    sity Press 2000
Caccia, Ivana. *Managing the Canadian Mosaic in Wartime: Shaping Citizenship
    Policy, 1939–1945*. Montreal & Kingston: McGill-Queen's University Press
    2010
Campbell, Annie. "' ... thousands of tiny fingers moving': The Beginning of the

Junior Red Cross Movement in New South Wales, 1914–1925." *Journal of the Royal Australian Historical Society* 90 (2004): 184–200

Campbell, Duncan. *The Voluntary Non-Profit Sector: An Alternative.* Kingston: Queen's University School of Policy Studies 1993

Canada in the Great World War: An Authentic Account of the Military History of Canada from the Earliest Days to the Close of the War of the Nations, vol. 2, *Days of Preparation.* Toronto: United Publishers of Canada 1917

Canada's Part in the Great War. Ottawa: Department of Public Information 1919

Canadian Cancer Society. "Fighting since 1938 – Our History." 2014 www.cancer.ca

Canadian Diabetes Association. "History." 2014 www.diabetes.ca

Canadian Patriotic Fund Association. "As you are doubtless aware." Form letter, 1900. CIHM no. 51948

Canadian Red Cross. 2013 www.redcross.ca

Canadian Red Cross Memorial Hospital – The Official Unofficial Cyberspace Shrine. 2013 www.crcmh.com

The Canadian Who's Who. Vol. 8, 1958–1960. Toronto: University of Toronto Press 1960

Canadian Year Book 1951. Ottawa: King's Printer 1951

CARE. "History of CARE." 2013 www.care.org

Carr, Iona. *A Story of the Canadian Red Cross Information Bureau during the Great War.* s.n.: s.i. [1930?]

"Charles A. Hodgetts: Fundamental to the Advancement of the First Aid Movement in Canada." [*Canadian Public Health Journal* 25 (1934)] Canadian Public Health Association CPHA 100 – Celebrating a Century of Public Health Leadership. http://cpha100/history/profiles-public-health/hodgetts

Chatelain, C., and C.A. Neukomm. "The Story of an Idea." [ICRC?] 1989

Christie, Nancy, and Michael Gauvreau. *A Full-Orbed Christianity: The Protestant Churches and Social Welfare in Canada 1900–1949.* Montreal & Kingston: McGill-Queen's University Press 1996

Clarke, Frank K. "'Keep Communism Out of Our Schools': Cold War Anti-Communism at the Toronto Board of Education, 1948–1951." *Labour/Le Travail* 49 (spring 2002): 93–119

Clements, Elsey V.N. *The Work of the Canadian Red Cross Society in the Province of New Brunswick during the Years of the Great War.* Saint John: The Saint John Globe Publishing Company 1919. CIHM no. 85840

Cole-Mackintosh, Ronnie. *A Century of Service to Mankind: A History of the St John Ambulance Brigade.* London: Century Benham 1986

Comacchio, Cynthia R. *Nations Are Built of Babies: Saving Ontario's Mothers and Children 1900–1940.* Montreal & Kingston: McGill-Queen's University Press 1993

Comacchio Abeele, Cynthia. "'The Mothers of the Land Must Suffer': Child and Maternal Health in Rural and Outpost Ontario, 1918–1940." *Ontario History* 80, no. 3 (1988): 183–205

Compton Brouwer, Ruth. *Canada's Global Villagers:* CUSO *in Development,*
    1961–86. Vancouver: UBC Press 2013
– *Modern Women Modernizing Men: The Changing Missions of Three Profes-*
    sional Women in Asia and Africa, 1902–69. Vancouver: UBC Press 2002
Connor, J.T.H. "'Medicine Is Here to Stay': Medical Practice, the Northern
    Frontier and Modernization in 1930s' Newfoundland." In Connor and Cur-
    tis, *Medicine in the Remote and Rural North, 1800–2000,* 129–51
– and Stephan Curtis, eds. *Medicine in the Remote and Rural North, 1800–*
    2000. London: Pickering and Chatto 2011
Cook, Ramsay. *The Regenerators: Social Criticism in Late Victorian English*
    Canada. Toronto: University of Toronto Press 1985
Cook, Sharon Ann. "Evangelical Moral Reform: Women and the War against
    Tobacco, 1874–1900." In *Religion and Public Life in Canada: Historical*
    and Comparative Perspectives, edited by Marguerite Van Die. Toronto:
    University of Toronto Press 2001
Cook, Tim. *Warlords: Borden, Mackenzie King, and Canada's World Wars.*
    Toronto: Allen Lane 2012
Cooper, Lois MacDonald. *Wartime Letters Home.* Nepean, ON: Borealis Press
    2004
Cooter, Roger. "Medicine and the Goodness of War." *Canadian Bulletin of*
    Medical History 7, no. 2 (1990): 147–59
Corfield, William E. *To Alleviate Suffering: The Story of the Red Cross in*
    London Canada 1900–1985. London, ON: CRCS 1985
Cormack, Barbara Villy. *The Red Cross Lady (Mary H. Conquest M.B.E.).*
    Edmonton: Institute of Applied Art 1960
Cortiula, Mark. "Collecting Blood for Battle: The Wartime Origins of the
    Transfusion Service in New South Wales." *Journal of the Royal Australian*
    Historical Society 85, no. 2 (1999): 105–19
– "Serum and the Soluvac: The Australian Approach to Whole Blood Substi-
    tutes and Blood Transfusion during the Second World War." *Journal of the*
    History of Medicine & Allied Sciences 54, no. 3 (1999): 413–38
CRCS. "Partnering to Build a Resilient Civil Society: Final Report, Auxiliary
    to Government Project." Ottawa: CRCS 2008
– *The Role of One Voluntary Organization in Canada's Health Services.*
    Toronto: CRCS 1962
– "Toward a Renewed Canadian Red Cross: Forging Stronger Partnerships in
    Support of a Humanitarian Agenda." Ottawa: CRCS 2007
– *What the Canadian Red Cross Society Is Doing in the Great War.* Toronto:
    CRCS [1918?]
CRCS Long Range Planning Committee. *And Who Is My Stranger: Exploring*
    Red Cross Policies, Strategies and Priorities for the Seventies. Toronto: CRCS
    1973
CRCS Vancouver Branch POW Department. *The Queen's Tea Party.* Vancou-
    ver: Sun Job Presses 1916. CIHM no. 83237

Creighton, Donald. *The Forked Road: Canada 1939–1957*. Toronto: McClelland & Stewart 1976

Crossland, James. "Expansion, Suspicion and the Development of the International Committee of the Red Cross: 1939–45." *Australian Journal of Politics and History* 56, no. 3 (2010): 381–92

Cruikshank, Ken, and Nancy B. Bouchier. "Dirty Spaces: Environment, the State, and Recreational Swimming in Hamilton Harbour, 1870–1946." *Sport History Review* 29 (1998): 59–76

Cuthbert Brandt, Gail, Magda Fahrni, Naomi Black, and Paula Bourne. *Canadian Women: A History*. 3rd ed. Toronto: Nelson 2011

A Cyclopaedia of Canadian Biography: Being Chiefly Men of the Time. Toronto: Rose Publishing Co. 1886

Darracott, Joseph, and Belinda Loftus. *First World War Posters*. London: Imperial War Museum 1972

Davison, Henry P. *Proposed Plan for World-Wide Coordination of Red Cross Activities*. Washington: American Red Cross 1919

Day, Francis Martin, Phyllis Spence, and Barbara Ladouceur, eds. *Women Overseas: Memories of the Canadian Red Cross Corps (Overseas Detachment)*. Vancouver: Ronsdale Press 1998

Dean, Wesley R. "Broken Promises: The Canadian Tainted-Blood Scandal." PhD diss., University of Alberta 2002

de Groot, Joanna. "'Sex' and 'Race': The Construction of Language and Image in the Nineteenth Century." In *Cultures of Empire: Colonizers in Britain and the Empire in the Nineteenth and Twentieth Centuries – A Reader*, edited by Catherine Hall, 37–60. New York: Routledge 2000

Desgrandchamps, Marie-Luce. "'Organising the Unpredictable': The Nigeria-Biafra War and Its Impact on the ICRC." *International Review of the Red Cross* 94, no. 888 (2012): 1409–32

Dictionary of Canadian Biography Online. 2013 www.biographi.ca

Dodd, Dianne. "Advice to Parents: The Blue Books, Helen MacMurchy, MD, and the Federal Department of Health, 1920–34." *Canadian Bulletin of Medical History* 8 (1991): 203–30

– "Helen MacMurchy: Popular Midwifery and Maternity Services for Canadian Pioneer Women," in Dodd and Gorham, eds. *Caring and Curing*, 135–62

– and Deborah Gorham, eds. *Caring and Curing: Historical Perspectives on Women and Healing in Canada*. Ottawa: University of Ottawa Press 1994

Domm, Elizabeth. "Called to Duty: Medical and Nursing Care at Saskatoon and Moose Jaw during the Northwest Rebellion in 1885." *Saskatchewan History* 58, no. 2 (2006): 15–23

– "From the Streets of Toronto to the Northwest Rebellion: Hannah Grier Coome's Call to Duty," in Rutherdale, *Caregiving on the Periphery*, 109–26

Duffin, Jacalyn. Review of *Tainted*, written by Kat Lanteigne and directed by Vikki Andersen. *Canadian Bulletin of Medical History* 31, no. 1 (2014): 229–31

Duley, Margot I. "The Unquiet Knitters of Newfoundland: From Mothers of the Regiment to Mothers of the Nation." In Glassford and Shaw, *A Sisterhood of Suffering and Service*, 51–74

Dulles, Foster Rhea. *The American Red Cross: A History*. Westport, CT: Greenwood Press 1971

Dunant, Henry. *A Memory of Solferino*. [1862] Geneva: ICRC 1986

Durand, André. *From Sarajevo to Hiroshima: History of the International Red Cross*. Geneva: Henry Dunant Institute 1984

Durflinger, Serge Marc. *Fighting from Home: The Second World War in Verdun, Quebec*. Vancouver: UBC Press 2006

Easton McLeod, Ellen. *In Good Hands: The Women of the Canadian Handicrafts Guild*. Montreal & Kingston: McGill-Queen's University Press for Carleton University 1999

Eayrs, James. *In Defence of Canada: Peacemaking and Deterrence*. Toronto: University of Toronto Press 1972

Edwards, Owen Dudley, and Jennifer H. Litster. "The End of Canadian Innocence: L.M. Montgomery and the First World War." In *L.M. Montgomery and Canadian Culture*, edited by Irene Gammel and Elizabeth Epperley, 31–46. Toronto: University of Toronto Press 1999

Eggleston, Wilfrid. *Scientists at War*. Toronto: Oxford University Press 1950

Elliott, Jayne. "Blurring the Boundaries of Space: Shaping Nursing Lives at the Red Cross Outposts in Ontario, 1922–1945." *Canadian Bulletin of Medical History* 21 (2004): 303–25

– "'Keep the Flag Flying': Medical Outposts and the Red Cross in Northern Ontario 1922–1984." PhD diss., Queen's University, Kingston 2004

– "A Negotiated Process: Outpost Nursing under the Red Cross in Ontario," in Rutherdale, *Caregiving on the Periphery*, 245–77

– "(Re)constructing the Identity of a Red Cross Outpost Nurse: The Letters of Louise de Kiriline, 1927–36," in Elliot, Stuart, and Toman, *Place and Practice*, 136–52

– Meryn Stuart, and Cynthia Toman, eds. *Place and Practice in Canadian Nursing History*. Vancouver: UBC Press 2008

Ellis, Jean M., with Isabel Dingman. *Face Powder and Gunpowder*. Toronto: S.J. Reginald Saunders & Company 1974

Epp, Marlene. *Mennonite Women in Canada: A History*. Winnipeg: University of Manitoba Press 2008

Evans, W. Sanford. *The Canadian Contingents and Canadian Imperialism: A Story and a Study*. London: T. Fisher Unwin 1901

Fahrni, Magda, and Essylt Jones, eds. *Epidemic Encounters: Influenza, Society, and Culture in Canada, 1918–1920*. Vancouver: UBC Press 2012

Fallis, Donna. "World War I Knitting." *Alberta Museums Review* (Fall 1984): 8–10

Favez, Jean-Claude. *The Red Cross and the Holocaust*. Edited and translated by John and Beryl Fletcher. Cambridge: Cambridge University Press 1999

Feasby, W.R., ed. *Official History of the Canadian Medical Services 1939–1945*, vol. 1, *Organization and Campaigns*. Ottawa: Queen's Printer 1956

Feldberg, Georgina M. *Disease and Class: Tuberculosis and the Shaping of Modern North American Society*. New Brunswick, NJ: Rutgers University Press 1995

– Molly Ladd-Taylor, Alison Li, and Kathryn McPherson, "Comparative Perspectives on Canadian and American Women's Health Care since 1945." In *Women, Health and Nation: Canada and the United States since 1945*, edited by Georgina Feldberg, Molly Ladd-Taylor, Alison Li, and Kathryn McPherson, 15–42. Montreal & Kingston: McGill-Queen's University Press 2003

Feldman, Eric A. "Blood Justice: Courts, Conflict, and Compensation in Japan, France, and the United States." *Law & Society Review* 34, no. 3 (2000): 651–702

Ferry, Darren. *Uniting in Measures of Common Good: The Construction of Liberal Identities in Central Canada, 1830–1900*. Montreal & Kingston: McGill-Queen's University Press 2008

Fielding, David. "The Dynamics of Humanitarian Aid Decisions." *Oxford Bulletin of Economics and Statistics* 76, no. 4 (2014): 536–64

Final Report by the Commission of Inquiry into Canada's Blood System. Vol. 3. Ottawa: Queen's Printer 1997

Forsythe, David P. *The Humanitarians: The International Committee of the Red Cross*. Cambridge: Cambridge University Press 2005

Friedland, Judith. *Restoring the Spirit: The Beginnings of Occupational Therapy in Canada, 1890–1930*. Montreal & Kingston: McGill-Queen's University Press 2011

Fussell, Paul. *The Great War and Modern Memory*. 25th Anniversary Edition. New York: Oxford University Press 2000

Gifford, Jim. *Hurricane Hazel: Canada's Storm of the Century*. Toronto: Dundurn Press 2004

Gill, Rebecca. "Networks of Concern, Boundaries of Compassion: British Relief in the South African War." *Journal of Imperial and Commonwealth History* 40, no. 5 (2012): 827–44

Glassford, Sarah. "Bearing the Burdens of Their Elders: English-Canadian Children's First World War Red Cross Work and Its Legacies." *Études canadiennes/Canadian Studies*, no. 80 (2016): 129–50

– "'The Greatest Mother of Them All': Carework and the Discourse of Mothering in the Canadian Red Cross Society during the First World War." *Journal of the Association for Research on Mothering* 10, no. 1 (2008): 219–32

– "'Marching as to War': The Canadian Red Cross Society, 1885–1939." PhD diss., York University 2007

– "Mobilisées, organisées, et aptes à s'occuper des autres: le travail sanitaire des femmes de la Croix-Rouge au Canada au XXe siècle." In *L'incontournable caste des femmes. Histoire des services de santé au Québec et au Canada,*

edited by Marie-Claude Thifault, 59–78. Ottawa: University of Ottawa Press 2012
– "Practical Patriotism: How the Canadian Junior Red Cross and Its Child Members Met the Challenge of the Second World War." *Journal of the History of Childhood and Youth* 7, no. 2 (2014): 219–42
– and Amy Shaw, eds. *A Sisterhood of Suffering and Service: Women and Girls of Canada and Newfoundland during the First World War.* Vancouver: UBC Press 2012
Gordon, Beverley. *The Saturated World: Aesthetic Meaning, Intimate Objects, Women's Lives, 1890–1940.* Knoxville: University of Tennessee Press 2006
Gordon, P.H. *Fifty Years in the Canadian Red Cross.* Toronto: CRCS 1967
Granatstein, J.L. *Canada 1957–1967: The Years of Uncertainty and Innovation.* Toronto: McClelland & Stewart 1986
– *Canada's War: The Politics of the Mackenzie King Government, 1939–1945.* Toronto: Oxford University Press 1975
– and Peter Neary, eds. *The Good Fight: Canadians and World War II.* Toronto: Copp Clark 1995
– and Peter Neary, eds. *The Veterans Charter and Post-World War II Canada.* Montreal & Kingston: McGill-Queen's University Press 1998
Grauer, A.E. *Public Health: A Study Prepared for the Royal Commission on Dominion Provincial Relations.* Ottawa: [s.i?], 1939
Greene, B.M., ed. *Who's Who.* Toronto: International Press 1920, 1931, 1946
Griffiths, N.E.S. *The Splendid Vision: Centennial History of the National Council of Women of Canada 1893–1993.* Ottawa: Carleton University Press 1993
Hamelin, Christine. "A Sense of Purpose: Ottawa Students and the Second World War." *Canadian Military History* 6, no. 1 (1997): 34–41
Hanes, Roy. "Linking Mental Defect to Physical Disability: The Case of Crippled Children in Ontario, 1890–1940." *Journal on Developmental Disability* 4, no. 1 (1995): 33–49.
Hasian Jr, Marouf Arif. *The Rhetoric of Eugenics in Anglo-American Thought.* Athens: University of Georgia Press 1996
Heart and Stroke Foundation of Canada. "National History." 2014 www.heartandstroke.com
Heath, Gordon L. *A War with a Silver Lining: Canadian Protestant Churches and the South African War, 1899–1902.* Montreal & Kingston: McGill-Queen's University Press 2009
Helleiner, Jane. "'The Right Kind of Children': Childhood, Gender and 'Race' in Canadian Postwar Political Discourse." *Anthropologica* 43, no. 2 (2001): 143–52
Henderson, Stuart. *Making the Scene: Yorkville and Hip Toronto in the 1960s.* Toronto: University of Toronto Press 2011
Historica Canada. The Memory Project. 2014 www.thememoryproject.com
Holmes, John W. *The Shaping of the Peace: Canada and the Search for World Order 1943–1957.* Vol. 1. Toronto: University of Toronto Press 1979

Hotson, J.W. "Sphagnum from Bog to Bandage." *Puget Sound Biological Station Publication* 2 (1919): 211–47

Humphries, Mark W. *The Last Plague: Spanish Influenza and the Politics of Public Health in Canada.* Toronto: University of Toronto Press 2013

Hutchinson, John F. *Champions of Charity: War and the Rise of the Red Cross.* Boulder, CO: Westview Press 1996

– "The Nagler Case: A Revealing Moment in Red Cross History." *Canadian Bulletin of Medical History* 9 (1992): 177–90

– "Rethinking the Origins of the Red Cross." *Bulletin of the History of Medicine* 63, no. 4 (1989): 557–78

Iacovetta, Franca. *Gatekeepers: Reshaping Immigrant Lives in Cold War Canada.* Toronto: Between the Lines 2006

ICRC. "1914–1918 War: International Prisoners of War Agency." 2015 www.icrc.org

– "The Fundamental Principles of the Red Cross and Red Crescent." Ref. 0513. Geneva: ICRC 1996

– "Prisoners of the First World War, The ICRC Archives." 2015 www.grande guerre.icrc.org

Iriye, Akira. *Cultural Internationalism and World Order.* Baltimore, MD: Johns Hopkins University Press 1997

Irwin, Julia. *Making the World Safe: The American Red Cross and a Nation's Humanitarian Awakening.* New York: Oxford University Press 2013

Isitt, Benjamin. *From Victoria to Vladivostok: Canada's Siberian Expedition, 1917–19.* Vancouver: UBC Press 2012

Joint Committee for Reappraisal of the Role of the Red Cross. *An Agenda for Red Cross.* Geneva: Henry Dunant Institute 1975

Jones, David C. *Empire of Dust: Settling and Abandoning the Prairie Dry Belt.* 2002 ed. Calgary: University of Calgary Press 2002

Jones, Essylt W. *Influenza 1918: Disease, Death and Struggle in Winnipeg.* Toronto: University of Toronto Press 2007

Jones, Kevin G. "Sport in Canada, 1900–1920," in *Proceedings of the First Canadian Symposium on the History of Sport and Physical Education,* 43–55

Judd, Denis, and Keith Surridge. *The Boer War.* London: John Murray 2002

Kahn Atkins, Irene. "Seeds of Destiny: A Case History." *Film and History* 11, no. 2 (1981): 25–33

Kapp, Richard W. "Charles H. Best, the Canadian Red Cross Society, and Canada's First National Blood Donation Program." *Canadian Bulletin of Medical History* 12 (1995): 27–46

Kealey, Gregory. *Toronto Workers Respond to Industrial Capitalism, 1867–1892.* Toronto: University of Toronto Press 1980

Kealey, Linda. "Delivering Health Care in Rural New Brunswick: Outpost Nursing in the Twentieth Century," in Connor and Curtis, *Medicine in the Remote and Rural North, 1800–2000,* 183–98

– *Enlisting Women for the Cause: Women, Labour and the Left in Canada, 1890–1920.* Toronto: University of Toronto Press 1998

– "Historical Perspectives on Nutrition and Food Security in Newfoundland and Labrador." In *Resetting the Kitchen Table: Food Security, Culture, Health and Resilience in Coastal Communities*, edited by C.C. Parrish, N.J. Turner, and S.M. Solberg, 177–90. New York: Nova Science Publishers 2008

– ed. *A Not Unreasonable Claim: Women and Reform in Canada, 1880s–1920s*. Toronto: The Women's Press 1979

Keough, Willeen G., and Lara Campbell. *Gender History: Canadian Perspectives*. Don Mills, ON: Oxford University Press 2014

Keshen, Jeffrey. *Saints, Sinners, and Soldiers: Canada's Second World War*. Vancouver: UBC Press 2004

Kinnear, Mary. *In Subordination: Professional Women, 1870–1970*. Montreal & Kingston: McGill-Queen's University Press 1995

Kipling, Rudyard. "The Absent-Minded Beggar." In *Rudyard Kipling's Verse 1885–1932 Inclusive Edition*. London: Hodder & Stoughton 1933

Klein, Naomi. *No Logo: Taking Aim at the Brand Bullies*. Toronto: Vintage Canada 2000

Kossuth, Robert S. "Dangerous Waters: Victorian Decorum, Swimmer Safety, and the Establishment of Public Bathing Facilities in London (Canada)." *The International Journal of the History of Sport* 22, no. 5 (2005): 796–815

Krebs, Paula M. *Gender, Race and the Writing of Empire: Public Discourse and the Boer War*. Cambridge: Cambridge University Press 1999

"Lady Grace Julia Drummond." *Prominent People of the Province of Quebec, 1923–24*. Montreal: Biographical Society of Canada, Limited [n.d.]

Lawrence, M.E. "Red Cross at Halifax, a Sketch," in Clements, *The Work of the CRCS in New Brunswick*, 46–7

The League of Red Cross Societies. Paris: Secretariat of the League 1929

Lenskyj, Helen. "Raising 'Good Vigorous Animals': Medical Interest in Children's Health in Ontario, 1890–1930." *Scientia Canadensis: Canadian Journal of the History of Science, Technology and Medicine* 12, no. 2 (1988): 129–49

LeRoy Miller, Gertrude. *Mustard Plasters and Handcars: Through the Eyes of a Red Cross Outpost Nurse*. Toronto: Natural Heritage Books 2000

Lifesaving Society. "Lifesaving Society Chronological Timelines." 2013 www.lifesaving.ca

Lowry, Donal. "'The Boers were the beginning of the end'?: The Wider Impact of the South African War." In *The South African War Reappraised*, edited by Donal Lowry, 203–46. Manchester: Manchester University Press 2000

MacDermot, H.E. *Sir Thomas Roddick: His Work in Medicine and Public Life*. Toronto: Macmillan 1938

MacDonald, Laura. *Curse of the Narrows: The Halifax Explosion 1917*. Toronto: HarperCollins 2006

Mackay, D.S.C., ed. "The North-West Rebellion, 1885: A Memoir by Colour

Sergeant (Later General) C.F. Winters [sic]." *Saskatchewan History* 35, no. 1 (1982): 1–16

MacKenzie, David, ed. *Canada and the First World War: Essays in Honour of Robert Craig Brown*. Toronto: University of Toronto Press 2005

– "Eastern Approaches: Maritime Canada and Newfoundland," in D. MacKenzie, *Canada and the First World War*, 350–76

Mackenzie, Hector. "Mapping Canada's World: Depicting Canada's International Relations in the Twentieth Century." *Canadian Issues/Thèmes Canadiens* (spring 2009): 39–44

Maclean Miller, Ian Hugh. *Our Glory and Our Grief: Torontonians and the Great War*. Toronto: University of Toronto Press 2002

Macleod Moore, Mary. *The Maple Leaf's Red Cross: The War Story of the Canadian Red Cross Overseas*. London: Skeffington & Son [1919?]

Macmillan, Margaret. "Canada and the Peace Settlements," in D. Mackenzie, *Canada and the First World War*, 379–408

MacNaughton, Colleen. "Promoting Clean Water in Nineteenth-Century Public Policy: Professors, Preachers, and Polliwogs in Kingston, Ontario." *Histoire sociale/Social History* 32, no. 63 (1999): 49–61

Macphail, Sir Andrew. *Official History of the Canadian Forces in the Great War 1914–19: The Medical Services*. Ottawa: King's Printer 1925

Mainville, Curtis. *Till the Boys Come Home: Life on the Home Front, Queens County, NB, 1914–1918*. Fredericton: Goose Lane Editions 2015

Mair, Robert Henry. "W. Burdett-Coutts (Westminster)." In *Debret's House of Commons and the Judicial Bench*. London: Dean & Son 1886

Manitoba Division CRCS. *Call 320: A Documentary Record of the 1950 Manitoba Flood and Red Cross Activities in the Disaster*. Winnipeg: CRCS 1950

Mann, Susan. *Margaret Macdonald: Imperial Daughter*. Montreal & Kingston: McGill-Queen's University Press 2005

Maroney, Paul. "'The Great Adventure': The Context and Ideology of Recruiting in Ontario, 1914–17." *Canadian Historical Review* 77 (March 1996): 62–99

– "'The Peaceable Kingdom' Reconsidered: War and Culture in English Canada, 1884–1914." PhD diss., Queen's University 1996

Marquis, Greg. *In Armageddon's Shadow: The Civil War and Canada's Maritime Provinces*. Montreal & Kingston: McGill-Queen's University Press 1998

Marr, Lucille. "Paying 'the price of war': Canadian Women and the Churches on the Home Front." In *Canadian Churches and the Great War*, edited by Gordon L. Heath, 263–80. Eugene, OR: Pickwick Publications 2014

Marshall, Dominique, and Julia Sterparn. "Oxfam Aid to Canada's First Nations, 1962–1975: Eating Lynx, Starving for Jobs and Flying a Talking Bird." *Journal of the Canadian Historical Association* 23, no. 2 (2012): 298–344

Massie, Merle. "Ruth Dulmage Shewchuk: A Saskatchewan Red Cross Outpost Nurse." *Saskatchewan History* 56 (Fall 2004): 35–44

McClung, Nellie. *The Next of Kin: Those Who Wait and Wonder*. Toronto: Thomas Allen 1917
– *The Stream Runs Fast: My Own Story*. Toronto: Thomas Allen 1946
– *In Times Like These*. Toronto: McLeod & Allen 1915
McCuaig, Katherine. "'From Social Reform to Social Service.' The Changing Role of Volunteers: The Anti-Tuberculosis Campaign, 1900–1930." *Canadian Historical Review* 61, no. 4 (1980): 480–501
McCullough, Alan. *Origin and History of the Restoring Family Links Program*. Ottawa: CRCS 2011
McIntosh, Robert. "The Boys in the Nova Scotian Coal Mines: 1873–1923." In *Histories of Canadian Children and Youth*, edited by Nancy Janovicek and Joy Parr, 77–87. Don Mills, ON: Oxford University Press 2003
McKay, Ian. "Sarnia in the Sixties (or the Peculiarities of the Canadians)." In *New World Coming: The Sixties and the Shaping of Global Consciousness*, edited by Karen Dubinsky et al., 24–35. Toronto: Between the Lines 2009
McKenzie, Andrea. "Women at War: L.M. Montgomery, The Great War, and Canadian Cultural Memory." In *Storm and Dissonance: L.M. Montgomery and Conflict*, edited by Jean Mitchell, 83–105. Newcastle: Cambridge Scholars Publishing 2008
McPherson, Kathryn. *Bedside Matters: The Transformation of Canadian Nursing, 1900–1990*. Toronto: University of Toronto Press 2003
A Memoir of the Life and Work of Hannah Grier Coome Mother-Foundress of the Sisterhood of St John the Divine Toronto, Canada. London: Oxford University Press 1933
Miller, Carman. *A Knight in Politics: A Biography of Sir Frederick Borden*. Montreal & Kingston: McGill-Queen's University Press 2010
– "The Montreal Militia as a Social Institution before World War I." *Urban History Review* 19, no. 1 (June 1990): 57–64
– *Painting the Map Red: Canada and the South African War, 1899–1902*. Montreal & Kingston: Canadian War Museum and McGill-Queen's University Press 1993
Minnett, Valerie, and Mary Anne Poutanen. "Swatting Flies for Health: Children and Tuberculosis in Early-Twentieth Century Montreal." *Urban History Review* 36, no. 1 (2007): 32–44
Mitchell, Miriam C., and Florence C. Deacon. *641: A Story of the Canadian Red Cross Corps, Overseas*. St Catharine's, ON: Advance Printing Inc. 1978
Mitchinson, Wendy. *The Nature of Their Bodies: Women and Their Doctors in Victorian Canada*. Toronto: University of Toronto Press 1991
Montgomery, L.M. *Rilla of Ingleside*. [1921] Toronto: Seal Books 1992
– *The Selected Journals of L.M. Montgomery*, vol. 2, 1910–1921, edited by Mary Rubio and Elizabeth Waterston. Toronto: Oxford University Press 1987
Moorehead, Caroline. *Dunant's Dream: War, Switzerland and the History of the Red Cross*. New York: Carroll & Graf Publishers 1998
Morgan, Henry James, ed. *The Canadian Men and Women of the Time: A*

Hand-book of Canadian Biography, Part 2. 1st ed. Toronto: William Briggs 1898

Morris, Phillip, ed. *The Canadian Patriotic Fund: A Record of Its Activities from 1914 to 1919.* s.n.: Canadian Patriotic Fund [1919?]

Morrison, David A. *Aid and Ebb Tide: A History of CIDA and Canadian Development Assistance.* Waterloo: Wilfrid Laurier University Press 1998

Morton, Desmond. "Colonel Otter and the First Canadian Contingent in South Africa, 1899–1900." In *Policy by Other Means: Essays in Honour of C.P. Stacey,* edited by Michael Cross and Robert Bothwell, 97–120. Toronto: Clarke, Irwin & Co. 1972

– *Fight or Pay: Soldiers' Families in the Great War.* Vancouver: UBC Press 2004

– *The Last War Drum: The North West Campaign of 1885.* Toronto: Hakkert 1972

– *A Peculiar Kind of Politics: Canada's Overseas Ministry in the First World War.* Toronto: University of Toronto Press 1982

– *Silent Battle: Canadian Prisoners of War in Germany 1914–1919.* Toronto: Lester Publishing 1992

– "Supporting Soldiers' Wives and Families in the Great War: What Was Transformed?" in Glassford and Shaw, *A Sisterhood of Suffering and Service,* 195–218

– *When Your Number's Up: The Canadian Soldier in the First World War.* Toronto: Random House 1993

– and Glenn Wright. *Winning the Second Battle: Canadian Veterans and the Return to Civilian Life 1915–1930.* Toronto: University of Toronto Press 1987

Morton, Suzanne. *Wisdom, Justice, and Charity: Canadian Social Welfare through the Life of Jane B. Wisdom 1884–1975.* Toronto: University of Toronto Press 2014

Mosby, Ian. *Food Will Win the War: The Politics, Culture, and Science of Food on Canada's Home Front.* Vancouver: UBC Press 2014

Moser Jones, Marian. *The American Red Cross from Clara Barton to the New Deal.* Baltimore, MD: Johns Hopkins University Press 2013

Mulvany, Charles Pelham. *The History of the North-West Rebellion of 1885.* Toronto: A.H. Hovey & Co. 1886

Munn Smith, Catherine. "Marion Moodie: From Proper Lady to New Woman." *Alberta History* 49 (Winter 2001): 9–15

Myers, Tamara. "Blistered and Bleeding, Tired and Determined: Visual Representations of Children and Youth in the Miles for Millions Walkathon." *Journal of the Canadian Historical Association* 22, no. 1 (2011): 245–75

– and Mary Anne Poutanen. "Cadets, Curfews, and Compulsory Schooling: Mobilizing Anglophone Children in WWII Montreal." *Histoire sociale/Social History* 76 (November 2005): 367–98

Nattress, William. "Field Hospitals and Climate in the North-West Territory." *Canadian Medical and Surgical Journal* 14 (1886): 197–204

Neary, Peter. *On to Civvy Street: Canada's Rehabilitation Program for Veter-*

ans of the Second World War. Montreal & Kingston: McGill-Queen's University Press 2011

Nicholson, G.W.L. *Canada's Nursing Sisters*. Toronto: Hakkert & Co. 1975

– *Seventy Years of Service: A History of the Royal Canadian Army Medical Corps*. Ottawa: Borealis Press 1977

– *The White Cross in Canada: A History of St John Ambulance*. Montreal: Harvest House 1967

Nielson, Carmen J. *Private Women and the Public Good: Charity and State Formation in Hamilton, Ontario, 1846–93*. Vancouver: UBC Press 2014

Nova Scotia Division CRCS. *Nova Scotia Red Cross during the Great War Nineteen Fourteen-Eighteen*. Halifax: CRCS [1918?]

Nowlan, Mary Elizabeth. "Junior Red Cross Volunteer Knitting in Winnipeg School Division No. 1 during and immediately after World War II (1939–1946)." Master's thesis, University of Manitoba 1996

Ontario Division CRCS. "Historical Review of the Canadian Red Cross Society." Toronto: CRCS 1934

Oppenheimer, Melanie. "'The Best P.M. for the Empire in War'? Lady Helen Munro Ferguson and the Australian Red Cross Society, 1914–1920." *Australian Historical Studies* 33 (April 2002): 108–24

– "Controlling Civilian Volunteering: Canada and Australia during the Second World War." *War & Society* 22, no. 2 (2004): 27–50

– "Control of Wartime Patriotic Funds in Australia: The National Security (Patriotic Funds) Regulations, 1940–1953." *War & Society* 18, no. 1 (2000): 71–90

– *The Power of Humanity: 100 Years of Australian Red Cross 1914–2014*. Sydney: HarperCollins Publishers 2014

Ormston, Randal Eric. "A Community Approach to Education: An Analysis of the Red Cross Youth Program with Recommendations for Change." Master's thesis, Simon Fraser University 1974

Overton, James. "Brown Flour and Beriberi: The Politics of Dietary and Health Reform in Newfoundland in the First Half of the 20th Century." *Newfoundland Studies* 14, no. 1 (1998): 14–20

Oxfam Canada. "Introduction to Oxfam – History." 2014 www.oxfam.ca

Page, Robert. *The Boer War and Canadian Imperialism*. Historical Booklet no. 44. Ottawa: Canadian Historical Association 1987

Parr, Joy. *The Gender of Breadwinners: Women, Men, and Change in Two Industrial Towns 1880–1950*. Toronto: University of Toronto Press 1990

Paterson, Timothy Murray. "Tainted Blood, Tainted Knowledge: Contesting Scientific Evidence at the Krever Inquiry." PhD diss., University of British Columbia 1999

Penny, Barbara R. "Australia's Reactions to the Boer War – A Study in Colonial Imperialism." *Journal of British Studies* 17 (1967): 97–130

Picard, André. *The Gift of Death: Confronting Canada's Tainted Blood Tragedy*. Toronto: HarperCollins Canada 1995

Pickles, Katie. *Female Imperialism and National Identity: Imperial Order Daughters of the Empire*. Manchester: Manchester University Press 2002

Pictet, Jean. *Development and Principles of International Humanitarian Law*. Dordrecht, Netherlands: Martinus Nijhoff Publishers 1985

Pierson, Ruth Roach. *"They're Still Women after All": The Second World War and Canadian Womanhood*. Toronto: McClelland and Stewart 1986

Polk, Jennifer Ann. "The Canadian Red Cross and Relief in Siberia, 1918–1921." Master's thesis, Carleton University 2004

Pomerleau, Daniel. "La Société canadienne de la Croix-Rouge et les prisonniers de guerre, 1939–1945." *Bulletin d'histoire politique* 16, no. 1 (2007): 177–88

Porter, Bernard. *The Lion's Share: A Short History of British Imperialism 1850–2004*. 4th ed. London: Pearson-Longman 2004

Porter, McKenzie. *To All Men: The Story of the Canadian Red Cross*. Toronto: McClelland & Stewart 1960

Poulter, Margaret. "The Archives of the British Red Cross." *Social History of Medicine* (Britain) 6 (1993): 143–7

Powell, Walter W., and Elisabeth S. Clemens, eds. *Private Action and the Public Good*. New Haven: Yale University Press 1998

Prentice, Alison, et al. *Canadian Women: A History*. 2nd ed. Toronto: Harcourt 1996

Proceedings of the First Canadian Symposium on the History of Sport and Physical Education. Ottawa: Fitness and Amateur Sport Directorate, National Department of Health and Welfare 1970

Proceedings of the Medical Conference Held at the Invitation of the Committee of Red Cross Societies, Cannes, France, April 1 to 11, 1919. Geneva: League of Red Cross Societies 1919

Pugh, Derek S., and David J. Hickson. *Writers on Organizations*. 5th ed. London: Sage Publications 1997

Putnam, Robert D. *Bowling Alone: The Collapse and Revival of American Community*. New York: Simon & Schuster 2000

Quiney, Linda J. "'Assistant Angels': Canadian Women and Voluntary Aid Detachment Nurses during and after the Great War, 1914–1930." PhD diss., University of Ottawa 2002

– "Borrowed Halos: Canadian Teachers as Voluntary Aid Detachment Nurses during the Great War." *Historical Studies in Education* 15 (2003): 79–99

– "'Bravely and Loyally They Answered the Call': St John Ambulance, the Red Cross, and the Patriotic Service of Canadian Women during the Great War." *History of Intellectual Culture* 5 (2005): 1–19

– "'Suitable Young Women': Red Cross Nursing Pioneers and the Crusade for Healthy Living in Manitoba, 1920–30," in Elliot, Stuart, and Toman, *Place and Practice*, 91–110

– "'We Must not Neglect Our Duty': Enlisting Women Undergraduates for the Red Cross during the Great War." In *Cultures, Communities, and Con-*

flict: Histories of Canadian Universities and War, edited by Paul Stortz and Lisa Panayotidis, 71–94. Toronto: University of Toronto Press 2012

Rabinow, Paul. "Artificiality and Enlightenment: From Sociobiology to Biosociality." In Essays on the Anthropology of Reason, edited by Paul Rabinow, chapter 7. Princeton: Princeton University Press 1996

Ramkhalawansingh, Ceta. "Women during the Great War." In Women at Work: Ontario, 1850–1930, edited by Janice Acton, Penny Goldsmith, and Bonnie Shepherd, 261–307. Toronto: Canadian Women's Educational Press 1974

Read, Daphne, ed. The Great War and Canadian Society: An Oral History. Toronto: New Hogtown Press 1978

"Reconnaissance de la Croix-Rouge canadienne." Bulletin International des Sociétés de la Croix-Rouge 58 (November 1927): 835–6

Red Cross Outpost Historic House Museum. 2015 www.redcrossoutpost.org

The Red Cross School of Nursing. Toronto: RCSN ca. 1912. CIHM no. 86895

Reinisch, Jessica. "Auntie UNRRA at the Crossroads." Past and Present 218, supplement 8 (2013): 70–97

Remembering Herbert Hoover and the Commission for Relief in Belgium. Brussels: University Foundation 2006

Report by the Central British Red Cross Committee on Voluntary Organisations in Aid of the Sick and Wounded during the South African War. London: His Majesty's Stationery Office 1902

Report of the Royal Commission on Dominion-Provincial Relations Book 1, Canada: 1867–1939. Ottawa: King's Printer 1940

Reznick, Jeffrey. Healing the Nation: Soldiers and the Culture of Caregiving in Britain during the Great War. Manchester: Manchester University Press 2004

Riegler, Natalie. "Sphagnum Moss in World War I: The Making of Surgical Dressings by Volunteers in Toronto, Canada, 1917–1918." Canadian Bulletin of Medical History 6 (1989): 27–43

Robinson, Danielle, and Ken Cruikshank. "Hurricane Hazel: Disaster Relief, Politics, and Society in Canada, 1954–55." Journal of Canadian Studies 40, no. 1 (2006): 37–70

Rodgers, Daniel T. Atlantic Crossings: Social Politics in a Progressive Age. Cambridge, MA: Harvard University Press 1998

Roland, Charles G. "Allied POWs, Japanese Captors and the Geneva Convention." War & Society 9, no. 2 (1991): 83–99

Rollings-Magnusson, Sandra. Heavy Burdens on Small Shoulders: The Labour of Pioneer Children on the Canadian Prairies. Edmonton: University of Alberta Press 2009

Routley, F.W. "Radio Talk Prepared for the Canadian Social Hygiene Council and Delivered at CKCL Broadcasting Studio, Toronto, April 19th, 1927 – Red Cross Outpost Hospitals." The Public Health Journal 18, no. 6 (1927): 280–3

Roy, Patricia E., J.L. Granatstein, Masako Lino, and Hiroko Takamura.

Mutual Hostages: Canadians and Japanese during the Second World War.
Toronto: University of Toronto Press 1990

Rutherdale, Myra, ed. *Caregiving on the Periphery: Historical Perspectives on Nursing and Midwifery in Canada.* Montreal & Kingston: McGill-Queen's University Press 2010

Rutherdale, Robert. *Hometown Horizons: Local Responses to Canada's Great War.* Vancouver: UBC Press 2004

Ryerson, George Sterling. *Looking Backward.* Toronto: Ryerson Press 1924

– *The Soldier and the Surgeon.* Toronto: William Briggs, 1899. CIHM no. 01395

Salamon, Lester M., S. Wojciech Sokolowski and Associates. *Global Civil Society: Dimensions of the Nonprofit Sector.* Bloomfield, CT: Kumarian Press 2004

Salvatici, Silvia. "'Help the People to Help Themselves': UNRRA Relief Workers and European Displaced Persons." *Journal of Refugee Studies* 25, no. 3 (2012): 428–51

Saskatchewan Division CRCS. *Red Cross in Saskatchewan, 1913–1959.* Regina: CRCS 1959

Scates, Bruce. "The Unknown Sock Knitter: Voluntary Work, Emotional Labour, Bereavement and the Great War." *Labour History* (Australia) 81 (November 2002): 29–49

Schneider, Eric F. "The British Red Cross Wounded and Missing Enquiry Bureau: A Case of Truth-Telling in the Great War." *War in History* 4 (1997): 296–315

Schneider, William H. "Blood Transfusion between the Wars." *Journal of the History of Medicine* 58 (April 2008): 187–224

Sellick, Patricia. "Responding to Children Affected by Armed Conflicts: A Case Study of the Save the Children Fund (1919–1999)." PhD diss., Bradford University 2001

Shaw, Robert. "The Peoples' Papers: The Rise and Fall of the Canadian Tabloid." *Broken Pencil* 42 (2009): 19–23

Shaw, Rosa L. *Proud Heritage: A History of the National Council of Women of Canada.* Toronto: Ryerson Press 1927

Sheehan, Nancy M. "Junior Red Cross in the Schools: An International Movement, a Voluntary Agency, and Curriculum Change." *Curriculum Inquiry* 17 (1987): 247–66

– "The Junior Red Cross Movement in Saskatchewan, 1919–1929: Rural Improvement through the Schools." In *Building beyond the Homestead: Rural History on the Prairies,* edited by David C. Jones and Ian MacPherson, 66–86. Calgary: University of Calgary Press 1985

– "The Red Cross and Relief in Alberta, 1920s–1930s." *Prairie Forum* 12 (1987): 277–98

Skocpol, Theda. *Diminished Democracy: From Membership to Management in American Civic Life.* Norman: University of Oklahoma Press 2003

Slater, David W., with R.B. Bryce. *War Finance and Reconstruction: The Role of Canada's Department of Finance 1939–1946*. Ottawa: privately printed 1995

Smart, Elizabeth. *By Grand Central Station I Sat Down and Wept*. London: Panther Books 1966

Smith, Barbara. "The Role of Nongovernmental Organizations in Responding to Health Needs Created by War." In *War and Public Health*, updated edition, edited by Barry S. Levy and Victor W. Sidel, 293–307. Washington: American Public Health Association 2000

Smith, Helen, and Pamela Wakewich. "'Beauty and the Helldivers': Representing Women's Work and Identities in a Warplant Newspaper." *Labour/ Le travail* 44 (Fall 1994): 71–107

Soares, John. "'Very Correct Adversaries': The Cold War on Ice from 1947 to the Squaw Valley Olympics." *International Journal of the History of Sport* 30, no. 13 (2013): 1536–53

Spencer, Emily. *Lipstick and High Heels: War, Gender and Popular Culture*. Kingston: Canadian Defence Academy Press 2007

Stanbury, W.S. *Origin, Development and Future of the Canadian Red Cross Blood Transfusion Service*. Toronto: CRCS 1961

– *Survey of Blood Transfusion Facilities in Canadian Hospitals and Proposed Plan for a Canadian National Blood Transfusion Service*. Toronto: CRCS 1945

Stephen, Jennifer A. *Pick One Intelligent Girl: Employability, Domesticity, and the Gendering of Canada's Welfare State, 1939–1947*. Toronto: University of Toronto Press 2007

Stevenson, Michael D. *Canada's Greatest Wartime Muddle: National Selective Service and the Mobilization of Human Resources during World War II*. Montreal & Kingston: McGill-Queen's University Press 2001

Stewart, Roderick, and Sharon Stewart. *Phoenix: The Life of Norman Bethune*. Montreal & Kingston: McGill-Queen's University Press 2011

Street, Kori. "Bankers and Bomb Makers: Gender Ideology and Women's Paid Work in Banking and Munitions during the First World War in Canada." PhD diss., University of Victoria 2001

– "Patriotic, not Permanent: Attitudes towards Women Being Bankers and Making Bombs," in Glassford and Shaw, *A Sisterhood of Suffering and Service*, 148–70

Strong-Boag, Veronica. "Home Dreams: Women and the Suburban Experiment in Canada, 1945–60." *Canadian Historical Review* 77, no. 4 (1991): 471–505

– *The New Day Recalled: Lives of Girls and Women in English-Canada, 1919–1939*. Toronto: Copp-Clark Pitman 1988

– "'Setting the Stage': National Organization and the Women's Movement in the Late 19th Century." In *The Neglected Majority: Essays in Canadian Women's History*, edited by Susan Mann Trofimenkoff and Alison Prentice, 87–103. Toronto: McClelland & Stewart 1977

"The Structure and Role of the Red Cross." Ottawa: CRCS 1992

Struthers, James. "How Much Is Enough? Creating a Social Minimum in Ontario, 1930–44." *Canadian Historical Review* 72 (1991): 39–83

Sutherland, David A. "Voluntary Societies and the Process of Middle Class Formation in Early Victorian Halifax, Nova Scotia." *Journal of the Canadian Historical Association*, new series, 5 (1994): 237–64

Sutherland, Neil. *Children in English-Canadian Society: Framing the Twentieth-Century Consensus.* Toronto: University of Toronto Press 1976

Sutphen, Molly. "Striving to Be Separate? Civilian and Military Doctors in Cape Town during the Anglo-Boer War." In *War, Medicine and Modernity*, edited by Roger Cooter, Mark Harrison, and Steve Sturdy, 48–64. Phoenix Mill, England: Sutton Publishing 1998

Szychter, Gwen. "The War Work of Women in Rural British Columbia: 1914–1919." *British Columbia Historical News* 27 (Fall 1994): 5–9

Tector, Amy. "A Righteous War? L.M. Montgomery's Depiction of the First World War in *Rilla of Ingleside*." *Canadian Literature* 179 (Winter 2003): 72–86

Tennant, Margaret. *Across the Street, Across the World: A History of the Red Cross in New Zealand 1915–2015*. Dunedin: New Zealand Red Cross 2015

Thomas, Debbie, and Margaret Dawson, eds. *My Grandmother's Wartime Diary*. Charlottetown, PEI: Veterans Affairs Canada 1999

Thompson, John Herd. *Ethnic Minorities during Two World Wars.* Canada's Ethnic Groups Booklet no. 19. Ottawa: Canadian Historical Association 1991

– and Allen Seager. *Canada 1922–1939: Decades of Discord*. Toronto: McClelland & Stewart 1985

Thorn, Brian T. "'Healthy Activity and Worthwhile Ideas': Left- and Right-Wing Women Confront Juvenile Delinquency in Post-World War II Canada." *Histoire sociale/Social History* 42, no. 84 (2009): 327–59

Tillotson, Shirley. *Contributing Citizens: Modern Charitable Fundraising and the Making of the Welfare State, 1920–1966*. Vancouver: UBC Press 2008

Tisdall, Frederick F. "Canadian Red Cross Food Parcels for British Prisoners-of-War in Germany." *The Canadian Medical Association Journal* 44 (1941): 77–8

– "Further Report on the Canadian Red Cross Food Parcels for British Prisoners-of-War." *Canadian Medical Association Journal* 50 (1944): 135–8

– et al. "Final Report on the Canadian Red Cross Food Parcels for Prisoners-of-War." *Canadian Medical Association Journal* 60 (1949): 279–86

Titmuss, Richard M. *The Gift Relationship: From Human Blood to Social Policy*, original edition with new chapters, edited by Ann Oakley and John Ashton. London: LSE Books 1997

Toews, J.A. *Alternative Service in Canada during World War II*. Winnipeg: Canadian Conference of the Mennonite Brethren Church 1959

Toman, Cynthia. "Crossing the Technological Line: Blood Transfusion and

the Art and Science of Nursing, 1942–1990." Master's thesis, University
of Ottawa 1998
– *An Officer and a Lady: Canadian Military Nursing and the Second
World War*. Vancouver: UBC Press 2007
– "Officers and Ladies: Canadian Nursing Sisters, Women's Work, and the
Second World War." PhD diss., University of Ottawa 2003
Toronto Branch CRCS, *History Toronto Branch The Canadian Red Cross
Society 1914–1948*. Toronto: CRCS [1949?]
Toxopeus, Deanna. "1951 Agreement between the Red Cross and St John
Ambulance: A Case Study of the Effect of Civil Defence on Canada's Health
Care System." Master's thesis, Carleton University 1997
Trepanier, James. "Building Boys, Building Canada: The Boy Scout Move-
ment in Canada, 1908–1970." PhD diss., York University 2015
Vallée, Stéphane. "Naissance et développement de l'affaire du sang contaminé
au Canada." Master's thesis, University of Ottawa 1999
Valverde, Mariana. *The Age of Light, Soap, and Water: Moral Reform in
English Canada, 1885–1925*. Toronto: McClelland & Stewart 1991
– "The Mixed Social Economy as a Canadian Tradition." *Studies in Political
Economy* 47 (Summer 1995): 33–60
Vance, Jonathan. "Canadian Relief Agencies and Prisoners of War, 1939–
1945." *Journal of Canadian Studies* 31, no. 2 (1996): 133–147
– *Death So Noble: Memory, Meaning, and the First World War*. Vancouver:
UBC Press 1997
– *Maple Leaf Empire: Canada, Britain, and Two World Wars*. Don Mills, ON:
Oxford University Press 2012
– *Objects of Concern: Canadian Prisoners of War throughout the Twentieth
Century*. Vancouver: UBC Press 1994
– "The Trouble with Allies: Canada and the Negotiation of Prisoner of War
Exchanges." In *Prisoners of War and Their Captors in World War II*, edited
by Bob Moore and Kent Fedorowich, 69–85. Oxford: Berg 1996
Wade, Susan. "Joan Kennedy and the British Columbia Women's Service
Corps." In *Not Just Pin Money: Selected Essays on the History of Women's
Work in British Columbia*, edited by Barbara K. Latham and Roberta J.
Pazdro, 407–28. Victoria, BC: Camosun College, 1984
Walker, Eric Keith. "Over the Top: Canadian Red Cross Fundraising during
the Second World War." Master's thesis, University of Ottawa 2011
The War Charities Act, 1917, and Regulations and Forms Thereunder, fore-
word by Martin Burrell. Ottawa: King's Printer 1918
Ward, Paul. "Empire and the Everyday: Britishness and Imperialism in
Women's Lives in the Great War." In *Rediscovering the British World*, edited
by Philip Buckner and R. Douglas Francis, 267–83. Calgary, AB: Calgary
University Press 2005
Warder, Maitland. *Fifty Years of Service: A Profile of a Small Red Cross
Branch in Ontario*. Lion's Head, Ontario: CRCS 1982

Watson, E.H.A. *History Ontario Red Cross 1914–1946.* Toronto: Ontario Division Headquarters [1947?]

Weindling, Paul, ed. *International Health Organisations and Movements, 1918–1939.* Cambridge: Cambridge University Press 1995

Whitton, Charlotte. *Canadian Women in the War Effort.* Toronto: Macmillan 1942

"Who Was C.-E. A. Winslow?" Yale School of Public Health, www.public health.yale.edu/about/history/winslow_award/biography.aspx

Willis, Ian. *Ministering Angels: The Camden District Red Cross 1914–1945.* Camden, Australia: Camden Historical Society 2014

Wilson, Catharine Anne, "Reciprocal Work Bees and the Meaning of Neighbourhood." In *Home, Work & Play: Situating Canadian Social History,* 2nd ed., edited by James Opp and John C. Walsh, 130–44. Don Mills, ON: Oxford University Press 2010

Winslow, C.-E.A. "Suggestions for a Red Cross Health Programme." *International Journal of Public Health* 2 (September–October 1921): 488–508

Winter, Jay. *Sites of Memory, Sites of Mourning: The Great War in European Cultural History.* Cambridge: Cambridge University Press 1995

World Vision Canada. "About Our History." 2013 www.worldvision.ca

Young, Alan R. "L.M. Montgomery's *Rilla of Ingleside*: Romance and the Experience of War." In *Myth and Milieu: Atlantic Literature and Culture, 1918–1939,* edited by Gwendolyn Davies, 95–122. Fredericton, NB: Acadiensis 1993

INDEX

Aboriginals, 31, 94, 177, 186, 304n29.
See also Métis
"Absent-Minded Beggar, The"
(Kipling), 57
Ador, Gustave, 139
Alberta: Blood Transfusion Service in,
236; CRCS branches in, 52, 83, 94,
98, 118, 185, 187, 188; CRCS Division of, 23, 76, 109, 115, 137, 143,
148, 152, 155, 159, 183, 214, 270,
317n79; and CRCS leadership,
299n80, 304n34; government of,
272; Great Depression in, 159. See
also Bennett, R.B.; Calgary; Duggan,
D.M.; Fort McMurray; Huckvale,
W.E.; McClung, Nellie; Waagen,
Mary
Aleta Dey (Beynon), 117
ambulances: as Red Cross assistance,
13, 62, 99, 105, 205; in wartime, 27,
31–2, 36, 77, 103. See also SJAA;
SJAB; VADS
American Civil War, 20, 29
American National Red Cross (ANRC),
29, 48, 71, 73. See also ARC
American Red Cross (ARC), 15, 16, 29,
73, 299n73; blood collection and,
234; and the CRCS, 8, 25, 44, 76,
108–9, 208–9, 222, 280, 284,
300n83; and the Great Depression,
159, 283–4, 318n85; and the Halifax

explosion, 125–6; and Junior Red
Cross, 93; peacetime mandate of,
70–1, 79, 133, 181, 216, 311n4;
publicity of, 88, 109, 122, 186; war
work of, 133, 183, 217, 229, 231,
312n18, 314n39. See also ANRC;
Barton, Clara; Boardman, Mabel;
Davison, Henry; disaster relief;
Foringer, A.E.; LRCS
Amnesty International, 21, 28
And Who Is My Stranger (report), 258,
264–7
Anglican Church, 43, 83, 90, 175,
292n21
Army Medical Department of Canada,
36, 44
Arsenault, Iphegenie, 221, 333n24
Association of Medical Officers of the
Militia of Canada (AMOMC), 39–40,
45, 72. See also Bergin, Darby
Auger, Madeleine, 176
Australia: blood donation system of,
198, 239, 271; Red Cross Society of,
16, 20, 87, 139, 208, 303n26,
311n4; war service of, 64, 294n11
Austria, 38, 105

Baby Boom, 221, 228, 230, 260
Bank of Montreal, 102, 170, 175
Baptist Convention of Ontario and
Quebec, 176